# The Vulnerable Brain and Environmental Risks

Volume 1
Malnutrition and Hazard Assessment

# The Vulnerable Brain and Environmental Risks

Volume 1
Malnutrition and Hazard Assessment

Edited by

**Robert L. Isaacson**
*Binghamton University*
*Binghamton, New York*

and

**Karl F. Jensen**
*U. S. Environmental Protection Agency*
*Research Triangle Park, North Carolina*

Plenum Press • New York and London

Library of Congress Cataloging-in-Publication Data

```
The Vulnerable brain and environmental risks / edited by Robert L.
  Isaacson and Karl F. Jensen.
     p.   cm.
  Includes bibliographical references and index.
  Contents: v. 1. Malnutrition and hazard assessment -- v. 2. Toxins
in food.
  ISBN 0-306-44148-9 (v. 1). -- ISBN 0-306-44165-9 (v. 2)
  1. Neurotoxicology. 2. Neurotoxicology--Environmental aspects.
I. Isaacson, Robert L., 1928-    . II. Jensen, Karl F.
  [DNLM: 1. Environmental Exposure. 2. Nervous System Diseases-
-chemically induced. 3. Neurotoxins. 4. Protein-Energy
Malnutrition--complications.   WL 100 V991]
RC347.5.V85  1992
616.8--dc20
DNLM/DLC
for Library of Congress                                        92-49396
                                                                    CIP
```

ISBN 0-306-44148-9

© 1992 Plenum Press, New York
A Division of Plenum Publishing Corporation
233 Spring Street, New York, N.Y. 10013

All rights reserved

No part of this book may be reproduced, stored in a retrieval system, or transmitted in any form or by any means, electronic, mechanical, photocopying, microfilming, recording, or otherwise, without written permission from the Publisher

Printed in the United States of America

# Contributors

*Robert J. Austin-LaFrance* • Trinity College, Hartford, Connecticut 06106

*Carey D. Balaban* • Department of Otolaryngology, University of Pittsburgh and the Eye and Ear Institute of Pittsburgh, Pittsburgh, Pennsylvania 15213

*William K. Boyes* • Neurophysiological Toxicology Branch, Neurotoxicology Division, Health Effects Research Laboratory, U.S. Environmental Protection Agency, Research Triangle Park, North Carolina 27711

*Joseph D. Bronzino* • Trinity College, Hartford, Connecticut 06106

*Helen B. Daly* • Department of Psychology and Center for Neurobehavioral Effects of Environmental Toxins, State University of New York at Oswego, Oswego, New York 13126

*Janina R. Galler* • Boston University School of Medicine, Boston, Massachusetts 02215

*M. E. Gilbert* • Mantech Environmental Technology Inc., Research Triangle Park, North Carolina 27709

*Ryan J. Huxtable* • Department of Pharmacology, College of Medicine, University of Arizona, Tucson, Arizona 85724

*Diane B. Miller* • Neurotoxicology Division, U.S. Environmental Protection Agency, Research Triangle Park, North Carolina 27711

*Peter J. Morgane* • Laboratory of Physiology and Pharmacology, Worcester Foundation for Experimental Biology, Shrewsbury, Massachusetts 01545

*Roger W. Russell* • Center for the Neurobiology of Learning and Memory and Department of Psychology, University of California, Irvine, California 92717

*Frank M. Scalzo* • Department of Pediatrics, University of Arkansas for Medical Sciences and Arkansas Children's Hospital, Little Rock, Arkansas 72205

*Mark E. Stanton* • Neurotoxicology Division, Health Effects Research Laboratory, U.S. Environmental Protection Agency, Research Triangle Park, North Carolina 27711

*John Tonkiss* • Boston University School of Medicine, Boston, Massachusetts 02215

*Gary L. Wenk* • Division of Neural Systems, Memory and Aging, University of Arizona, Tucson, Arizona 85724

# General Introduction

This series was undertaken because of our awareness that environmental pollution is adversely affecting brain function and behavior. The degree and nature of these effects in many instances remain uncertain but are active targets of investigation by scientists working in many domains of neuroscience. Different techniques, approaches, and conceptual frameworks are being used, many of a specialized nature. As a result, it is difficult for experts or for students in any one field to gain an overview of these various efforts and to be aware of points of convergence among investigations. We believe that the sharing of information among those using different approaches is necessary to a full understanding of the nature of the problems confronting the human species. We believe that gaining a more complete understanding of the effects of environmental toxins and pollutants is essential to world health.

As demonstrated in the chapters of these books, pollutants affect sensory, motor, and emotional functions, as well as learning, memory, and intellectual capacities. These effects can range from the subtle to the profound. Very little is known about the mechanisms by which pollutants affect the nervous system, and little is known about the number of compounds causing such effects. According to the U.S. Congress's Office of Technology Assessment, "The number of neurotoxic substances that pose a significant public health risk is unknown because the potential neurotoxicity of only a small number of chemicals has been evaluated adequately."*

There is an urgent need for understanding the effects of pollutants on the nervous system at every level of analysis. By bringing together contributions from scientists in both basic and applied neuroscience, we hope that investigators of all ages and disciplines, including graduate and undergraduate students, will become interested in these problems and their solutions. These books demonstrate the fruitfulness of using diverse methods to study the effects of environmental pollutants, and by so doing suggest new ways in which scientists of many persuasions can join in the attempt to understand the vulnerability of the brain and the behavioral sequelae of this vulnerability.

Unfortunately, almost all of the chapters assume some degree of familiarity with the topics being presented. With a few exceptions, the chapters have been written so as to be credible to those working in the field and may be difficult for the nonspecialist in some aspects. But how else can current science be presented in a faithful manner? We believe

*U.S. Congress, Office of Technology Assessment, 1990, *Neurotoxicity: Identifying and Controlling Poisons of the Nervous System,* OTA-BA-436 U.S. Government Printing Office, Washington, DC.

that it is wisest to present the best and most current information as seen by leaders in the field. Even though the books may be considered to be "samples of ideas and methods," we believe they sample the best.

These volumes reflect our belief that an adequate description of current risk from environmental pollutants requires full use of current knowledge of behavior, physiology, anatomy, biochemistry, and pharmacology to assess the integrity of the nervous system. Thus, for all types of toxins we have tried to put together an interdisciplinary body of information from closely related, but distinct, arenas of research. In a number of cases, we have intentionally selected topics or perspectives that are controversial, since it is controversy that often reveals the most interesting facets of scientific investigation.

We hope the reader, on finishing these books, will have a better understanding of a number of issues concerning the effects of nutrients and pollutants on brain and behavior, that is, the many substances in our environment that endanger our functional capabilities. The goal of adequately assessing large numbers of substances for potential effects on brain and behavior faces substantial challenges. These challenges can be addressed only by appropriately focused and interdisciplinary research efforts in neurotoxicology.

Robert L. Isaacson<br>Karl F. Jensen

*Binghamton, New York*
*Research Triangle Park, North Carolina*

# Introduction to Volume 1

The first two volumes of this series contain 28 chapters concerning the risks to optimal brain function arising from food: its quantity and appropriateness, its adulteration, its processing, and its contamination. The authors of 27 of these chapters are experts in fields of direct scientific relevance to these topics. The authors of the 28th chapter (the last chapter of Volume 2) are authorities in the field of legal regulation and federal oversight of food substances, a topic of great practical significance to everyone.

Originally, we had intended these first two volumes to be a single book, but as we began to consider the field in all aspects, it became apparent that our original plan had to be enlarged and the concept of a single book abandoned.

Perhaps a few words about the origin of the first two volumes would be appropriate. About 2 years ago, over 100 letters were sent to active researchers working in various neuroscientific disciplines related to environmental toxins. In these letters, suggestions about topics and authors to be included in a book about food-related toxins were solicited. From the replies, a consensus was compiled and letters were sent to scientists in the domains selected for representation. Over 90% of those asked to contribute chapters responded favorably, and their chapters are in these first two volumes. Their contributions were important and timely. The difficult decision was how to divide up the contributed chapters into the two books. After considerable thought and discussion, we decided to cover the effects of malnutrition and general methods of assessment of toxicological damage in the first volume. The second volume contains sections on metal and toxicant toxicity, certain mechanisms whereby toxins exert their effects, and, last, how courts and agencies are involved in the regulation of pollutants and toxins.

One of the major environmental risks in the world today is not getting enough to eat. Everywhere people are concerned about food. The nature and intensity of concern differ in different parts of the world. In some regions the question is whether or not sufficient food can be bought, stolen, or scavenged to sustain life for just one more day. The seemingly simple matter of gaining access to an adequate number of calories may override all other concerns. Starvation remains the greatest human tragedy of our time. The numbers are striking. Every day over 35,000 people die from starvation. Over 10 million will die of starvation this year. Of course, the absolute number of people dying from

---

The material presented in this introduction has not been submitted to the Environmental Protection Agency's peer and administrative review; therefore, the views and opinions expressed are those of the editors and should not be construed to reflect the policy of the agency.

starvation is related to the world population, which now exceeds over 5 billion. By 2050, it will be over 10 billion. The irony is that there is currently, and will continue to be in 2050, enough food to go around. The distribution of food represents major moral, economic, and political issues for all of the world's governments to which there are no easy solutions.*

Extensive nutritional rehabilitation, "catching up," after periods of undernutrition early in life is only partial and incomplete. The overall behavioral signs of early malnutrition seem to be hyperactivity, impulsiveness, and poor abilities to anticipate events, even when part of a daily routine. Inadequate nutrition during development also puts the individual at risk, with a greater susceptibility to all types of "insults" (e.g., those produced by infections, toxins, and pollutants).

In Part I of this volume, the chapter by Peter Morgane, Robert Austin-LaFrance, Joseph Bronzino, John Tonkiss, and Janina Galler addresses the effects of malnutrition on the development of brain and behavior, while the chapters by Frank Scalzo and Gary Wenk address the neural and behavioral effects of malnutrition during adulthood. Ryan Huxtable describes various psychoactive and neurotoxic compounds occurring naturally in wild and cultivated plants, some of which are consumed for their food value and others for their psychoactive effects. Roger Russell then discusses the effects of apparently minor alterations in a basic dietary substance, choline, that result in its being turned into a toxin with a delayed onset of toxic effects. The result of this alteration is both neural and behavioral changes. The alterations of the choline molecule are ones that could occur during food processing or preparation for consumption.

Morgane and his colleagues point out that we should not be misled into thinking that the development of the brain or behavior is altered only by privations or insults occurring during a single, limited critical period of development. There are many critical periods during development. The times of susceptibility depend on the particular species under observation. This chapter emphasizes the need for understanding differences in nervous system development between different species. Some developmental milestones are achieved prenatally in some species but well after birth in others. Morgane and his colleagues point out that while the manifestations of early deprivation may be subtle, they are in most cases permanent. The efforts of this group directed toward the study of undernutrition or malnutrition using anatomical and electrophysiological techniques are excellent examples of the need for a multidisciplinary approach to characterizing impairments induced by developmental nutritional privations. (For other examples of electrophysiological approaches for characterizing neurotoxicity, see the chapters by Boyes and Gilbert in Part II.)

Turning to the effects of undernourishment in the adult, Frank Scalzo describes investigations addressing the effects of caloric restriction in adulthood. There has been a great deal of interest generated by the increased longevity found in animals that are subjected to enforced caloric reductions relative to those that are allowed to eat freely. Not only is life prolonged in animals on restricted diets, but many of their biological functions are well preserved, even ones that usually decline or fail with aging. It is as if the reduction in food intake causes the body to shift its overall goals from growth and cellular proliferation to maintaining the "status quo." Bodily resources become directed toward repair and maintenance. This redirection of resources is reflected in a number of biolog-

---

*See J. Maddox, 1972, *The Doomsday Syndrome*, McGraw-Hill, New York; and D. Goulet and M. Hudson, 1971, *The Myth of Aid*, IDOC North America, New York.

ical changes at molecular and systems levels. The aged animals with dietary restrictions have enhanced immune functions and greater resistance to the growth of tumors. Results like these bring many questions to mind. Are the results applicable to all species? What are the mechanisms by which nutritional deficiencies cause such large and important changes? Is longevity itself so important—especially in the absence of a reasonable quality of life? What *is* the quality of life associated with longer existence? Do the brain and mental activities shift from growth-directed goals (learning and seeking new experiences) to ones of a more vegetative nature?

Gary Wenk addresses a more specific hypothesis. He discusses the effects of altering relative intake of proteins, fats, or carbohydrates on learning and remembering. He argues that specific neurochemical pathways mediating cognition, learning, and memory are altered by nutritional status. Wenk points out, however, that, in addition to the major classes of nutrients he has studied, our food also contains certain substances that may be pharmacologically potent, even at low levels. This theme is extended in other directions by Ryan Huxtable in his elegant discussion of neuroactive and neurotoxic substances that occur naturally in plants. His "ethnopharmacological" approach stresses how cultural factors have influenced the use of plants for their neuroactive properties, even sometimes in spite of their neurotoxic potential.

We think of food as providing calories for energy and materials for growth and repair of our bodies. Several of the foregoing chapters demonstrate that foods also provide us with substances that can, through pharmacological or toxicological effects, influence the way in which our nervous systems function. People select certain foods for special reasons. For example, having a warm glass of milk may help some people sleep. On the other hand, people avoid foods that produce unpleasant effects. Roger Russell has investigated how close the molecular structure of nutrients and poisons may be. In his chapter, he describes experiments on the effects of a compound almost identical to choline, differing only in one minor modification. When laboratory animals have this modified choline incorporated into their diet, there are dramatic changes in brain and behavior. These studies have many ramifications, one of which is that use of similarities in chemical structure to predict the safety or toxicity of a compound is inappropriate and potentially dangerous. In many cases, a substantial similarity of structure can obscure a small, but biologically significant, alteration that confers unwanted potencies on certain drugs and poisons.

In Part II, a number of different approaches to the study of neurotoxicity and neurotoxic effects on behavior are presented. It should be emphasized that the development of methods to detect and characterize the effects of neurotoxicants remains one of the most troublesome areas in neurotoxicology. There are several reasons for this. The hazards posed by a toxicant to the human population are often identified on the basis of epidemiological studies in which there are numerous complications, making it difficult to associate particular human disorders with exposure to specific environmental pollutants.

Many neurologic diseases progress very slowly. The earliest symptoms, such as those found in patients with Alzheimer's or Parkinson's disease, may appear as confusion, minor lapses in memory, or disturbances in coordination that are barely noticeable. They may appear intermittently, as in multiple sclerosis, where there are periods of remission in which the patient may be almost symptom free. Therefore, it is extremely difficult to identify some neurological disorders in their early stages, a time when they could be more easily associated with exposure to a poison. With the human, we are limited to retrospective studies beginning at the time of diagnosis, which can be early or late in the development of the disease. Since the time between the onset and the detection of the disease is variable, a specific association of a disease with a previous exposure to an environmental pollutant may be almost impossible to establish with certainty.

The initial symptoms of neural malfunctions may not appear to be particularly important to an outside observer, since they may not appear to be of a physically debilitating nature. As with other forms of neural insult, the past history and the socioeconomic conditions of the individual play a significant role in determining the nature of the behavioral or physiological anomalies. The first symptoms to appear may not be devastating in themselves, but can lead to problems with family, friends, and co-workers. The deterioration of such relationships may be very important to those suffering the neurotoxic insult.

Many of the early symptoms of neurological diseases are not definitive for one particular disorder. The effects of neurotoxicants may be diffuse and general, affecting various functions of the brain, both by direct toxic actions and through secondary influences of other organs of the body that, in turn, affect the nervous system. The resulting symptoms may appear vague and nonspecific. These include such things as fatigue, irritability, depression, difficulties with concentration, memory disturbances, headaches, and slight impairments of motor coordination. Such symptoms are referred to as "soft signs." While the difficulty of diagnosis based on such uncertain symptomatology is obvious, it should be borne in mind that the diagnosis of a variety of common diseases is made on the basis of combinations of soft signs such as fever, stomach disorders, rashes, and so forth that over the years have been shown to converge on a common disease. The relatively new study of neurological syndromes associated with pollutant exposure presents significant and novel challenges for the future.

Given the difficulty of establishing a relationship between a neurological impairment and exposure to a pollutant, it is not surprising that those neurological syndromes that have historically been associated with neurotoxic exposure are those that exhibit dramatic alterations in sensorimotor functions. A collection of neurological syndromes in which cognitive, emotional, or autonomic functions are the dominant impairment may not be as obvious. Experimental studies, however, have demonstrated a variety of cognitive, autonomic, and sensorimotor deficits in experimental animals following exposure to pollutants. The long-term value of these studies goes beyond the demonstration that pollutants can induce impairments in brain and behavior. Their greatest utility may lie in helping to develop more certain methods to detect the neurotoxic properties of compounds.

A formidable set of problems must be overcome to develop methods that will unequivocally identify neurotoxic compounds. Some of these problems are practical. What kind of alterations are likely to be observed? Which agents or substances should be studied? How can effects of the thousands of compounds in our environment be examined for neurotoxicity in a cost-effective manner? Other problems are conceptual. How should alterations in specific aspects of behavior, physiology, anatomy, or chemistry be interpreted? What kinds of alterations in the structure or function of the nervous system produce adverse effects?

Very few current answers to these questions are satisfactory. One of the least tenable solutions has been the idea of a tiered testing system. This notion holds that "primary screening tests" could be found that would provide practical approaches for the widespread screening of compounds of possible neurotoxic potential. Ideally such primary screens would be inexpensive and quick while still giving some reasonably accurate indication of whether a compound should be evaluated further for any neurotoxic potential. The problem is that no single test has been demonstrated to detect wide varieties of neurological deficits. In reality an interdisciplinary approach is necessary. No one discipline, be it behavioral, anatomical, physiological, or biochemical, has proved itself capable of adequately detecting neural insults or neurological deficits.

Another problem with current assessments of neurotoxicity is that large numbers of animals or humans often are required to detect small changes. This is particularly important, since a toxicant may induce a small alteration in function, rather than a dramatic one. In other words, it is unlikely that a pollutant will produce the inability to think, talk, or walk. Instead, a pollutant may produce a slight, but measurable, impairment in the performance of one or several types of activities. Experimental designs must be rigorous and an adequate number of subjects must be included in an experiment. Using too small a number of subjects in an assessment test is not cost-effective, since the experiment will contribute little or nothing to the knowledge of the agent or substance being tested.

In Part II, we have included chapters that address behavioral, physiological, and structural approaches to assessing the integrity of the nervous system. We hope these chapters assist the reader in critically appraising and formulating their own opinions about the relative value of different ways neurotoxicity can be assessed.

There are a number of toxicants that when consumed during pregnancy can have adverse effects on the neurological development of the offspring. Mark Stanton describes a number of variables that must be considered in trying to evaluate the effects of pollutant exposure on the development of the ability to learn and remember.

In her chapter, Helen Daly demonstrates how essential the behavioral approach is to a complex problem such as assessing the neurotoxic consequences of eating contaminated freshwater fish (salmon) from Lake Ontario. She summarizes many studies, a substantial number of them done in her laboratory and with faculty in her department. The most direct, and indeed essential, evidence of neurotoxicity comes from animal studies. It would be unethical and irresponsible not to warn people of the danger of eating these fish, although many people do. Only indirect, correlational evidence can come from studies of fish consumption and behavioral changes in people—the fundamental problems found in all epidemiological investigations. The correlational studies with people she cites are difficult to interpret by themselves, but Daly has done an excellent job in indicating where comparable results have been found in animal and human investigations.

In her own work, she has used a number of different testing paradigms. The interpretation of many, if not all, of her results from her animal studies can be based on the assumption that the animals had greater than normal reactions to aversive events and situations. Further, she has found evidence that the effects of the adulteration of the animals' food with the salmon can lead to long-term, if not permanent, impairments. This is the case even when the animals were born from mothers eating the contaminated diets and never ate the fish-contaminated food themselves. Her data are convincing and frightening. It is also distressing to note that she had to use the West Coast ocean salmon as her control food. She could find no uncontaminated source of freshwater salmon inside the country.

Turning to physiological approaches to assessing the functional integrity of the nervous system, Mary Gilbert describes the phenomena of "kindling" in the central nervous system. *Kindling* is the term used to describe the increase in the responses recorded in one portion of the brain evoked by repeated stimulation, usually electrical stimulation, of another region. The recorded, evoked electrical response to the same stimulus gradually increases as the result of repeated stimulation, often to the point of inducing electrical seizures. Because kindling can result in the development of such seizures, it can be viewed as a pathological counterpart of the nervous system's ability to alter itself in response to repeated stimulation. Gilbert describes her work with several pollutants that induce or alter kindling. While such an approach might ultimately implicate pollutants in neurological disorders such as epilepsy, Gilbert's work also suggests pollutants might interfere with normal neural processing, such as the changes that occur during low-level repetitive stimulation (e.g., long-term potentiation), which may be involved in the process of how we learn and remember.

Pollutants can also affect our ability to see, hear, feel, taste, and smell. William Boyes reviews a large body of data on a variety of neurotoxicants and how they may interfere with our ability to see. Boyes points out that such toxicants can interfere with vision both by directly affecting the eye and by affecting the brain. In addition, toxicants can simultaneously affect several sensory systems, and our ability to detect such effects on the nervous system as a whole may depend on the sensitivity of the methods applicable to particular sensory systems.

One of the oldest and most well-established cornerstones of neurotoxicity assessment is the neuropathological and neurohistological evaluation of brain tissue. Such evaluations vary in thoroughness and may entail the examination of a couple of histological sections of human or animal brain or the examination of intensive histological reconstructions of entire regions of the nervous system based on the examination of brains of many patients or animals. Even with the use of new methods and extensive examinations, however, there are no certain histological indicators of irreversible damage to the nervous system. Ironically, one of the most promising approaches appears to be the application of techniques that have been in use for over 50 years, silver stains that are selective for neural degeneration. These stains and their application to neurotoxicology are described in the chapter by Carey Balaban (their application to assessing the effects of organophosphates is described in the chapter by Tanaka and his coauthors in Volume 2). By doing a sequential study of the brains of animals at different times after administration of a toxicant, it is possible to determine areas first affected and those that are altered at later times. Areas in which transneuronal degeneration occurs can also be identified. Such characterization is important to the distinction between primary and secondary damage made in a number of chapters, and this distinction may be important for characterizing possible modes of action of toxicants in general. The silver degeneration procedure also has the advantage of determining the particular cells within a nuclear group that are being affected by a toxin based on the study of changes in cell processes. Not all the cells of a region or a nucleus within the brain have cells that project to the same areas. It is important to determine the subgroups of such areas that are being affected by any particular agent.

Converging data from functional and structural assessments are often considered unequivocal evidence of neurotoxicity. There are, however, conditions under which such alterations may occur that are not the direct result of the action of a toxicant on the nervous system. An example of such a condition is when a toxicant may excessively activate or inhibit the adrenal gland. Diane Miller reviews the importance of considering the effects of such hormonal influences in the interpretation of structural, biochemical, and functional changes induced by neurotoxicants. The understanding of the interactions among toxins and endogenous hormones may prove to be a necessary key to unraveling the mechanisms of action of many toxins and pollutants.

We conclude this volume with these methodological considerations. In Volume 2, the consideration of food-related toxins continues, beginning with common metals and moving on to the man-made toxicants and poisons.

Robert L. Isaacson<br>
Karl F. Jensen

# CONTENTS

## Part I. Malnutrition

**Chapter 1**
**Malnutrition and the Developing Central Nervous System**
*Peter J. Morgane, Robert J. Austin-LaFrance, Joseph D. Bronzino, John Tonkiss, and Janina R. Galler*

| | |
|---|---:|
| 1. General Introduction and Overview | 3 |
| 2. Concepts of Malnutrition Related to Mental Development | 5 |
| 3. Basic Principles and Concepts in Malnutrition in Relation to Developmental Sequences in the Brain | 6 |
| 4. The Concept of Critical Periods | 12 |
| 5. Vulnerable-Period Hypotheses Related to Insults to the Brain | 13 |
| 6. Species Differences in the Brain Growth Spurt | 14 |
| 7. Normal Developmental Events in the Brain | 17 |
| 8. Neuropathology of Mental Retardation and Diffuse Neuronal Insults | 21 |
| 9. Specific Pathologies of Insults to the Developing Brain | 23 |
| 10. Animal Models of Prenatal Retardation | 25 |
| 11. Brain Models for Studies of Insults to the Brain and Concepts of Selective Vulnerability | 27 |
| 12. The Hippocampal Formation as a Brain Model System | 29 |
| 13. Recent Physiological Studies: Emphasis on Hippocampal Neuronal Activity | 31 |
| 14. Recent Behavioral Studies: Emphasis on Hippocampally Related Behaviors | 36 |
| 15. General Conclusions | 38 |
| References | 39 |

**Chapter 2**
**Prolonged Dietary Restriction and Its Effects on Dopamine Systems of the Brain**
*Frank M. Scalzo*

| | |
|---|---:|
| 1. Introduction | 45 |
| 2. General Benefits of Dietary Restriction | 47 |

3. Methodology ................................................... 48
   3.1. Terminology .............................................. 48
   3.2. Methods of Caloric Restriction ............................ 48
   3.3. Caloric Restriction, Aging, and Toxicology ................ 49
4. Biomarkers for Neurotoxicity ................................... 49
   4.1. Neurochemical Assessment of Aged Animals .................. 50
   4.2. Effects of Chronic Caloric Restriction on Neurochemistry in Aged Animals .................................................. 50
   4.3. Behavioral Assessment of Aged Animals ..................... 54
   4.4. Effects of Chronic Caloric Restriction on Behavior of Aged Animals .................................................. 56
5. Interaction of Chronic Caloric Restriction with Trimethyltin Toxicity in Aged Animals ............................................. 58
6. Dopamine Agonists, Aging, and Neurotoxicity .................... 60
7. Chronic Caloric-Restriction Effects and Implications for Toxicity Testing .. 61
8. Summary and Conclusions ........................................ 61
   References ..................................................... 62

## Chapter 3
### Dietary Factors That Influence the Neural Substrates of Memory
*Gary L. Wenk*

1. Introduction ................................................... 67
2. Behavioral Effects of Specific Dietary Nutrients ............... 68
   2.1. Dietary Proteins ......................................... 68
   2.2. Dietary Fats ............................................. 69
   2.3. Dietary Carbohydrates .................................... 70
   2.4. Caffeine and Benzodiazepines in Food ..................... 71
3. Effects of Specific Nutrients on Timing Behavior ............... 72
   3.1. The Timing Behavior Task ................................. 72
   3.2. The Role of Acetylcholine ................................ 72
4. Summary ........................................................ 73
   References ..................................................... 74

## Chapter 4
### Neurotoxins in Herbs and Food Plants
*Ryan J. Huxtable*

1. Introduction ................................................... 77
2. Mammalian Defenses Against Plant Toxins ........................ 78
3. Plant Neurotoxins .............................................. 79
   3.1. Neurotoxic Alkaloids ..................................... 82
   3.2. Neurotoxic Amino Acids in Plants ......................... 95
   3.3. Neurotoxic Monoterpenes and Terpenoids ................... 98
   3.4. Other Plant Neurotoxins .................................. 101
4. Conclusions .................................................... 103
   References ..................................................... 105

## Chapter 5
### "Malnutrition" and the Vulnerable Brain: What a Difference a Molecule Makes
*Roger W. Russell*

| | |
|---|---|
| 1. From Molecules to Behavior | 109 |
| 2. Differences in Molecular "Configuration" | 111 |
| 3. A Missing Molecule: Genetic Errors of Metabolism | 111 |
| 4. A Single Change in Molecular Structure | 113 |
| 5. Functional Receptors | 114 |
| 6. Biotransformation | 115 |
| 7. Natural Toxicants | 116 |
| 8. A Human Error in Synthesis | 118 |
| 9. Neurobehavioral Effects of Food Processing | 118 |
| 9.1. Energy and Molecular Changes | 118 |
| 9.2. Food Additives and Contamination | 120 |
| 10. Defense Against Food Toxicants | 122 |
| 11. In Conclusion | 123 |
| References | 124 |

## Part II. Methods

## Chapter 6
### Animal Models of Cognitive Development in Neurotoxicology
*Mark E. Stanton*

| | |
|---|---|
| 1. Introduction | 129 |
| 2. Criteria of Animal Model | 130 |
| 3. Spatial Delayed Alternation as a Rodent Model System | 132 |
| 4. Conceptual/Operational Approach to Behavioral Capacity | 132 |
| 5. Developmental Profile of Behavior | 135 |
| 6. Neural Substrates of Behavioral Development | 136 |
| 7. Neurotoxicant Effects on Developing Brain and Behavior | 140 |
| 7.1. Early Detection of Neurobehavioral Impairment | 141 |
| 7.2. Special Effects of Developmental Exposure | 144 |
| 7.3. Special Sensitivity of Early Assessment | 145 |
| 8. Summary and Conclusions | 146 |
| References | 146 |

## Chapter 7
### The Evaluation of Behavioral Changes Produced by Consumption of Environmentally Contaminated Fish
*Helen B. Daly*

| | |
|---|---|
| 1. Introduction | 151 |
| 2. Research Approaches | 152 |

3. Research Results ............................................. 153
   3.1. Human Offspring ....................................... 153
   3.2. Adult Humans .......................................... 154
   3.3. Adult Rats ............................................ 154
   3.4. Rat Offspring ......................................... 163
4. Interpretations .............................................. 166
5. Which Chemicals Are Responsible? We Do Not Know ............... 167
6. Summary and Conclusions ...................................... 168
   Appendix ..................................................... 169
   References ................................................... 170

Chapter 8
**Neurotoxicants and Limbic Kindling**
*M. E. Gilbert*

1. Toxicants and Neurological Disease ........................... 173
2. Toxicants and Convulsions .................................... 174
3. Electrical Kindling .......................................... 174
4. Kindling as a Model of Plasticity ............................ 178
5. Acute Generalized Seizure Tests and Electrical Kindling ...... 178
6. Proconvulsant Kindling Studies ............................... 182
7. Chemical Kindling ............................................ 182
8. Endosulfan Chemical Kindling ................................. 184
9. Clinical Relevance ........................................... 187
   References ................................................... 188

Chapter 9
**Testing Visual System Toxicity Using Visual Evoked Potentials**
*William K. Boyes*

1. Introduction ................................................. 193
   1.1. Need for Tests of Visual Function ..................... 194
   1.2. Examples of Visually Toxic Compounds .................. 195
   1.3. Current Neurotoxicity Testing ......................... 203
2. Visual Evoked Potentials ..................................... 204
   2.1. Advantages of Sensory Evoked Potentials ............... 204
   2.2. Types of Visual Evoked Potentials ..................... 204
3. Strain and Species Considerations ............................ 210
4. Overview of Compounds Tested ................................. 212
   4.1. Metals ................................................ 214
   4.2. Solvents .............................................. 214
   4.3. Pesticides ............................................ 214
   4.4. Industrial Compounds .................................. 215
   4.5. Anesthetics ........................................... 215
   4.6. Gases ................................................. 215
5. Conclusions .................................................. 216
   References ................................................... 217

## Chapter 10
**The Use of Selective Silver Degeneration Stains in Neurotoxicology: Lessons from Studies of Selective Neurotoxicants**
*Carey D. Balaban*

| | |
|---|---:|
| 1. Introduction | 223 |
| 2. Distinguishing Primary and Secondary Neuronal Degeneration | 224 |
| 3. Visualizing Neuronal Degeneration: Origin and Role of Silver Degeneration Stains | 225 |
|     3.1. Anterograde (Direct Wallerian) Degeneration: Role in Development of Selective Degeneration Stains | 226 |
|     3.2. Axon Reaction, Retrograde Somatic Degeneration, and Indirect Wallerian Degeneration | 227 |
|     3.3. Transneuronal Degeneration | 229 |
|     3.4. Summary: Role of Silver Stains in Demonstrating Neuronal Degeneration | 229 |
| 4. Interpretation of Silver Degeneration Stains in Neurotoxicology | 229 |
|     4.1. Identification of Neuronal Populations | 230 |
|     4.2. Interpreting Neuronal Degeneration: Time Course and Patterns of Degeneration | 232 |
| 5. Summary: The Role of Suppressive Silver Stains in Toxin Assessment | 235 |
| References | 236 |

## Chapter 11
**Caveats in Hazard Assessment: Stress and Neurotoxicity**
*Diane B. Miller*

| | |
|---|---:|
| 1. Introduction and Overview | 239 |
| 2. Adrenal Axis Interaction with Behavioral Measures | 242 |
| 3. Adrenal Axis Interactions with Electrophysiological Measures | 249 |
| 4. Morphological and Biochemical Measures Used in Neurotoxicity Assessment | 253 |
| 5. Suggestions | 258 |
| References | 259 |

**Index** ............ 267

# Part I

# Malnutrition

# Chapter 1

# Malnutrition and the Developing Central Nervous System

*Peter J. Morgane, Robert J. Austin-LaFrance, Joseph D. Bronzino, John Tonkiss,* and *Janina R. Galler*

## 1. GENERAL INTRODUCTION AND OVERVIEW

During the past three decades there has been a tremendous increase in awareness of the importance of adequate nutrition for brain development and behavior, with recent marked increases in both animal and human research in the field. As a result of this investigative activity, we now have considerable information on some of the major issues that have been raised in the past, e.g. (1) It is now clear that nutrition plays a critically important role in the development and functional organization of the nervous system and that malnutrition adversely affects nervous system maturation and functional development, (2) malnutrition is usually only one of a group of factors affecting development of the nervous system, and (3) appropriate dietary restitution and environmental stimulation may help prevent and, in certain cases, partly ameliorate these effects. Overall, in considering the arguments presented below, it must be kept in mind that the proper maturation of the brain and development of optimal mental capacities depends on three essential factors, namely, the genetic or inborn directives, the stimulus properties or complexity of the environment, and adequate nutritional intake. With regard to nutritional intake, it is necessary to take into account five main factors in evaluating the effects of malnutrition. The first is the type of malnutrition, i.e., whether the deprivation is lack of proteins, calories, vitamins, trace elements, etc., or various combinations of these. The second aspect of malnutrition is the

---

*Peter J. Morgane* • Laboratory of Physiology and Pharmacology, Worcester Foundation for Experimental Biology, Shrewsbury, Massachusetts 01545. *Robert J. Austin-LaFrance* and *Joseph D. Bronzino* • Trinity College, Hartford, Connecticut 06106. *John Tonkiss* and *Janina R. Galler* • Boston University School of Medicine, Boston, Massachusetts 02215.
*The Vulnerable Brain and Environmental Risks, Volume 1: Malnutrition and Hazard Assessment,* edited by Robert L. Isaacson and Karl F. Jensen. Plenum Press, New York, 1992.

timing of the insult, i.e., the period in the organism's development, gestational or postnatal, at which the malnutrition occurs. The third factor to be considered is the duration of the period of malnutrition, while the fourth is the severity of the malnutrition. Finally, a fifth factor is consideration of other environmental stressors, e.g., infection, which increase the severity of the effects.

This chapter does not aim to be a broad overview or review of the great mass of information on the effects of malnutrition on development of the central nervous system. Instead, an attempt will be made to discern patterns and to clarify concepts, and to suggest some principles that may be useful for future work in this field. It is necessary at the outset to consider a few basic concepts and definitions related to interpretation of the effects of malnutrition on the developing brain. In terms of definitions, the word *malnutrition* encompasses all forms of insufficient nutrition and can include a general reduction in calories (often referred to as *undernutrition*), of proteins, carbohydrates, vitamins, or various trace elements. In the usual situation, humans generally experience a combination of several deficiencies, whereas in experimental studies a specific type of malnutrition can be individually investigated. In recent years it has become apparent that malnutrition may either delay or retard the maturation of the brain or permanently stunt its development. Thus, in many instances, depending on timing and other factors, various degrees of damage to brain structures may occur as a consequence of malnutrition. Further, in relation to the chronology of brain development (see text below), it is important to examine the effects of malnutrition insult at the molecular, cellular, systems, and behavioral (especially cognitive) levels in order to fully interpret the basis and ultimate significance of the effects. In the field of malnutrition insult to the brain, the term *retardation* tends to be misleading, since it suggests a pathogenesis in which normal, but slower, processes predominate. Thus, it indicates a development that is tardy but otherwise normal, and in this sense suggests a "catch-up" potential. In this regard, a developmental process that ceases at a certain age is deficient, but perhaps may be normal for that particular functional age. Additionally, the term *growth,* without further qualification, is often misconstrued and probably a better term is *development* or *maturation,* these latter referring to a series of developmental events taking place in the brain or body. Any of these developmental events are often not simply retarded by the insult to the brain, but rather are actually disrupted or made aberrant.

Nutrition is probably the single most important environmental influence on the developing organism. An appropriate supply of essential nutrients is required for the maintenance of growth, as well as the normal development of all physiological functions. It appears likely that the basic cause of fetal brain developmental retardation will in most instances ultimately be malnutrition in one form or another. Maternal malnutrition, including placental insufficiency, may well prove to be one of the principal causes of perturbed development of the fetal brain. In fact, numerous types of insults to the developing brain appear to produce their various effects by ultimately altering nutrient intake. For example, Balázs et al. (1975) report that the effects of undernutrition on the biochemical maturation of the brain are similar to those observed in hypothyroid animals. Additionally, considerable evidence now shows that selective fetal malnutrition is a primary result of the fetal alcohol syndrome (Fisher, 1988).

The goal of this chapter is to integrate some of our knowledge regarding nutrition and brain developmental events with an emphasis on the effects of prenatal protein malnutrition. All nutrients, to a certain extent, have some influence on brain maturation, but protein appears to be the component most critical for the development of neurological structure and functions. Amino acids, the building blocks of proteins, are precursors of enzymes, peptide hormones, and peptide neurotransmitters or, in other instances, are themselves neurotransmitters. They are also the precursors of the structural proteins essential for the growth of body tissues, including the brain. From this, it is obvious that the overall involvement of amino acids in the functional organization of the central nervous system goes far beyond simple support of protein synthetic function.

## 2. CONCEPTS OF MALNUTRITION RELATED TO MENTAL DEVELOPMENT

An understanding of the complex relationship between nutrition and mental development depends on the accuracy with which we can define and measure nutritional status of the child or experimental animal, their mental development or performance, and the importance of other concomitant or interfering phenomena, such as poverty, sociocultural deprivation, understimulation, and infection. The evidence in humans that early malnutrition, i.e., from conception through the first two or so years of life, causes deficits in brain and behavioral function has been well documented (Galler, 1984). However, in most human studies, diet and environmental conditions are inseparable in their multiplicative effects on the developing brain and its performance. Moreover, malnutrition and certain sociocultural factors appear to act synergistically to depress both development and organization of the brain. On the whole, then, nutrition is usually but one of a constellation of factors that interact with developmental and functional maturation of the central nervous system (Coursin, 1975; Fleischer and Turkewitz, 1984; Galler and Kanis, 1987; Smart, 1977, 1987). In this regard, there is some indication that the anatomic, biochemical, and electrophysiological changes seen with deprivation of environmental stimulation are, in some ways, similar to those resulting from nutritional deprivation.

Deficits in environmental stimulation tend to characterize societies showing a continuum of a significant incidence of impaired brain development, performance, and behavior. Of special interest is that these deficits collectively contribute to the perpetuation of developmental problems from one generation to another, producing biologic features that may be transmitted intergenerationally and providing continued environmental conditions that foster them.

In general, intrauterine (gestational) malnutrition tends to be more common in developed countries than postnatal malnutrition and is clearly related to long-term mental handicaps in children (Rosso, 1987). The etiology of inadequate intrauterine nutrition is complex and multifactorial, but appears to be related to factors altering placental passage of nutrients, including poor placental blood supply to the fetus, maternal undernutrition, multiple fetuses in a pregnancy, maternal disease, including intrauterine infections, and genetic disturbances (Chase *et al.*, 1971). The types of maternal malnutrition that affect brain growth most extensively are chronic, severe malnutrition and combined prepregnancy and gestational malnutrition, especially early in gestation. In this regard, it is of interest to point out that a permanently "immature" brain does not simply mean a "small" brain, but rather one that is not adequately developed, i.e., the change is qualitative and not simply a smaller, normal brain.

## 3. BASIC PRINCIPLES AND CONCEPTS IN MALNUTRITION IN RELATION TO DEVELOPMENTAL SEQUENCES IN THE BRAIN

In defining prenatal malnutrition we are concerned with the insult occurring in part of or over the entire fetal period, during which there are many critical periods of peak neurogenesis in different areas of the brain (Fig. 1). We are less concerned with the earlier stage of organogenesis or embryonic period (Fig. 2) in which the developing organism is considerably more vulnerable to harmful external factors. In this period severe insults result either in resorption of the embryo or in marked distortions of shape and form of the developing organism, including the brain. This largely relates to the field of teratology but must be considered as one early critical phase when an entire organism or organ can be deformed. In these cases, provided the organism survives, there are such marked abnormalities that their consideration in a study of malnutrition becomes largely inappropriate. Hence, the present discussions will concentrate on the effects of malnutrition insults that occur primarily during the fetal and early postnatal periods of the life cycle (Fig. 2).

The development of the mammalian nervous system involves a series of highly regulated, sequential changes, which include cell division (neurogenesis and gliogenesis), cell migration to target areas in the brain, cellular differentiation (including dendritic arborization, axonal extensions, and formation of circuits), deposition of myelin into sheaths surrounding axons, formation of synapses (synaptogenesis), synthesis and release of neurotransmitters, and selective cell death during the entire developmental period. The functional result of these maturational events is an overall increase in sensorimotor and higher brain activity. These various neurological processes have different time tables in different species, with many beginning prenatally and extending well beyond birth, while

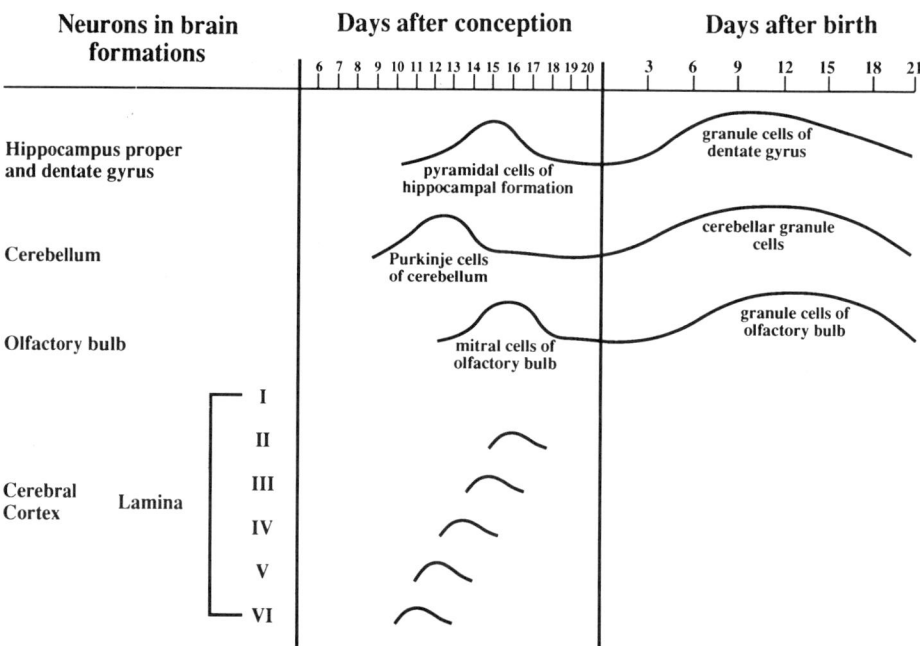

**FIGURE 1.** Times of origin of neurons in four structural areas of the mouse brain.

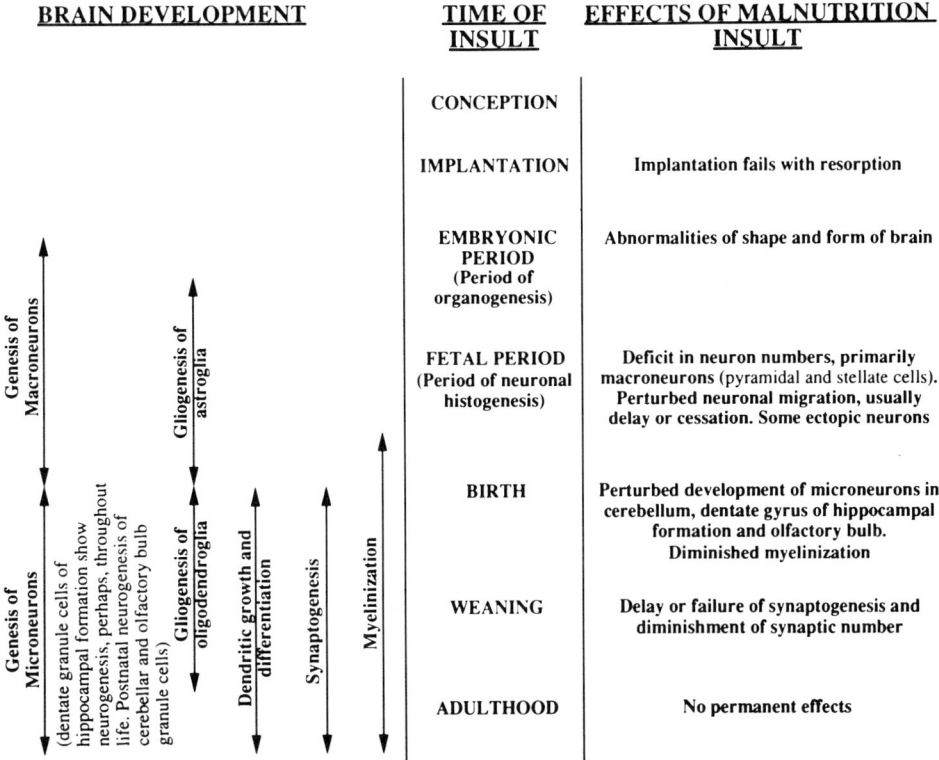

**FIGURE 2.** Maturational events in the rat brain indicating the effects of malnutrition insult at different developmental stages.

others occur primarily during the postnatal period (Figs. 2–5). All of these aspects of brain development may be affected selectively by prenatal and/or postnatal insults, depending on the timing of the insult in relation to developmental events in the brain, as well as on the duration, severity, and type of insult.

The effects of maternal malnutrition on cell acquisition during brain development include: (1) damage to the proliferative cell pools, resulting in distortion of the cell generation cycle; (2) interference with the rate of cell division, resulting in a permanent deficit in brain cells; (3) increase in numbers of degenerate postmitotic cells in germinal zones; (4) reduction of germinal cells postnatally; and (5) lasting changes in the cellular composition of the brain, thereby affecting ratios of the different cell types. Relative to the primary causes of the above-mentioned alterations in brain development reported following malnutrition, some aspects specific to delivery of nutrients to the fetus need to be outlined. The mother is capable of supplying nutrients to the fetus even when she herself is malnourished but, for various reasons, the fetus does not receive sufficient nutrients. As is well known, all mammals adapt to pregnancy by markedly expanding their blood volume, increasing cardiac output, and importantly, increasing uterine blood flow, which reflects not only the increased vascularity of the uterus itself but also the growth of the highly vascularized placenta (Rosso, 1984). Maternal malnutrition curtails these adaptive responses, resulting in a placenta with an overall reduced blood flow. This, in turn, retards

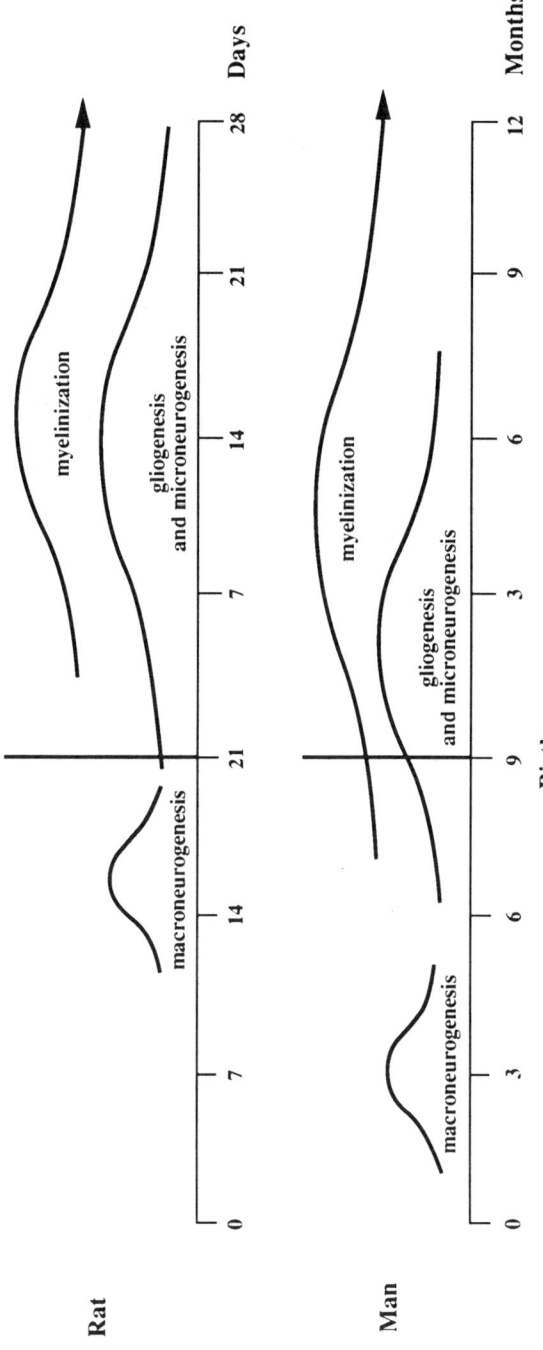

**FIGURE 3.** Comparison of major developmental events in the brain of the human and rat during pre- and postnatal periods. Arrows on myelinization curves indicate that in some areas of the brain myelinization continues late into postnatal life.

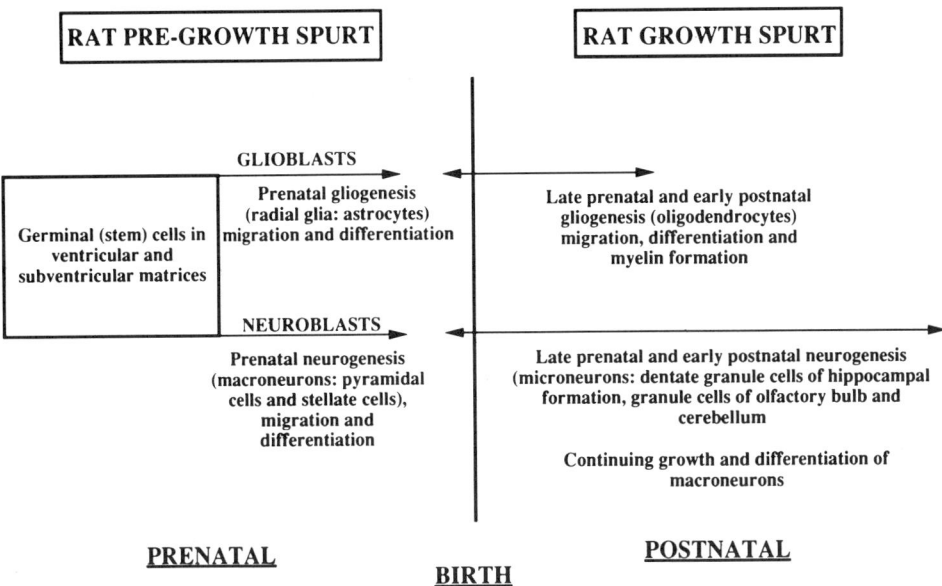

**FIGURE 4.** Major developmental events occurring in the pre-brain growth spurt and brain growth spurt periods in mammalian brain.

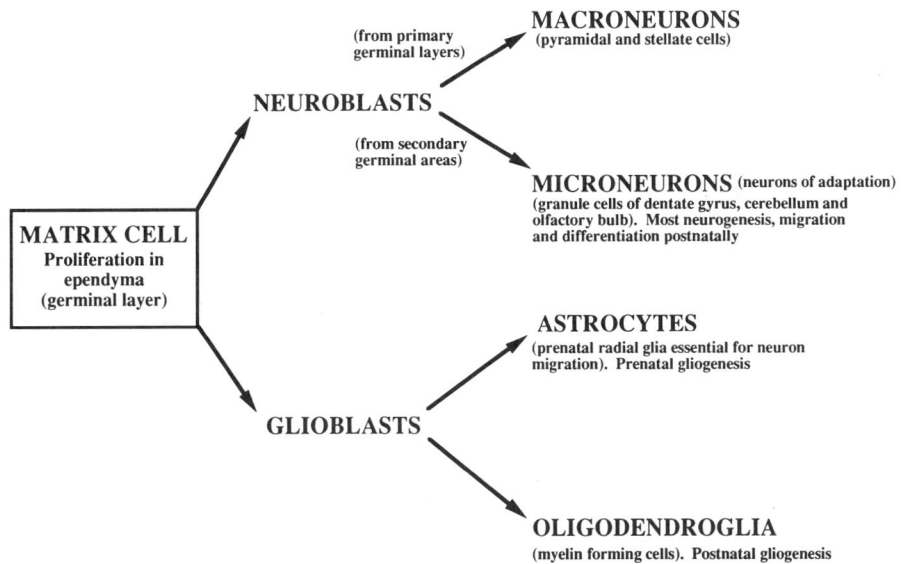

**FIGURE 5.** Histogenetic events involved in the production of neurons and glia.

placental growth and reduces the overall capacity of the placenta to transport nutrients to the fetus. Thus, fetal malnutrition resulting from a malnourished mother may not only be due to lack of nutrients in the maternal blood supply but also from an inability of the placenta to deliver adequate nutrients to the fetus. This results in a proportional growth failure, characterized by a decrease in the rate of cell division in all fetal organs, including the brain (Winick and Noble, 1966; Winick, 1969). In these latter studies all areas of the fetal rat brain examined showed a reduced number of cells by day 16 of gestation. In this regard, multiple regulatory factors control the complex flow of nutrients to sites of synthesis of components of the proliferating neurons, and insults can affect any of these factors and thereby derange the system.

Winick and Noble (1966), Winick (1969), Chase et al. (1971), Chow (1974), Zamenhof and van Marthens (1978), Tonkiss and Galler (1990), and Tonkiss et al. (1990a, 1990b, 1991) have all emphasized that rats malnourished only during pregnancy give birth to pups that show behavioral abnormalities that persist into adult life. It is clear that malnutrition affects brain growth largely by interfering with the rate of cell division and permanently retards growth by causing a reduction in the total number of cells (Winick, 1969; Zamenhof et al., 1968, 1971). Thus, fewer cells are produced overall and the effect is permanent, i.e., there is no recovery in those organs, including the brain, where cell division has been curtailed even when adequate nutrition is restored. If any reversal of these effects is to occur, rehabilitation must begin during the period of active cell division. In this sense the prenatally malnourished fetus is already irreversibly damaged by the time of birth.

We are not yet able to directly connect many biochemical, structural, and physiological abnormalities resulting from malnutrition to specific dysfunctions of the brain. However, animal models of malnutrition are revealing abnormalities in certain aspects of behavior that are characteristic of damage to particular brain structures, e.g., the hippocampal formation and cerebellum. Not only do we have to consider the effects of insults to the brain as affecting brain anatomy, physiology, biochemistry, and behavior, but we also must recognize that malnutrition affects the manner in which the developing organism interacts with its mother, siblings, and the external environment, resulting in different amounts of stimulation, which, in turn, affects brain development (Fig. 6).

In considering the "diffuse" brain effects of a malnutrition insult, it is commonly reported, both in humans and experimental animals, that apathy is a usual sign of protein/calorie and/or protein malnutrition. There is a general loss of curiosity and initiative, along with a lack of desire for exploring and investigating the environment and an actual progressive diminished responsivity and withdrawal from the environment. Attention deficits are also common, particularly the ability to maintain sustained attention. Relative to these usual behavioral findings in both humans and animals, the brain substrates of these types of global activities have been particularly difficult to determine. It is obvious, then, that there is a marked gap between our knowledge of biochemical and structural "maturity" of the brain and what we call the process of achieving mental maturity. Relative to this, biochemical changes associated with prior malnutrition, with correlated changes in behavior, have been reported to be partially ameliorated by an enriched, generally stimulating environment (Barnes, 1976).

There are several issues that relate restitution of function following malnutrition insult that need to be outlined. The major question relative to rehabilitation following malnutrition insult is whether damage inflicted on the brain of developing animals or humans at a critical developmental period, of which the so-called brain growth spurt (see

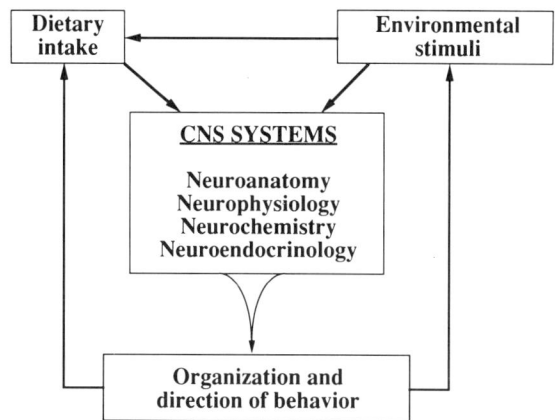

**FIGURE 6.** Interactions of diet and environment affecting central nervous system function and behavior.

below) is but one, heals with time and nutritional rehabilitation. Here, again, confusion reigns in that the literature is full of statements such as "the critical period for human babies begins with the second half of fetal life and ends about 18 months after birth" (Dobbing, 1972). In the rat this brain growth spurt period has been defined as being almost entirely postnatal. However, this is only one critical period and does not account for other even more important critical periods in brain development, such as peak periods of neurogenesis, which vary in every brain structure (Fig. 1), and periods of neuronal migration. These fundamental, largely prenatal, periods in brain development are perhaps of greater significance for subsequent brain function than the "differentiation" period. By the time of macroneuron differentiation (Figs. 2–5), the neurons have already been born and have migrated into their target areas in different regions of the brain. Of course, as discussed below, the differentiation period for macroneurons is also the period of peak microneurogenesis and differentiation. It appears that undue emphasis has been placed on the brain growth spurt period, as though it were the only or principal critical period of importance. Too much attention to this period in experimental malnutrition studies has deemphasized the importance of prenatal malnutrition, particularly in the rat model, and in some cases has given false hopes for restoration of function following the institution of adequate diets. Relative to this, it is important to point out that some brain structural growth may be reinstituted as a result of dietary rehabilitation, whereas topological distortions, such as derangements of dendritic networks and altered cell ratios, tend to remain permanently affected. Morphogenesis of dendritic arborizations is tightly controlled by interactions with all other types of cells that establish contact with particular cells under study, which is, no doubt, a general phenomenon in the developing nervous system. For example, a reduction in the number of maturation of dentate granule cells, together with asynchronous alterations in maturation of pyramidal cells, results in distortions of spatio-temporal relationships between pyramidal and granule cells, both in malnutrition and in thyroid-deficient animals (Balász et al., 1977, 1979). It is important to understand that if there is a permanent loss of neurons due to disruptions of the cell cycle, such as slowed or failed neurogenesis or a failure of the start of neuronal migrations or migrations that begin but then cease prematurely, resulting in ectopic neurons, then these effects are not reversed by subsequent dietary rehabilitation.

## 4. THE CONCEPT OF CRITICAL PERIODS

Before discussing normal brain development, some further elaboration of so-called critical periods is needed. Considerable importance has been placed on "critical periods" in brain development, which generally refer to highly circumscribed changes in many parameters (Colombo, 1982; Herschkowitz and Rossi, 1972; Scott, 1979). However, this concept is valid only so long as it does not distract from the overlapping and sequential nature of the various patterns of events taking place in the central nervous system (Rodier, 1976, 1980). It should be kept in mind that a single exposure to an insulting agent or toxin delivered at different times can alter various brain structures, focally or diffusely, and thus result in different functional deficits. These particular time frames during which an insult exerts more marked effects are termed *critical* or *vulnerable periods*. They are not simply associated with times of rapid gross brain-weight changes, as Dobbing (1970, 1984, 1985, 1990) would have us believe, but rather refer to multiple periods in each brain area when neurogenesis, gliogenesis, or neuronal migration is at its summit. In humans, where life span is comparatively long and the developmental processes are correspondingly slow, there are less obvious suggestions of such "critical periods." It is only in the more commonly studied laboratory species, in which the same developmental processes follow each other more rapidly, that there appears to be a simultaneous occurrence of many different events. Our frequent failure to characterize the sequential rather than the simultaneous nature of these events in these species is due mainly to the technical difficulty of separating them in rapidly developing brains. There is, therefore, a great need for accurate information about the relative timing of events in developmental neurobiology so that components of "critical periods" can be more firmly visualized and separated into a sequential series.

Relative to these issues, several pitfalls are apparent in the field of developmental neurobiology. Among these is a failure to standardize the environmental conditions of developing litters from one laboratory to another, and even within the same laboratory, so that animals of the same chronological age acquire widely different developmental ages. When the brain is growing rapidly, even small differences in litter size are sufficient to produce a wide variation in values from individuals of the same chronological age, thus leading to considerable confusion in determining the sequence of developmental events. Another problem is the assumption that because a number of changes are occurring over the same period, they are necessarily causally linked, which may or may not be the case. Neuron populations showing very short periods of neurogenesis are especially vulnerable to insults that occur during select time frames. For example, the longer the periods of mitosis in proliferative cell pools, the less the chance for limited period insults to exert irreparable deficits. In seeking to define windows of special vulnerability, i.e., critical periods, in the experimental situation, it is essential to know the periods of peak neurogenesis in different brain structures and of the different cell types within particular brain structures. In malnutrition, however, the deficiency is most frequently continuous, i.e., chronic over the entire prenatal period, rather than consisting of brief acute episodes. Chronic malnutrition may, nonetheless, vary in degree at particular times. Consequently, many critical periods within and across a range of brain structures are concomitant with the chronic insult. Accordingly, following such insult, most anatomical or biochemical effects are widespread, though many brain areas may be more selectively vulnerable based on their special intrinsic properties (see below).

In this same context, it is also necessary to consider the issues of brain plasticity in relation to insults to the brain and compensations the organism may be able to make. The compensatory capacities of the brain, particularly during development, must be taken into account when attempting to correlate various levels of anatomical defects with mental dysfunction. Developmental plasticity manifests itself both prenatally and postnatally in a variety of ways and does so along with adaptive (reactive) plasticity. In this manner, compensatory processes may offset the effects of insults to the developing brain (Altman, 1970). For example, Balázs et al. (1975) showed that in thyroid deficiency, cell numbers in the cerebellum ultimately reach normal levels as a result of prolongation of the period of extensive cell proliferation. Further, the deletion of a fraction of cells of a particular type may be, in part, functionally compensated for by the convergence of the remaining cells of the same type on the relevant postsynaptic cells. In certain brain regions, especially the hippocampal formation, there is apparently some capacity for restitution of neuronal circuit functioning and, hence, a greater chance for sparing of function. Hence, it is clear that there are numerous safety factors built into the structural design of the central nervous system. Activity-dependent plasticity may play a role in the partial compensation for the effects of malnutrition and other insults. Thus, the stimulated brain remains more flexible and is thereby better able to develop multiple complex relations with the environment.

## 5. VULNERABLE-PERIOD HYPOTHESES RELATED TO INSULTS TO THE BRAIN

One basic idea that has come to underlie considerable work on malnutrition and the developing central nervous system is the vulnerable-period hypothesis of the brain growth spurt put forth by Dobbing and his group (1968b, 1970, 1972). This hypothesis states that developmental processes in the brain are more vulnerable to dietary restriction and other insults at the time of their fastest growth rates. However, in these studies the growth rates take into account only total brain weights using velocity curves to show rates of increasing weight and then decay. In general, the concept has caused considerable confusion in the field, since it has often been misinterpreted as to precisely what it postulates and what the ultimate uses of these curves are for various species, especially since they do not include the periods of early neurogenesis. One main problem with this concept is that it deals only with velocity curves of gross brain weights, which are notoriously unreliable as indicators of brain development and shed little or no light on local brain changes or alterations of particular cell types in various brain areas. Further, as noted above, the brain is vulnerable to insult in varying degrees during the entire period of its development, and hence, focusing only on one brain growth spurt period may be quite misleading in that it deemphasizes important developmental events occurring in the brain before the so-called brain growth spurt period, i.e., during the pre-growth spurt period (Fig. 4).

In a long series of papers, Dobbing (1968a, 1968b, 1972, 1990) has defined the brain growth spurt period as one in which brain vulnerability to insult is maximal due to the fact that this is the period when the brain gains weight fastest. In Dobbing's studies, curves of brain growth, i.e., increases in wet weight, were developed for a variety of species, including humans, and these, of course, differ markedly across species. As discussed below, this difference is but one of many factors that must be considered when assessing periods of special vulnerability in animal models compared to humans. In the rat, this brain growth spurt relates mainly to the stage of postnatal neuronal differentiation of cell populations that were generated prenatally, oligodendroglial genesis, and differentiation, and especially, production of myelin. As indicated in Figure 3, the brain growth spurt in the human incorporates both the late prenatal and early postnatal periods. Exceptions to the prenatal neurogenesis in both rats and humans are the microneuron populations of the dentate gyrus of the hippocampal formation, cerebellum, and olfactory bulb, which largely show postnatal neurogenesis (see further below). Dobbing (1968b, 1971, 1985, 1990) emphasized that the brain growth spurt in humans extends from the last trimester of gestation, reaches a maximum before birth, and then falls off at a slower rate for the first 18 months or so of postnatal life. In the rat, this period encompasses the initial 3 weeks following birth. In all species the brain growth spurt begins at the time when the adult number of neurons has been reached, with the exception, as noted, of the microneurons, which are largely produced postnatally in the rat and in the human during the last trimester of pregnancy and in the early postnatal period (Figs. 1–4). During the postnatal period in the rat, there is an explosive multiplication of glial cells along with microneurogenesis, and in the human there is continuing gliogenesis and microneurogenesis. In terms of absolute numbers, the glial cell production is much greater than in the "pre-growth spurt" period, which largely involves multiplication of macroneurons (Figs. 2–5). Following gliogenesis of oligodendroglia, there occurs the formation of myelin (myelinization phase) over a period of time that, again, differs from one brain system to another. It has been presumed that if an insult occurs over a considerable period of the brain growth spurt, a "once-and-for-all" opportunity for normal development and function of the brain is missed. Hence, the effect of the insult during this period has been stressed by Dobbing as persisting into adulthood and is likely to be permanent.

## 6. SPECIES DIFFERENCES IN THE BRAIN GROWTH SPURT

The event of mammalian birth, which is of such profound significance to the development of cardiovascular and respiratory structure and function, apparently has considerably less significance for the developing central nervous system. However, though parturition does not mark a significant break in the biological development of the brain, at birth external stimulation (brain–environment interaction) now comes into play to affect further brain maturation and function. In terms of timing, rats and mice are born before the so-called brain growth spurt has begun, while guinea pigs have almost completed this stage at the time they are born. The brain growth spurt of the rhesus monkey occurs somewhat earlier than in humans, being mainly prenatal, all of which accords well with their greater behavioral maturation at birth than is found in humans. Relative to this, in the scheme of Dobbing, animal species can be divided somewhat arbitrarily, with respect to their brain growth patterns, into prenatal, perinatal, and postnatal brain developers. This concept does have some utility in experimental malnutrition as to the appropriate period for experimental application of insults relative to the known chronology of select, mostly postnatal, developmental neural events in each species. The point that needs reiterating is the very different timing of the brain growth spurt in relation to birth in different species. It then follows that such terms as *fetal brain, neonatal brain,* or *postnatal brain* are, in reality, of little value unless we know both the species being considered and the particular developmental characteristics of its brain. Such considerations are frequently ignored when interspecies extrapolations are being made and, in particular, when they are related to comparisons of human brain development with that of other species. However, it is the examination of the many components that underlie the velocity curves of brain growth spurts that would provide more useful information concerning the rapidly changing anatomical, physiological, neurochemical, and behavioral patterns across species.

In reality, there are as many brain growth spurts, and thus vulnerable periods, as there are parameters to measure in the developing brain. Further, given the emphasis on velocity curves of brain weight changes, it is interesting to point out that dietary restrictions initiated even before the brain growth spurt may, in some instances, have nearly as great an effect on adult body weight and brain weight as malnutrition during the Dobbing brain growth spurt itself. Ultimately, and perhaps most important, is the "cell division growth spurt," particularly of neurons, loss of which results in altered brain circuitry. Nonetheless, the brain growth spurt curves of Dobbing have been used in two regards: (1) to categorize species into prenatal, perinatal, and postnatal brain "developers" from the positions of their peak velocities of brain growth in terms of weight relative to birth and (2) to present a general visual impression of the proportion of the brain growth spurt in each individual species that is prenatal or postnatal, as determined by the relative size of the two areas beneath the velocity curves on either side of birth.

The brain growth spurt period has also been defined by Dobbing as a critical period during the growth of the brain when metabolic changes resulting from malnutrition markedly affect all future brain development and function. Investigations of malnutrition during the brain growth spurt in rats have repeatedly pointed to the reduced brain myelinization, decreased dendritic proliferation, diminished synaptogenesis, deficits in brain protein, and even reduced brain cell size, all resulting in various abnormalities in behavioral development (Bass *et al.*, 1970; Morgan and Naismith, 1984). The studies of Cragg (1972) suggest that the number of synapses associated with each neuron determines the complexity of neuronal circuitry, and hence, in his view, may indirectly govern mental performance or intelligence. Actually, it appears that either pre- or postnatal malnutrition imposes some limitations on the complexity and organization of neuronal circuits, but by entirely different mechanisms (see below). This, in part, seems a reasonable explanation for the effects of early postnatal malnutrition on learning in humans. It would apply, perhaps even more so, in prenatal malnutrition that results in loss of nerve cells due to perturbed neurogenesis or failed neuronal migration, since this results ultimately in diminished numbers of synapses and alterations in the complexity of neuronal circuitry.

The question of the validity of extrapolation of results from animal studies to humans is a critically important one, since the majority of research has been carried out in laboratory animals. Thus, we need to question to what extent does normal brain development in humans resemble that of commonly studied mammalian species such as the rat. In general, as discussed below under normal brain development, all mammalian brains pass through a similar sequence of developmental processes (Fig. 2). Early organogenesis is almost identical, neurogenesis and migration of neurons are essentially similar, and there is a relatively early establishment of adult numbers of neurons. In all species so far studied, there follows a great proliferation of neuronal and glial stem cells, and subsequently, largely postnatally, the laying down of myelin sheaths. In regard to the latter, myelin may represent some 25% of brain weight and thus would account for a significant proportion of the brain growth spurt. Interestingly, in all species the brain growth spurt occurs relatively early compared to that of the body. The precise relation between the timing of the most rapid period of brain growth relative to the period of malnutrition insult is of some importance. However, it would be more useful to relate velocity curves of maturation of specific brain structures and cell types to the period of malnutrition insult. Hence, as noted above, it is essential to take into account one marked difference between species, i.e., the timing of multiple brain growth spurt periods in relation to birth. From examining brain growth spurt curves, representing a variety of underlying parameters across species, it can be seen that the insult would have to be applied at distinctly different times in relation to birth if similar developmental processes are to be affected in the same manner. Provided, however, that such different time scales are taken into account, it is, of course, valid to examine the effects of malnutrition on various developmental processes in animal models.

Since neuronal proliferation in the rat brain is largely prenatal, we would speculate that decreased brain weight resulting from prenatal malnutrition is primarily associated with a deficit in neuronal numbers, as first shown by Zamenhof et al. (1968). Postnatal malnutrition would not be expected to markedly interfere with neuronal numbers in most brain areas, other than those special regions showing postnatal neurogenesis (see below). Rather, the neuropil tends to be deficient in postnatal malnutrition, resulting in a lowered index of neuronal connectivity. It appears that most forms of postnatal experimental malnutrition do not markedly affect those nerve cells produced prior to birth, other than reducing their perikaryal size and dendritic/axonal branching.

It is obvious from the above remarks that postnatal malnutrition must clearly be distinguished from prenatal malnutrition in terms of its main effects on the central nervous system. In this regard, it is well to stress again that the brain is a subtle series of organ subsystems that are exquisitely integrated and mutually interdependent, especially during early development, when timings of multiple events have to occur in sharply limited periods for functional links to develop between neurons and for the formation of functional circuits to occur. In fact, sequential production of classes of neurons is likely to be a prime mechanism for the orderly growth of neuronal circuitry. Thus, prenatal failures of neuron production, disturbances or mistimings in neuronal migration, and inabilities to properly organize and laminate columns of cells, as in cortical structures, may underlie some behavioral and learning deficiencies later in life. These prenatal insults may be far more decisive than so-called growth spurt insults, since these prenatal events are clearly "once-only," time-limited processes with almost no "catch-up" potential. In this sense, we stress that too much attention has been given to the "brain growth spurt," whereas more microevents, including molecular processes occurring prenatally, would appear to be of even greater significance for the development of primary processes in the brain related to all subsequent organization. Related to aspects of prenatal malnutrition insult is the issue of brain "sparing," which is a view that has also resulted in numerous misconceptions in this field. In the older views of Dobbing, for example, "sparing" was based primarily on sparing of brain weight, which told little or nothing about critical internal events in the brain whose disruptions would not manifest themselves at so gross a level as overall weight. Basically put, prenatal malnutrition of moderate severity and duration affects many different aspects of neurogenesis. It also affects the fundamental organizing underpinnings of brain structure by interfering with neuronal migration. Dobbing (1968a, 1968b, 1972), in particular, has stressed repeatedly that there is marked brain "sparing" during the fetal period in the face of malnutrition insult. He has also expressed the view that, even if there were limited brain "sparing," cell loss per se may not be important for later mental development. Some of this type of misconception may stem from the fact that in normal development neurons are constantly "turning over," with cell death in most brain structures being a normal aspect of brain organization and development. Cell death is most certainly a fundamental process taking place during development (Oppenheim, 1991) but should not be taken to mean that it is an event similar to cell loss induced by malnutrition and other types of brain insults. Some misconceptions relative to "sparing" in the prenatal period appear to derive from the literature on postnatal malnutrition, where prolonged starvation in human adults results in only small losses of bulk in the brain and heart, whereas muscles, liver, and spleen lose from one third to two thirds of their bulk. General conclusions that have been drawn from this latter type of malnutrition led to views that essential organs are "spared," meaning that tissues tend to be sacrificed in inverse order to their importance. Extrapolating this type of "sparing" to the prenatal brain situation is, however, clearly not warranted.

The above remarks should not be construed to imply, however, that there are no mechanisms engaged during prenatal malnutrition, some of which could compensate, in part, for the insult. In fact, if brain weight, a factor in which we put limited stock, is calculated as a proportion of body weight, it is clear that the brain is reduced less in weight than other organ systems by malnutrition during various prenatal periods (Winick and Noble, 1966). In this regard, it should also be kept in mind, relative to the time of insult, that if brain components are in a period of slow growth, including slower cell proliferation, then the insult will have less of an effect and, ultimately, be reflected in smaller losses of brain weight. This would not appear to represent an example of true brain "sparing" in terms of overall "protection" of the brain. The issue of the effects of cell loss in the brain on behavioral functioning has been variously argued, often in a counterproductive manner. Dobbing, in a series of papers (1968a, 1968b, 1970, 1971, 1972, 1985), and Davison and Dobbing (1968) maintained that cell loss in the brain may be meaningless in terms of behavioral function, since huge numbers of cells would have to be lost to alter function. The absence of a pathological "lesion" (see further below) probably brought on this type of thinking. On the other hand, Rodier (1977, 1980, 1988), in an elegant series of papers, observed that cell loss need not be massive to alter function. It is difficult to imagine, in critical brain structures such as the hippocampal formation, that marked cell loss would not manifest itself in altered function, even given the remarkable plasticity of this structure and the redundancy within its components, such as in the dentate gyrus. Relative to the issue of cell loss and its significance, the precision of regulation of neuron number apparent during the development of most neuronal populations strengthens the proposition that neuron number does matter a great deal. For example, there is considerable evidence that ratios of interconnected cells are regulated in a highly precise manner by naturally occurring cell death. In this way, neuron numbers can be adjusted by changes in proliferative potential and the extent of cell death. Thus, it appears that cell numbers are critical. Many tissues, including the brain, cannot recover from a restriction of cell number due to malnutrition and other insults, but certainly can recover from a restriction of cell size, this latter parameter being far less important for overall brain functioning.

## 7. NORMAL DEVELOPMENTAL EVENTS IN THE BRAIN

Understanding the sequences of events in central nervous system development is essential to interpreting behavioral assessments of any insults to the brain. This view has been most clearly expounded by Rodier (1977, 1980, 1988) and Rodier et al. (1979) in a series of studies on the chronology of brain development and the impact of precisely timed insults. Stages when interference with development leads to gross defects of the central nervous system, such as anencephaly or exencephaly, are seen very early in gestation during the period of organogenesis. In fact, most teratogens do not affect the developing brain, leading to gross abnormalities after the middle third of gestation. On the other hand, in the middle third of gestation teratogens or other insults may lead to functional changes with little or no evidence of a morphological lesion or damage. Since insults may interfere with cell proliferation, neuronal migration, and differentiation, knowledge of the timing of these processes in different areas of the central nervous system in species under study can provide important clues to aspects of altered anatomy, physiology, and behavior likely to be affected by a given insult. The fundamental tenant here is that there is in each species a quite rigid schedule on which the nervous system forms, and interference with basic developmental processes will selectively damage specific parts of the nervous system if delivered at different stages of development. Generally, with dose and agent held constant, the behavioral effects appear to be dependent on the time of insult.

The essential time table of brain development does not differ significantly among mammals, maturation of the brain in all species being a series of overlapping anatomical and physiological processes that provide the basis of function and behavior (Fig. 1). Therefore, it is possible to describe a general pattern of brain development that is applicable to all mammalian species. Accordingly, we use animal models to examine the effects of insults on the brain, since there are clearly corresponding events in the broad sequence of neuroontogenesis that do not vary fundamentally among different mammalian species. It is conventional to divide gestation into embryonic and fetal periods, the embryonic period lasting through the seventh week in humans, followed by the fetal period until birth. The embryonic period in humans is largely one of organogenesis, which is complete at about 3 months, while the fetal period is largely one of histogenesis and functional maturation. The fetus, in the face of insult, is relatively resistant to lethality or gross organ defects of shape and form but, as noted above, is susceptible to subtle, but important, histogenetic abnormalities and functional disturbances, which become apparent at subsequent stages of development.

We will now outline some of the major sequences of developmental events that occur in the organization and maturation of the brain as a basis for understanding how perturbations of these processes result in disturbed function and altered behavior. The cellular events during histogenesis of the brain are varied and complex and include: (1) neurogenesis, which involves proliferation of germinal cells to produce neurons and glia in the ventricular and subventricular zones; neural progeny sequentially leave the mitotic cycle after the terminal mitotic division and then migrate, a neuron birth date being defined as the time it leaves the cell cycle (Fig. 5); (2) migration of neurons to their final target destinations; (3) aggregation of neurons to form organized nuclear groups or cortical plates, the neuronal populations developing as both interacting and interdependent communities; (4) differentiation and maturation of neurons with branching and elongation of axons and dendrites and myelinization of axons; (5) synaptogenesis, including elaboration of axonal pathways and circuits, and development of mature (functional) synapses, including biosynthesis of chemical transmitters, a major task during this period being to produce the correct pattern of connections during a limited period of time; (6) regression and ultimate degeneration of cells, there being a programming of cellular death in all brain subsystems, with physiological cell death of excess neuroblasts and glioblasts at all stages of development.

We cannot possibly begin to interpret the mechanisms of developmentally restricting insults, such as prenatal protein malnutrition, on the brain without considering several of the above aspects of brain development, in particular, mechanisms controlling normal maturation of the brain at the cellular level. It is also clear that we must develop more knowledge of the genetic control of brain developmental events, the biosynthetic enzymes concerned with the production of proteins and lipids, and the distribution of their incorporation into various functional structures. In this regard, genetic regulation of brain development must also be considered to possibly be affected by malnutrition. Malnutrition during pregnancy appears to affect a variety of cellular processes. These include reducing the number of cells formed, perturbing and desynchronizing cellular migration from the original germinal zones, which may relate to failed or altered cellular interactions, and, if neurons do not get "in place," i.e., reach the target zone in a given time frame, they may not receive the necessary activation from inducing neurons moving in to synapse on them, and finally, delaying or blocking cellular growth and differentiation, and increasing cellular death. Disruption of these precise timing cycles by malnutrition may result in long-lasting and, in many cases, permanent changes in brain function.

While neurogenesis is only one of many events in the development of the nervous system, it is obviously an important one, since a nervous system lacking a full complement of neurons could hardly proceed to develop normally. The first thing to be emphasized about overall neuron production in different parts of the brain is that it occurs over an extremely long period, with various neuron types forming at different times and with different brain areas showing peaks of neurogenesis at particular times (Fig. 1). It is thus important in interpreting the effects of insults to understand the schedule of production of various cell types across subareas of the central nervous system. Accordingly, the stage of developmental events in the brain at the time of an insult such as malnutrition is the major determinant of the functional characteristics of brain-damaged animals. We should reiterate that no single species is an ideal model for human brain development if we consider only absolute time schedules. However, as noted, all mammalian species so far studied have proven to be remarkably similar in the sequence in which neurons form. The degree of functional maturity at birth differs from species to species, with the human more advanced in this regard than the rat and mouse, but considerably less advanced than the monkey. Since so many studies of neurogenesis have been carried out in the mouse and rat, it is of interest that developmental events in the rat are usually about 2 days later than in the mouse. In all mammals some neurons in the brain are generated very early, while others are produced throughout the remainder of gestation, with production levels becoming relatively low as birth approaches (Figs. 1 and 4). Following birth there is a return to high rates of cell proliferation in several brain areas, in particular, the microneuron (granule cell) populations of the dentate gyrus, olfactory bulb, and cerebellum, as well as the oligodendroglia, which are mostly generated postnatally in all areas of the brain (Figs. 2–5). A striking feature of the genesis of most cell types in specific brain subareas is that proliferation in a given brain area is completed in a very short time in all species (Figs. 1 and 3). What varies between species is the period of the crest of neurogenesis in each brain subdivision, meaning that an insult to the brain must overlap with particular peaks of neurogenesis in each region to produce a maximal deleterious effect on that particular area. Of interest is that species with longer periods of gestation show longer periods of neurogenic inactivity, rather than extensions of neuron proliferative periods for each neuron group (Rodier, 1980). This is important for the understanding of insults to the developing human brain, since it indicates that even brief insults can result in substantial neuron loss, just as in rats and mice. The more extended proliferative periods are associated with some medium-sized neurons and with all of the microneurons.

The major period of gliogenesis occurs largely postnatally, involving the oligodendroglia, which produce the myelin sheaths for axons (Figs. 2–4). However, there is also an early embryonic stage of gliogenesis involving the radial glia (astroglia), which are involved in directing the migration of neurons into the cerebral cortex, cerebellum, and various other brain areas. These proliferate in rodent embryos (Swarz and Oster-Granite, 1978) and multiply again in neonates (Basco et al., 1977). Both the early and late periods of gliogenesis are subject to disruption by malnutrition, with disturbances in the early period of radial glial proliferation related to conditions in which failures in neuron migrations occur (Choi and Lapham, 1978). Keeping in mind that considerable postnatal migration of neurons occurs in cerebellum, dentate gyrus, and olfactory bulb, usually from secondary germinal zones, postnatal insults could rather selectively affect these latter migrations. With respect to the migration of granule-cell precursors in the dentate gyrus of the hippocampal formation, Altman and Bayer (1990a, 1990b, 1990c) have questioned a role of radial glia in this structure. But, whatever the mechanism of this migration, it may be perturbed by postnatal malnutrition insult. In this regard, Seress (1977) has emphasized that the polymorph layer of the dentate gyrus is a secondary germinal layer that forms cells for the granular layer. Relative to heightened effects of insults to this region, Stanfield and Cowan (1988) point out that granule cells destined for the dentate gyrus divide on their way, or even after their arrival, in the granular layer.

The second major event in brain development is neuronal migration. During development of the brain, neurons migrate from the periventricular mitotic zones toward surfaces before further differentiation takes place. In most instances, with the exceptions given above, migrations are guided by a structural framework of radial glial fibers laid down early in development. Radial glial development is followed by both neuronal proliferation and proliferation of mature glia. The young neurons must move according to a rigid temporal schedule along specific pathways so as to arrive at their final locations in synchrony with their afferent synaptic partners (Rakic, 1975). Timing is of the utmost importance since, if migration rates are diminished, the young neurons would arrive at their ultimate destinations too late to recognize a specific target fiber. In considering target dependence of neurons, it is important to note that neuronal populations develop as both interacting and interdependent communities so that perturbations in migration result in disruptions of these precisely time-dependent processes. Ultimately, the reason for these migrations of nerve cells is to facilitate the formation of complex synaptic circuits, which are achieved by the precise spatial position and orientation of neurons in relation to neighboring neurons, both of similar and different types. In the normal developmental process, one result of these major shifts in position of nerve cell groups is that the architecture of the fetal brain bears only a rudimentary resemblance to that of the adult.

The third major phase of brain development is that of differentiation, involving all components of neurons and glia. Relative to final circuit formation, developing neuronal circuits in the central nervous system depend on the proliferation, migration, and differentiation of nerve cells being closely coordinated in both time and space. Normal development also depends on the formation and differentiation of both nerve cells and glial cells occurring in a highly interrelated fashion. Additionally, since catecholaminergic neurons are formed and differentiate at early stages of brain development, there is evidence that these neurons may influence the differentiation of nerve cells that they innervate. Any insults that affect early-developing serotonergic, noradrenergic, and dopaminergic systems may, therefore, produce effects on later differentiating nerve cells throughout the brain. In reality, prenatal malnutrition insult has been shown to affect these neurotransmitters dating from the time of birth (Morgane *et al.*, 1978, 1979). Finally, it is of interest, especially in light of our previous anatomical studies (Cintra *et al.*, 1982; Diaz-Cintra *et al.*, 1981a, 1981b, 1984), that many normal developmental processes in the brain involve a tendency for some parameters to actually diminish, such as is seen with the pruning of dendritic spines. In normal brain growth, there is not always a simple accumulation of more or larger units. In our studies we found that malnutrition insult actually appears to block the normal pruning of spines on dendrites in several brain areas, so that spine numbers remain higher than in normal controls (Diaz-Cintra *et al.*, 1981a, 1981b, 1984). This failure of normal pruning of dendritic spines may be one mechanism by which malnutrition insult perturbs brain development. In any event, it needs to be kept in mind, since the usual tendency is to look for various "deficits" in the insulted brain.

## 8. NEUROPATHOLOGY OF MENTAL RETARDATION AND DIFFUSE NEURONAL INSULTS

In considering the morphological bases of mental retardation, we should at the outset separate "degenerative" changes in the brain, which are the more usual "lesion"-type process, from "developmental" deviations, which are far more subtle and require special techniques to assess. Diffuse "lesions" of the central nervous system, as produced by insults that affect multiple brain areas, appear to have no focal neuropathology, as determined by the usual neuropathological assessments. Many of these "lesions" are at a biochemical or molecular level. Indeed, the general cytoarchitecture of the brain may appear relatively normal following such diffuse insults as malnutrition. Only quantitative neuroanatomical studies are capable of bringing out such subtle pathologies as, for example, shown in the series of experiments we have carried out on the brains of malnourished animals (Cintra *et al.*, 1990; Diaz-Cintra *et al.*, 1981b, 1984, 1991). Thus, elucidating the neuroanatomy of diffuse insult and "mental retardation" is a difficult task, though it is clear that the types of studies needed require animal models, given the obvious limitations of human brain material. Additionally, a brain model system is required, particularly one in which interdisciplinary studies can be effectively brought to bear. This is one reason why the hippocampal model system (see below) has proven to be so valuable in studies of many types of insults to the developing brain. Nonetheless, it should not be assumed that malnutrition or other insults affect only the hippocampal formation, or even that this complex structure is preferentially affected. This structure does offer a "window" on the brain, enabling multidisciplinary studies to be carried out. Many aspects of behavior associated with this formation have been defined, particularly its association with the expression of learned behaviors. Likewise, its anatomy, including the internal circuitry and various inputs and outputs, is also fairly well known. In addition, the hippocampal formation demonstrates a remarkable form of plasticity, exemplified by long-term potentiation, which appears to represent a principal substrate of learning and memory (see below). Its various components develop both pre- and postnatally and, therefore, specific neuronal assemblies of this system can be manipulated differentially to study both prenatal and postnatal insults. The known vulnerability of the hippocampal formation to a variety of insults is also well documented. Further, the formation plays a major role in arousal, motivational, emotional, and attentional processes, which can best be examined in an interdisciplinary manner.

We do not believe that forms of mental retardation resulting from insults to the brain arise form purely localized structural brain lesions, but rather subscribe to the view of a distributed (diffuse) lesion involving wide areas of the neuraxis. Though we do not know the anatomical structures associated with so-called higher mental functions, it is clear that systems involved in such functions are distributed at several integrative levels in the central nervous system. This does not in any way preclude examining specific brain model systems that form vital links in overall neuronal functioning and whose altered development and subsequent functioning has widespread manifestations related to higher order processing, including learning and memory. Dobbing (1985) has pointed out that undernutrition does not produce brain "damage," in the proper sense of the word, and therefore does not result in identifiable "scars." Thus, it merely distorts development and, in this manner, alters quantitative relationships within the brain so that quantitative histology is needed to elucidate the effects. As noted above, this is what our group (Diaz-Cintra et al., 1981b, 1984, 1991) has done, thereby shedding light on some local pathologies resulting from malnutrition insult. In Dobbing's view, early malnutrition has not been shown to cause "damage" to brain tissue but, rather, modifies brain growth without specific lesions. However, he points out that relevant brain structures show deficits because neurons have failed to arrive in sufficient numbers at the correct time in development. Thus, there results distortion of quantitative relationships between neuron types, and that is why developmental malnutrition has been described by Dobbing (1984) as one of deficits and distortions rather than brain lesions. Distortions of cellular elements cannot usually be seen but, rather, only measured using quantitative histological techniques.

One of the more common ways of assessing central nervous system damage following "diffuse" insults such as malnutrition has been to examine brain weight as a proportion of body weight. With toxic agents and insults such as malnutrition having systemic effects on cell proliferation, this ratio, however, becomes largely inappropriate. Only insults that damage the central nervous system and spare other body systems will lower the brain/body ratio. Interestingly, the whole idea of adjusting brain weight according to body weight rests on the assumption that the two measures are highly correlated in normal animals, an assumption for which there appears to be little or no evidence. The simple use of brain weight as an index of damage is probably logical as long as there is reason to suspect damage that affects large regions of the central nervous system. We would not weigh brains to confirm damage such as electrolytic lesions and would not expect weight differences in small samples after lesions to be confined to a small structure or two. Obviously, direct quantitative measurements of the structure itself are more sensitive and provide more information. We mention this again since brain weight has frequently been taken as an indicator of neuronal insult.

Interference with cell proliferation during central nervous system development has been shown to have permanent effects on both brain anatomical organization and behavior, and can often lead to a wide variety of brain damage syndromes. However, cell loss is not usually obvious in gross measures of the central nervous system such as "thickness" or area of entire brain regions, or brain weights, etc. As noted, changes in anatomy of the central nervous system following insults also do not necessarily appear as the absence of structures or as scars or alterations of normal form. Rather, they usually appear as small reductions or distortions of cell arrangement, e.g., irregular distribution of neurons in specific subregions, with simplified dendritic arborization and with altered spine densities, all of which require morphometric methods, including radioautographic measures, to be judged as abnormal. With regard to neuronal connectivity and circuitry, it is difficult to imagine that neuronal linkages, including circuit arrangements, could be normal when neuron numbers are abnormal.

## 9. SPECIFIC PATHOLOGIES OF INSULTS TO THE DEVELOPING BRAIN

Insults to the fetus result in developmental deviations in the fetal brain through diverse pathogenetic mechanisms, such as mitotic interference, chromosomal defects, enzyme inhibition, and alterations in energy sources, among others. Of interest is that the same pathogenetic mechanisms may not be operative at all stages of gestation. Clearly, to interpret the effects of malnutrition insult on the brain we must have an understanding of normal structural organization, including cellular patterns of arrangements, as well as developmental events during gestation, both at the cellular and molecular levels. Experimental studies have shown that clearly a variety of "molecular" pathologies exist following malnutrition insult (Balázs et al., 1977, 1979; Lewis et al., 1975; Shimada et al., 1977).

It appears likely that selective loss of proliferating cells is the mechanism by which most insults, including malnutrition, alter brain development (Fig. 7). As noted, many characteristics of brain damage may relate to perturbations of the sequence of neuronal production, and such a sequence of production of different classes of neurons appears to be a mechanism for the orderly growth of neuronal circuitry (Altman, 1986, 1987). While interfering with neurogenesis is only one way in which the central nervous system may be injured, it appears to be a major factor in some syndromes produced by insults to the brain. Reduced cell numbers may result in changes in the size of structures and can be more appreciated in laminar structures, where thickness of the laminae partially reflects cell numbers more clearly than in nucleate- or reticulate-type neuronal organizations. Given that there are transient periods of vulnerability related to transient periods of cell division, it is important to distinguish between direct destruction of stem cells and simple changes in the proliferation rates later on. In either case, any later developmental processes that depend on the earlier completion of events that have been disturbed will themselves be secondarily affected.

The effects of prenatal protein malnutrition on the kinetics of cell proliferation are of special interest. A major approach has been identification of the phases of the cell cycle

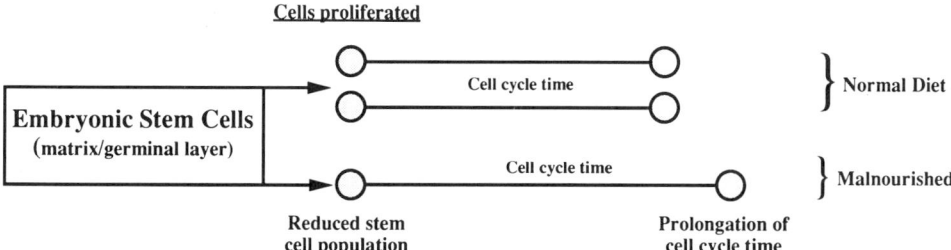

**FIGURE 7.** Malnutrition effects on cell kinetics altering cell cycle time and the number of cells generated in well-nourished compared to malnourished animals.

that are affected in the replicating cells of the developing brain. It has been shown by Balázs and his colleagues (1975, 1977, 1979) and by Lewis *et al.* (1975, 1979) that malnutrition caused distortions within each of the different phases of the cell generation cycle. These effects are illustrated in Figure 8, taken from various data of the above-mentioned authors and from that of Shimada *et al.* (1974) and Shimada and Morikawa (1978), the latter authors showing that the generation times of matrix cells (precursors of neurons) are prolonged by approximately 3 hr in malnourished animals compared to nonmalnourished controls. These effects on cell-cycle kinetics can result not only in reductions in final cell numbers, but also, importantly, in the cellular composition of the developing brain. These alterations induced by malnutrition would appear to play a major role in modifying neuronal maturation and eventual function. It should be stressed that the effects on cell formation are only one of the factors contributing to the behavioral anomalies that develop following various insults in early periods of development. Metabolic balance, for example, is important not only for nerve-cell proliferation, but also for the maintenance of existing cells (Balázs *et al.*, 1977). Thus, there is evidence that committed cells are lost in malnutrition, as well as in other types of insults, such as thyroid deficiency (Balázs *et al.*, 1977, 1979). Effects on neuronal differentiation and, importantly, on the consecutive development of neuronal interconnections are also of particular significance. An apparently paradoxical result has been of particular value in identifying the phases of the cell cycle that are affected in the replicating cells of the developing brain. It was found that the rate of cell acquisition is depressed throughout the brain of malnourished rats, but that the decrease is considerably less than that of the rate of DNA synthesis (Balázs *et al.*, 1975; Lewis *et al.*, 1975). It appears that such a discrepancy is due to a distortion of the different phases of the cell generation cycle. Malnutrition results in a marked prolongation in the length of the DNA synthetic (S) phase, but cell cycle time is much less affected, since the length of the G1 phase is severely curtailed (Fig. 8). This may have important

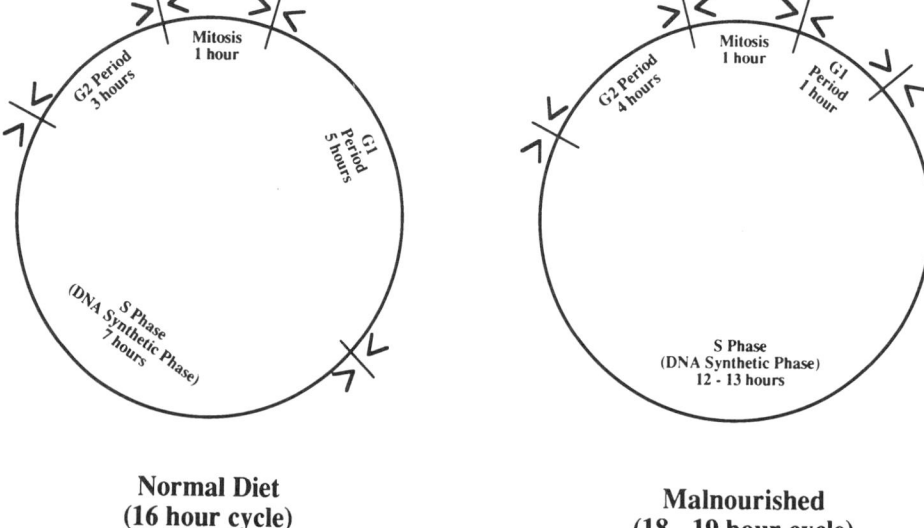

**FIGURE 8.** Schematic illustration of the effects of malnutrition on different phases of the cell cycle in the rat. Data for this figure were derived from studies of Lewis *et al.* (1975), Shimada *et al.* (1977), and Shimada and Morikawa (1978).

consequences for the progeny of the dividing cells, since molecular processes occurring during part of the G1 phase may be critical in terms of cell differentiation. As noted by Balázs et al. (1975) and Lewis et al. (1975), these effects on the kinetics of cell proliferation appear to be rather specific for tissues, such as the developing brain, where extensive cell replication is restricted to a limited period. Nutritional deprivation in other tissues also results in marked prolongation of the cell cycle time, including both the S and G1 phases, and a similar situation exists in the residual subependymal layer of malnourished adult rats. This indicates that, in contrast to the well-documented resistance of differentiated cells in the adult brain, the replicating cells are as vulnerable to nutritional insults as most other cells in the body. Neural cell differentiation is also affected by prenatal malnutrition, including distortions in the normal pattern of brain development, for example, affecting the coordinated development of neurotransmitter systems. In view of the importance of chronological programming in development and its relationship to the ultimate integrative organization of the central nervous system, such distortions, including resulting imbalances in cell types and neurotransmitter activity, would appear to contribute significantly to the functional impairments.

## 10. ANIMAL MODELS OF PRENATAL RETARDATION

Investigations using animal models of mental retardation (Thompson et al., 1986, 1987) have to date had limited success in elucidating neuroanatomical correlates of generalized cognitive impairments. These cognitive defects appear to involve such "diffuse" processes as information processing, vigilance, attention, and arousal, and such global activities obviously cannot be centered in particular brain structures; nor do overall learning systems of the brain correspond to any clearly defined multisynaptic functional pathways. As noted by Thompson et al. (1986, 1987), the learning system in the brain appears to be hierarchically organized and may have the potential to influence the activities of widespread regions throughout the neuraxis and, thereby, serves to form new associations and facilitates the organization and execution of appropriate behavioral responses. Many studies indicate that the hippocampal formation and its widespread input and output systems are important for several types of memory, although pinning down its precise activities in this regard has not yet been possible.

Among the psychological models developed to account for learning impairments in mentally retarded humans have been the so-called defect theories reviewed by Thompson et al. (1986, 1987). Three of these defect theories are clearly applicable to animal models featuring generalized learning impairments. The first of these theories assumes the presence of a defect in inhibitory processes, the second a defect in attentional processes, and the third a defect in short-term memory processes. The review of Thompson et al. (1986, 1987) noted that retarded brain-damaged rats can be well differentiated into subgroups based solely on the constellation of impaired and intact inhibitory, attentional, and short-term memory functions. This is of immediate interest, since our own work using the hippocampal model system following prenatal protein malnutrition shows alterations in many of these same processes (Austin et al., 1986, 1991; Bronzino et al., 1991a, 1991b). In interpreting diffuse brain damage induced by malnutrition insult during various critical periods of brain development, we consider the learning system in the brain to be an aggregate of interconnected neural regions whose combined activities are responsible for rather broad functions in learning. The organization of neural circuits in such a system are thought to be both diffuse and specific. We may consider this overall learning system as being composed of core subsystems, such as the hippocampal formation and basal ganglia, which function as generators or executive systems that coordinate and sequence activities of many local brain regions in carrying out planned behaviors. Types of cognitive functions of the hippocampal formation may be put in the context of this structural complex as playing a role in general activation, sequencing of behaviors, attentional processes, and similar activities (Altman, 1986, 1987). In our studies, as reviewed below, we have used the hippocampal model system to examine the effects of prenatal protein malnutrition on various hippocampally mediated aspects of behavior.

Studies on experimental animals have provided strong evidence that certain aspects of behavior are permanently altered following nutritional insults experienced during the perinatal period of brain development (Morgane et al., 1978; Smart, 1987, 1990). Developmental psychologists originally turned to animal models to elucidate the effects of early malnutrition on learning ability and behavior, since it was thought that the confounding variables associated with human malnutrition, i.e., a combination of social and environmental factors in the so-called deprived environment, could be better controlled in the laboratory. The procedures currently used to produce nutritional deficiency, such as separation of the young from the mother and increased litter size, also induce major changes in the suckling rat's social and environmental conditions; these changes no doubt play an important part in the determination of later behavior (Frankova, 1974; Galler et al., 1984; Galler and Kanis, 1987). Early malnutrition and the variables associated with it also affect subsequent size, motor ability, behavior toward food, ability to absorb and use food, as well as to adjust to food deprivation and, importantly, responses to environmental stimuli. It is, therefore, likely that the influence of early malnutrition may involve effects on these other variables that can affect learning performance, rather than directly upon learning capacity per se. These are all-important considerations, given that the overwhelming majority of studies relating nutrition and cognitive functioning have been conducted in the rat. Even with this species, however, Fleischer and Turkewitz (1984) have pointed out that several of the various techniques for producing malnutrition, i.e., raising animals in large litters, maintaining dams on inadequate diets pre- and/or postnatally, and periodically separating the litter from the dam, result in considerable extranutritional effects on the animals that may contribute to the deviations in development. The extranutritional environmental factors that have been most studied are the infant animal's social relations, e.g., mother–pup interactions (Galler et al., 1984). A number of methods of inducing malnutrition have been shown to affect those mother–pup interactions so that, to some extent, these factors cannot be completely eliminated, even in experimental animal models. However, since social and nutritional factors are so closely related in both rats and humans, the rat is a most useful model of human malnutrition. It is clear, nevertheless, in both species that malnutrition produces its effects by both direct and indirect mechanisms, with one principal mode of indirect effect being via alterations in mother–pup interactions.

All experimental studies of the effects of insults to the brain must recognize that the brains of different species show the maximum rates of development at different times in relation to birth (Fig. 4). As noted, interspecies extrapolations compare the relative "ages" of brains. Most interspecies comparisons can avoid difficulties if developmental progress is divided into stages according to neural events, rather than to their timing in any single species. Accordingly, appropriate comparisons can be made on the basis of events, i.e., developmental age, rather than on chronological age. Since major difficulties arise in making analogies between the effects of intrauterine malnutrition on the brains of laboratory animals and humans based on the wide range of brain maturation in relation to birth, some specific examples should be noted. Human brain development is approximately between that of the guinea pig and rat in terms of several parameters, including weight, myelin lipid formation, and total DNA at birth. The percentage of brain cells, as represented by total DNA, varies at birth in the three species, since most cells are present at birth in the guinea pig, approximately 75% are present in the human, while only 17% are present in the rat (Chase et al., 1971). A variety of evidence indicates that most of the postnatal increase in DNA in the human brain represents an increase in glial cells. The human brain initiates a period of rapid weight gain during the last half of fetal life, with a peak near the time of birth, which then decreases over the first year or so of postnatal life. Approximately two thirds of the human brain cells, as represented by DNA content, accumulate prior to birth, and one third accumulate between birth and age 5 months (Winick and Noble, 1966). On the other hand, less than one fifth of rat brain cells are normally present at birth (Chase et al., 1971). These types of developmental parameters are important to keep in mind when making assessments of how an insult affects a particular species in relation to its specific brain developmental events.

Consideration of interspecies and time-scale differences in parameters of brain development is critical for extrapolation of animal data to the human condition. Thus, parameters in which age-equivalent periods of development between species are matched is essential, i.e., it is necessary to first determine the periods during development when a parameter in question is equivalent for the two species. In this regard, the complex relationships between gestation time, brain weight, and advancement at birth have been thoroughly discussed by Sacher and Staffeldt (1974). Overall, they showed that gestation time increases with neonatal brain size and with advancement of brain weight at birth and decreases in litter size. These taxonomic patterns of fetal development are important factors to consider in relating animal nutritional deprivations to those in humans in terms of effects on brain and body weights. It is apparent that brain growth proceeds at the maximum rate allowed by its nutrition, i.e., if nutrition is not rate limiting, and its intrinsic growth rules.

When considering overall brain weights as a rough "indicator" of brain "development," the following two points should be considered: (1) what is the value of brain weight as an indicator of brain function in higher order processing, and (2) the correspondence between brain weight and actual cellular composition and the degree of connectivity is most certainly not a direct one. The functional significance of actual total "cell numbers" may be less clear with regard to neuron numbers in relation to later disturbances in brain function and behavior. There is little doubt, however, that the remarkable burst of gliogenesis, which occurs mostly postnatally to produce oligodendroglia, results directly in brain myelinization, with myelin eventually comprising some 25% of brain weight. In terms of myelogenesis affecting brain function, this process is of the utmost importance, but no more than the original production of nerve cells, which, of course, has much less significance on total brain weight as expressed by the so-called brain growth spurt.

## 11. BRAIN MODELS FOR STUDIES OF INSULTS TO THE BRAIN AND CONCEPTS OF SELECTIVE VULNERABILITY

The question of truly "selective" vulnerability is how generalized insults affect localized populations of neurons. Aspects of these so-called selective types of vulnerability in various diffuse brain insults have always been puzzling. The pathogenesis of selective damage or deviations in the programs of development still remain largely unknown. However, in the hippocampal formation alterations in amino-acid transmitter systems appear to play a major role in selective damage to this structure. There is considerable evidence that selective regional insults are reflected in measurable biochemical alterations at different stages of development (Balázs et al., 1979; Coursin, 1975). Some toxins certainly damage all nerve cell types, but failures of repair mechanisms, involving altered restorative plasticity, may be responsible for the persistence of microdamage in select brain regions.

Special vulnerability of the brain results from a complex, programmed chronology of development, and interference with any part of this developmental sequence may produce irreversible effects on structure and function. For example, Balázs et al. (1979) reported an abnormally high rate of cell degeneration occurring in the brain germinal layers in malnutrition. It is clear that nutritional deficiency affects the structural and biochemical development of the central nervous system, with some indices appearing to be reversible following dietary rehabilitation. However, because of the programmed chronology in development in relation to the ultimate integrative organization of the brain, the apparently "reversible" nature of some of the alterations produced by malnutrition does not preclude various distortions, such as alterations in cell ratios, which lead to abnormalities in brain function.

There is clearly selective vulnerability of neuronal subpopulations during ontogeny that reflect discrete molecular events associated with normal brain development. Many aspects of the molecular bases for selective vulnerability and its variations during ontogeny are not well understood but, in any event, ontogenetic changes in selective vulnerability are often associated with many striking biochemical changes, and this association frequently suggests a pathogenic mechanism. To appreciate some of these, it should be emphasized that neuronal death and inhibition of mitotic activity are not the only expressions of vulnerability in the developing brain. For example, the establishment of synaptic connections, the competition for fields of innervation by axons from different neuronal populations, as well as programmed elimination of excess synaptic terminals are all normal growth processes that can be affected by insults to the developing brain (Wasterlain et al., 1990). It is of interest that selective vulnerability of discrete neuronal populations to a variety of metabolic insults undergoes dramatic changes during ontogeny. Interestingly, selective vulnerability may appear with the induction of a protein in a specific region of the brain. For example, in newborn rats the CA3 pyramidal neurons of the hippocampus proper contain only trace amounts of glutamate receptors of the kainic acid type, which are quite resistant to systemic administration of kainic acid in spite of its good penetration into the brain. However, after induction of kainic-acid receptors during development, the vulnerability of CA3 neurons to this excitotoxin increases dramatically (Wasterlain et al., 1990). Similarly, the vulnerability of CA1 pyramidal neurons to ischemic damage is not seen during the first postnatal week in the rat, which is a time when the immaturity of the Schaffer collaterals precludes the liberation of large amounts of excitotoxic transmitters, presumably glutamate, during ischemic insults. Interestingly, with maturation of the Schaffer collaterals during the second week of life, this is accompanied by a dramatic increase in ischemic vulnerability of the CA1 pyramidal neurons. Further, selective vulnerability may also disappear with the induction of a protein. Thus, in week-old rats, granule cells in the inner layers of the dentate gyrus are particularly vulnerable to hypoxic ischemia. However, as these cells acquire the calcium-binding protein calbindin D28k, which are thought to buffer intracellular calcium, they then become resistant to hypoxic-ischemic insults (Wasterlain et al., 1990). There are other interesting examples of selective vulnerability disappearing with some developmental events. Thus, the inhibition by seizures of mitotic activity, DNA, and protein synthesis has its most persisting consequences at the end of the so-called brain growth spurt period, which is a time when little mitotic potential is left to compensate for the results of this transient seizure-induced inhibition. Selective vulnerability may also peak with the hyperinduction of a protein; for example, NMDA-mediated damage peaks in rats during the second week of life, which is a time of peak expression of NMDA receptors. Selective vulnerability may also reflect a transient imbalance between metabolic pathways induced at different times during brain development. In this regard, in neonates of several species seizures and hypoxia profoundly deplete brain glucose, with severe developmental consequences. The ability of the brain at that age to utilize glucose appears to be greater than its capacity for transport across the blood–brain barrier, perhaps related to the low capillary density of the immature brain. These processes have important implications for the understanding and treatment of neonatal seizures, and suggest that normal brain development may result in transient windows of vulnerability when neurotransmitter circuitry or metabolic capacity are stressed by pathological processes (Collins, 1987).

Relative to selective vulnerability of the hippocampal formation to malnutrition insults, there is a growing body of evidence that malnutrition alters the development and functions of this structure with differential effects on its various subregions (Altman, 1986, 1987). A variety of anatomical and behavioral alterations have been reported in components of the hippocampal formation, particularly following postnatal malnutrition (Castro and Rudy, 1987; Fish and Winick, 1969; Katz and Davies, 1983; Noback and Eisenman, 1981; Shoemaker and Bloom, 1977). Especially, spatial memory deficits have been correlated with hippocampal anatomical changes following combined pre- and postnatal malnutrition. Further, Lewis et al. (1979) showed that prenatal malnutrition reduced the thickness of the granule-cell layer of the dentate gyrus in rats and moderately prolonged the cell cycle time, in particular, substantially lengthening the DNA synthetic phase and curtailing the G1 phase of the cell cycle. The cell acquisition rate in the dentate gyrus was markedly diminished, resulting in profound deficits in granule-cell numbers by the second postnatal week. Such changes may exert their effects by altering the normal afferent and efferent relationships of the dentate gyrus, which may underlie some of the functional changes seen in malnutrition. As reviewed further below, relative to physiological changes in hippocampal activity resulting from prenatal protein malnutrition, we have shown marked changes in ontogeny of the EEG, in particular aspects of theta rhythm maturation (Bronzino et al., 1983; Morgane et al., 1985), development and maintenance of long-term potentiation (Austin et al., 1986), alterations in the development of kindling (Bronzino et al., 1986, 1990), changes in patterns of input to the hippocampal formation that are vigilant-state dependent (Austin et al., 1989, 1991), and changes in paired-pulse inhibition of granule-cell excitability (Bronzino et al., 1991a, 1991b). Before reviewing the altered physiology of the hippocampal formation induced by prenatal protein malnutrition, we will briefly discuss the hippocampal formation as a brain model system for assessing insults.

## 12. THE HIPPOCAMPAL FORMATION AS A BRAIN MODEL SYSTEM

The hippocampal formation is a prominent archicortical structure that comprises a major neural complex in the brain of all mammals. It forms a division of the limbic system that consists of a large number of neural components thought to be involved in the regulation of autonomic and somatic behaviors, and has widespread connections with many regions of the forebrain and brainstem. The functional role of the hippocampal formation is complex, and analysis of its activity in overall nervous system function has so far not yielded clear-cut answers. Being the subject of intensive investigations in recent years at the anatomical, physiological, biochemical, and behavioral levels, it has become a common model system in which to study the effects of a wide variety of insults to the brain. Its role in motivational, attentional, and emotional behaviors, and especially, in learning and memory processing, have implicated the hippocampal formation as a key structure whose abnormal functioning reveals elements in animal models closely related to certain forms of human mental retardation (Altman, 1986, 1987).

This emphasis on the hippocampal model has been due primarily to its special anatomical organization, including lamination of its inputs and stereotyped geometry of synaptic relationships, as well as its physiological and functional characteristics and special developmental history, with different components showing either predominantly prenatal or postnatal neurogenesis. Thus, the hippocampal formation has become one of the most intensively studied areas of the central nervous system. Perhaps more importantly, it has become the structure of greatest relevance for investigations of neuronal plasticity, a central theme in considering the effects of insults to the brain and possibilities for potential restitution of function. Conceptually, the hippocampal formation has been especially exploited as a model system for furthering concepts of brain–environmental interactions, and various such considerations are examined in this chapter in relation to alterations resulting from malnutrition insult.

The hippocampal formation is a brain model system of special choice in various behavioral studies, since lesions of this structure are associated with some distinctive behavioral consequences. Moreover, since it has several neuronal cell types with different times of neurogenesis, it is also possible to separate the structure anatomically by varying the time of neuronal insult. With regard to use of the hippocampal brain model system to study insults to the brain, it should be pointed out that there are many cell types comprising the hippocampal formation, even though the two principal cell types are the pyramidal neurons of the hippocampus proper and the dentate granule cells of the dentate gyrus. Additionally, there are many types of interneurons in the hippocampal formation, including ones using GABA as a transmitter, as demonstrated by the studies of Ribak and Seress (1983). The separation of the structure into pyramidal cells and granule cells is clearly an inadequate description of the anatomical separation of functions in the hippocampal formation.

Activity in the internal circuitry of the hippocampal formation is, in turn, under modulation of local and projection-type inhibitory neurons and, largely, via the medial septal area, monoaminergic fibers from the brainstem and cholinergic pathways from the ventral forebrain (Fig. 9). Direct GABA projection neurons from the medial septal area synapse on the inhibitory interneurons (Freund and Antal, 1988; Schwerdtferger, 1986) and, importantly, along with cholinergic projections from the medial septal area, play a major role in pacing theta activity in the hippocampal formation. These complex interneuronal involvements, along with monoamine modulation of cellular activity, is an integral factor in the mechanism by which the hippocampal formation may process and gate incoming stimuli (Austin *et al.*, 1989). In this regard, one of the most important aspects of attempts to understand hippocampal function relates to the studies showing that the efficacy of neuronal transmission through the hippocampal formation varies with the vigilance state of the animal (see Section 13).

Though one theory of hippocampal function is that it is involved in the formation of

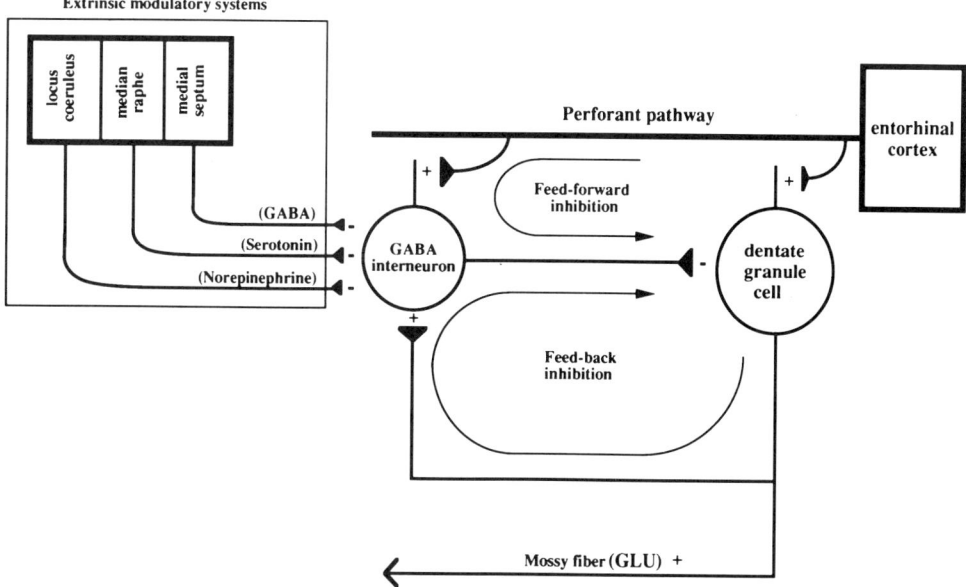

**FIGURE 9.** Illustration of circuits of the hippocampal dentate gyrus showing pathways of feedforward and feedback inhibition. The GABA interneuron is shown to be under the modulatory influence of three extrinsic systems known to synapse on the interneuron. See discussion in the text.

cognitive spatial maps, i.e., creating a neural map of the environment (O'Keefe and Nadel, 1978), a distillation of work to date indicates the functional role is not a simple one and certainly is not unitary in nature. Probably a most useful "generic" summary of its function is that it plays a major role in regulation of an animal's interaction with its environment. Thus, it appears to be involved in the integration and classification of incoming stimuli from the environment, both internal and external. If such functions are deranged by neuronal insults, the implications are that the organism experiences a failure of adequate interactions with the surrounding environment, which, in turn, would affect various aspects of learning and memory, possibly leading to developmental disabilities, failure of cognitive functions, and mental retardation. A key concept that relates to overall use of the hippocampal model in studies of insults to the brain is that, for example, in malnutrition there may be a functional isolation from its surroundings in that the animal either cannot fully receive or fully utilize information from its environment. Since malnutrition affects the vigilance-state-dependent gating of information input into and through the hippocampal formation (Austin et al., 1991), this vigilance-state dependence may prove to be a most useful way to interpret some of the disruptive effects of malnutrition in certain aspects of learning and memory.

## 13. RECENT PHYSIOLOGICAL STUDIES: EMPHASIS ON HIPPOCAMPAL NEURONAL ACTIVITY

Having considered some of the results of various types of nutritional insults on the proliferation, migration, and differentiation of cellular components of the central nervous system, the next question is to relate these alterations in cellular anatomy to bioelectric

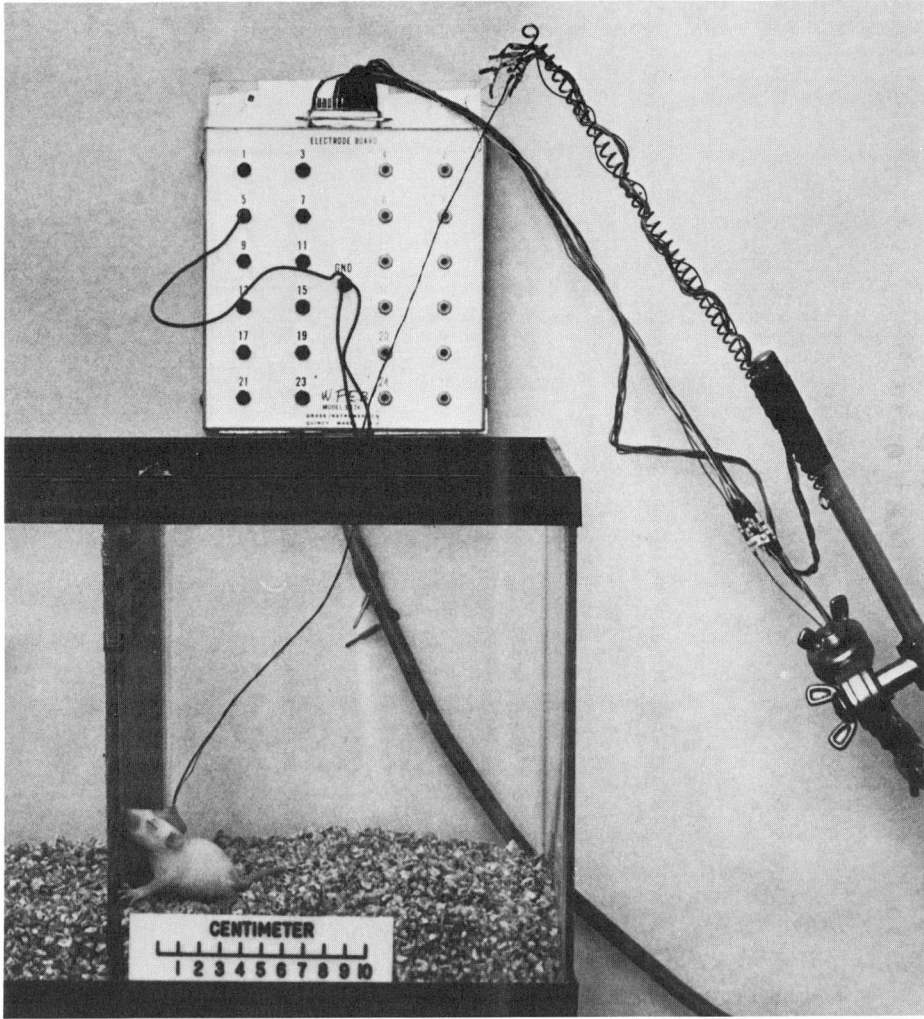

**FIGURE 10.** Photograph of a preweaning rat with eyes still closed being chronically recorded across the vigilance states. Electrodes within the hippocampal formation record EEG activity as a means of investigating the development and maturation of the theta rhythm.

measures of brain function and, ultimately, to behavior. Early studies in both rats (Gramsbergen, 1974, 1976) and humans (Schulte *et al.*, 1972) established that perinatal forms of malnutrition result in retarding the maturation of age-related EEG patterns. Data from our own examination of the development of EEG frequency components in the hippocampal formation (Bronzino *et al.*, 1983; Morgane *et al.*, 1985) established that concurrent protein malnutrition (combined pre- and postnatal protein malnutrition employing either an 8% or 6% casein diet) results in delaying the maturational shift in peak theta frequency recorded during REM sleep. These studies traced the ontogenetic development of the peak theta frequency measure from postnatal day 14 through day 45. Figure 10 shows the type of chronic recording apparatus we use to record hippocampal electrical activity from preweaning rats. In the rat, the first appearance of the theta rhythm is highly correlated with the initiation of basic exploratory behaviors and the opening of the eyes. This suggests that theta activity plays some critical role in the gating of environmental information very early in development. Although the peak theta frequency measure does reach values equivalent to that of normally nourished controls by about the 45th day of age, the change in the developmental synchrony between theta activity and the animal's early experience of and interaction with the environment during this critical formative stage may be of considerable consequence to the manner in which the animal interacts with the environment in later life. Given the role ascribed to theta activity in the modulation of hippocampal function (Vanderwolf and Leung, 1983; Winson, 1975), any change in the functional status of the theta rhythm, especially during the period of initial experience of and interaction with the environment, could be expected to have an impact, albeit perhaps a subtle one, on the manner in which the animal responds to the environment later in life. On a more mechanistic level, one of the more conceptually interesting functions suggested for theta is that it serves to gate information flow through the hippocampal formation (Bennett, 1975; Black, 1975). As such, the theta rhythm could be considered an attending signal, in waking states, focusing the attention of the animal upon biologically relevant stimuli within the environment, and during sleep states (REM) gating information flow through hippocampal neural systems, which play a role in the consolidation of memory. Nutritionally induced retardation in frequency maturation of REM theta activity would result in changes in this gating function, either interrupting or significantly altering information processing during critical periods of behavioral development.

An indication that this early developmental lag in peak theta frequency maturation may have implications in later life comes from the recently reported work of Austin *et al.* (1991). The high- and low-frequency components of this theta rhythm have been shown by pharmacological manipulation to depend upon separate neurotransmitter systems for their activity (Monmaur *et al.*, 1981). The slow or tonic component, associated with REM sleep, is characterized by a fixed-frequency peak in the adult, which is paced by cholinergic innervation arising from cells of the medial septum. The peak frequency of the phasic or mobility-related component of theta activity is variable, depending upon the specific behavior, and is generally of higher frequency than the tonic component. It is noncholinergic, as indicated by its resistance to atropine, and strong evidence indicates that this portion of the theta rhythm is GABA-ergic and also of septal origin. In normally nourished animals the peak frequency component of this theta activity is highly correlated with the specific behavioral state and shows a distinctive frequency shift between active waking behaviors and REM sleep. In contrast, the peak frequency component of mobility-related (active waking) theta recorded from protein-malnourished rats does differ significantly from that seen during REM sleep, i.e., there is no shift from slower to faster frequencies as the animal engages in various locomotory behaviors (Morgane *et al.*, 1990). These results suggest that the prenatal dietary insult results in enduring alterations to the noncholinergic theta-generating mechanisms associated with certain voluntary movement behaviors. Such behaviors would necessarily require the animal to be acquiring and processing information about its interaction with the immediate environment. The fact that these results were obtained in adult animals following an extended period of dietary rehabilitation indicates the long-lasting impact of a dietary insult instituted during the prenatal period.

Of particular significance to questions concerning the impact of dietary insults on information flow and processing within the hippocampal formation are the findings of

Winson and Abzug (1978). These indicate that the efficacy of neuronal transmission through the entire hippocampal formation is dependent upon the vigilance state of the animal. The efficacy of transmission is highest during slow-wave sleep, relatively suppressed during active waking behaviors, and variable, depending upon the phase of theta, during REM. These findings have provided the bases for our investigations of behaviorally mediated information flow through specific limbs of the hippocampal trisynaptic circuit in malnourished animals. As we have reported (Bronzino et al., 1991a), although there appears to be no significant difference in granule-cell input/output measures between normally nourished and malnourished animals, investigations utilizing paired-pulse stimulation of the perforant pathway, a technique designed to elucidate the effects of net modulatory influences on the level of granule-cell excitability, have revealed a significant increase in both the magnitude and duration of the early inhibitory phase of granule-cell modulation (Austin et al., 1989, 1991). In addition, these studies have revealed significantly higher levels of inhibitory control of granule-cell activity during the theta behaviors of active waking and REM sleep. These results again point out the special vulnerability to nutritional insult of systems involved in the generation of hippocampal theta activity.

In our studies (Austin et al., 1986) we have also investigated the effects of dietary insults on the phenomenon of long-term potentiation (LTP). LTP is defined as the long-lasting enhancement of synaptic transmission efficacy induced by high-frequency electrical stimulation. LTP has received much attention as a model of memory formation because it shares many characteristics with memory formation, including rapid onset, long duration, and strengthening with repetition (Teyler and DiScenna, 1984). In addition, pharmacological treatments that interfere with the induction of hippocampal LTP can also interfere with hippocampal-dependent learning (Morris et al., 1982, 1986). Thus, an enhanced understanding of LTP may lead to a greater knowledge of the neurobiology of memory formation. Studies of the LTP phenomenon in both anesthetized (Austin et al., 1986) and freely moving rats (Austin-LaFrance et al., 1991) indicate that prenatal protein malnutrition, followed by dietary rehabilitation commencing at the time of birth, results in significant alterations in specific measures of this phenomenon. In prenatally malnourished rats tested in adulthood, tetanic stimulation of the perforant pathway results in significant potentiation of the population EPSP component of the granule-cell field response. However, this enhancement is not translated into enhanced granule-cell discharge to the level seen in normally nourished controls. In addition, the decay rate in the level of enhancement of the population spike measure is markedly greater in malnourished animals. In a recent preliminary study, our group (Austin-LaFrance et al., 1991) has examined the ability of adult rats that were protein malnourished only during gestation and subsequently underwent dietary rehabilitation commencing at birth, to establish and maintain LTP of the perforant path/dentate granule-cell synapse. Results of this study indicate that malnourished animals show immediate potentiation of the population EPSP measure that occurs concomitant with a decline in the amplitude of the population spike amplitude measure. The population spike amplitude measure fails to show significant potentiation effects until 12–18 hr after tetanization. In contrast, normally nourished controls show an initial decline in both EPSP and population spike measures followed by a continuous rise in both measures out to 18 hr post-tetanization when this enhancement begins to decline. After tetanization the measures of both EPSP slope and population spike amplitude remain significantly enhanced in controls, whereas only the EPSP slope measure retains significant enhancement in malnourished animals. Again, enhanced inhibition of granule-cell output may be responsible for the overall decline in granule-cell response measured in this paradigm. In combination, the results of these studies suggest that, while the granule-cell network is capable of undergoing significant enhancement in synaptic activation measures (potentiation of the EPSP), mechanisms responsible for both the establishment and long-term maintenance of potentiated granule-cell activity are severely impacted by the nutritional insult.

Extending the results of these studies, we have performed studies utilizing a second model of hippocampal neuroplasticity, i.e., perforant path kindling (see Chapter 8). In the kindling model, regularly applied electrical activation of the perforant pathway with trains of biphasic stimulation results in the progressive intensification of both the electrographic and behavioral correlates of seizure activity. In malnourished animals, we have reported that the stimulus threshold necessary to evoke the afterdischarge activity indicative of electrographic seizure is significantly reduced, while the number of kindling stimulations required to elicit the first generalized seizure is significantly increased (Bronzino et al., 1986, 1990). In fact, under the conditions of this investigation, nearly 20% of all malnourished animals failed to progress to the generalized convulsive stage. So, while malnourished animals appear to be more susceptible to electrographic seizure activity, they are highly resistant to the development of fully generalized convulsive activity. Interpretation of these results was facilitated by follow-up investigations utilizing single- and paired-pulse stimulation of the perforant path in conjunction with daily kindling (Bronzino et al., 1991a, 1991b). Results of this work indicated that, although measures of granule-cell field potentials recorded in response to single-pulse stimulation showed significant enhancement as a result of the kindling process, paired-pulse responses showed that a significant rise in both the magnitude and duration of inhibitory modulation of granule responsiveness accompanied the kindling in malnourished animals. These results suggest that, although granule-cell synaptic responsiveness rises in response to kindling, the conversion of this rise to enhanced cellular discharge is over-ridden by a comparatively larger rise in inhibitory modulation of the granule-cell population. Such an effect would result in the creation of a localized "surround-type" inhibition, which would effectively limit the spread of epileptiform activity beyond the seizure focus and retard the development of the more intensive behavioral manifestations of seizure.

Results of each of our investigations noted above indicate that malnutrition occurring during gestation results in significantly enhanced levels of inhibitory control exerted on granule-cell activity. Thus, the single-most consistent result of investigations into the effects of malnutrition on the functional capabilities of the dentate gyrus can be seen, not so much at the level of the granule cells themselves, the majority of which are generated during the early postnatal period of development, but, more probably, at the level of systems modulating granule-cell excitability. These include the intrinsic GABAergic basket cells, which arise during the prenatal developmental period, but do not become functional until the early postnatal period, as well as major extrinsic projection systems encompassing the serotonergic system arising from the median raphé, the noradrenergic innervation originating from the locus coeruleus and the cholinergic and GABAergic inputs from the septal nuclei (Fig. 9). A number of studies (Bilkey and Goddard, 1987; Dahl and Winson, 1985; Frotscher and Leranth, 1988; Freund and Antal, 1988; Freund et al., 1990) have established that a primary action of each of the above-mentioned extrinsic modulatory systems is the inhibition of the intrinsic basket-cell population within the dentate gyrus. This is indicated by the fact that activation of each of the extrinsic nuclei has been shown to result in enhanced output of the granule-cell population. With this in mind, we can develop several testable hypotheses concerning the manner in which a gestational malnutrition insult would result in significantly enhanced levels of granule-cell inhibition. First, at the level of the basket cells themselves, the insult may result in heightened sensitivity to activation of either feedforward or feedback inhibition of the granule-cell population, malnutrition may impair GABA reuptake mechanisms, providing a longer duration of effective inhibition, or it may impair the activity of extrinsic modulatory systems, including the medial septal GABAergic projection, the serotonergic or norepinephrinergic projection systems arising from the brainstem, acting to inhibit the inhibitory basket cell output, i.e., resulting in disinhibition, leading to greater inhibition at the level of the granule cell (Fig. 9). In this regard, the extrinsic GABAergic input from the medial septum would appear to be a logical starting point for future investigation, based on the effects of malnutrition insult on aspects of noncholinergic theta generation. Since the granule cells of the dentate gyrus constitute the entry point for a sizable portion of information into the hippocampal formation, any change in the response level of the granule-cell population would result in altering the manner in which information flows through the entire hippocampal formation, possibly compromising the informational input and resulting processing of such information. These results indicate the necessity of future interdisciplinary methods of investigation, carried out in the same animals, as the approach that should be taken regarding the impact of malnutrition on cellular function of the central nervous system and the translation of these changes in function to altered behaviors.

## 14. RECENT BEHAVIORAL STUDIES: EMPHASIS ON HIPPOCAMPALLY RELATED BEHAVIORS

There have been recent reports of impaired development of various hippocampally mediated behaviors in rats malnourished over the first 18 days of postnatal life. Distal-cue utilization in the Morris water maze (Castro and Rudy, 1987), conditional spatial discrimination and short-term memory (Castro et al., 1989), and Pavlovian trace conditioning to a visual stimulus (Rudy and Castro, 1990) are all delayed by the nutritional insult. These findings are consistent with a retardation in the development and/or maturation of the hippocampal formation. In a series of studies from our own group focusing on the effects of prenatal protein malnutrition in the mature rat, significant behavioral changes have also been demonstrated (Tonkiss and Galler, 1990; Tonkiss et al., 1990a, 1990b, 1991). Of these, the finding of increased resistance to extinction during reversal of a food-rewarded alternation task on an elevated T-maze (Tonkiss and Galler, 1990) and retarded acquisition of a differential reinforcement of a low-rates (DRL-18 sec) operant task (Tonkiss et al., 1990a) are notable as consistent with the view that some, but certainly not all (see below), hippocampally mediated behaviors are compromised in the previously malnourished adult. DRL is a task that requires the rat to postpone pressing a lever until a specific interresponse time (the DRL requirement) has elapsed, the first response thereafter yielding reward. Early responding is not rewarded and simply restarts the DRL requirement. Impaired performance in this test is one of the most reliable findings following hippocampal lesion damage, as is difficulty in reversing a previously learned response (Gray and McNaughton, 1983; Schmaltz and Isaacson, 1966).

In order to explore the generality that hippocampally mediated behaviors may be impaired by prenatal and/or early postnatal malnutrition, an in-depth consideration of spatial learning in such animals follows. Interest in relating malformations or even microlesions of certain brain structures, as a result of diffuse insults, to their behavioral consequences has existed ever since this area of research began. However, as reviewed above, few direct relationships have been conclusively proven. Early work showed an apparent link between cerebellar susceptibility to both pre- and early postnatal malnutrition (Culley et al., 1968; Chase et al., 1969; Wallingford et al., 1980) and motor incoordination (Lynch et al., 1975; Jordan et al., 1979), though other workers were unable to replicate the findings of motor dysfunction in animals that had experienced early-life malnutrition (Galler and Turkewitz, 1977; Guthrie, 1968; Slob et al., 1973). Systematic alteration of the test conditions has also failed to reveal evidence of impaired motor coordination in previously undernourished rats (Smart and Bedi, 1982). The hippocampal formation shows a particular vulnerability to malnutrition (Cintra et al., 1990; Diaz-Cintra et al., 1991; Jordan et al., 1982) and exhibits marked alterations in physiological activity (Austin et al., 1986, 1991; Bronzino et al., 1991a, 1991b). Since this structure has been strongly implicated in spatial learning (O'Keefe and Nadel, 1978; Morris et al., 1982) and short-term working memory (Olton, 1983; Olton et al., 1979; Olton and Fuestle, 1981) many researchers have attempted to document whether these aspects of behavior might be adversely affected in animals with a history of early malnutrition. Initial reports from Jordan and his group (1982) suggested an abolition of spontaneous alternation behavior and a profound inadequacy in spatial navigation performance on 8- and 16-arm radial mazes (Jordan et al., 1981) in rats deprived of adequate nutrition during the prenatal and early postnatal periods. Subsequent work cast doubt upon whether these findings should be interpreted as evidence of a spatial deficit per se and pointed to the likelihood that the performance deficits may have reflected suboptimal motivational conditions existing during testing (Hall, 1983) and an inequality of motivation in the experimental groups (Halas and Sandstead, 1980; Halas et al., 1980; Smart et al., 1973; Tonkiss et al., 1990b). In our recent experiments, the open-field water test of spatial navigation (Morris water maze test) has been utilized, this test having the advantage over the radial-arm maze of avoiding the use of appetitive motivation. The test involves placing the animal in a large circular tank of milky water, with the requirement that it find a small platform located just below the water surface in the center of one of four quadrants. Since the platform cannot be seen or detected by smell, the only way the rat can locate it is via distal cues (e.g., cabinets, shelves, posters, etc.) in the vicinity of the tank. Goodlett et al. (1986) conducted such tests on rats with chronic mild protein malnutrition. In one test, the malnourished rats took longer to acquire the task, i.e., they showed an acquisition deficit. However, in other tests in which the rats were given extensive swim pretraining, such a deficit was not observed, the conclusion being that the ability to locate places in space was intact in malnourished rats. Thus, only when the rats were completely unfamiliar with the stressful test conditions did a performance deficit appear reflecting slower emergence of an appropriate search behavior. The results of Campbell and Bedi (1989) for rats nutritionally rehabilitated from postnatal malnutrition at the time of testing confirm the conclusions of Goodlett et al. that there is relatively sound spatial navigation ability in animals with a history of malnutrition. In that study, no evidence was found for spatial deficits, whether the rats were naive to the test conditions or had received swim pretraining. Since all of the above experiments were conducted on adult animals, in the available literature there appears to be little to encourage the notion that spatial abilities in the mature animal are consistently affected adversely by early or continuing (concurrent) malnutrition. Recently, Castro and Rudy (1987) conducted an ontogenetic analysis of proximal- (platform visible) and distal- (platform invisible) cue utilization in rats malnourished over the first 18 days of life. It was found that distal-cue utilization was delayed, i.e., the age of appearance of this ability was increased by early malnutrition. The authors concluded that these findings probably represented a delay in the development of the hippocampal formation and related structures. Unfortunately, the rats had minimal opportunity to rehabilitate from the physically debilitating effects of the malnutrition. Since the distal-cue task is more difficult than the proximal-cue task, requiring more searching behavior, it is likely to be the more tiring and stressful test to an animal that was undergoing malnutrition only a short period before. Thus, physical debilitation may have been a factor implicated in these findings. We are currently studying the ontogeny of proximal and distal-cue utilization in the open-field water test following exclusively prenatal malnutrition so that these rats will not be debilitated at the time of testing. Preliminary analysis has shown that there is a much greater impact upon the ontogeny of proximal-cue utilization than on distal-cue utilization.

## 15. GENERAL CONCLUSIONS

The findings we have reviewed and discussed suggest that malnutrition, especially when instituted prenatally, is a prime nongenetic factor influencing the developing central nervous system and, ultimately, behavior. This conclusion has important bearing on preventive medicine and also helps to provide the scientific foundation for action at the social and political level for eradication of a major human scourge. As indicated in this chapter, it appears that various perturbations of prenatal brain development in humans may result in mental retardation. But, perhaps more numerous and, therefore, more important, for society are the borderline cases produced by chronic, low-level malnutrition, resulting in suboptimal brain development and nonfulfillment of the genetic potential of the individual.

In examining the multiple effects of malnutrition insult on the central nervous system, the developmental approach is essential in furthering our understanding of the relationship between altered brain and behavior, particularly with regard to learning and memory function. It is clear that a full understanding of these relationships will not result from the application of a single approach, but rather will require the integration of various approaches in interdisciplinary studies.

Continuing studies in animals and humans are needed to identify and document more clearly the interacting effects between nutrition and other environmental factors in terms of brain development and behavior. The subtleties of these interrelationships, their prevalence, and their consequences for the individual and for the community need to be more precisely defined. By these approaches we hope to identify underlying mechanisms and to improve means of prevention of these derangements. It proves very difficult to propose a useful general hypothesis of "recovery" from developmental insults such as malnutrition because of the extraordinarily complex nature of brain development, with different processes dependent upon one another.

The brain growth "program" of the organism can be seriously and permanently upset during early development and its body and brain dimensions replanned in a permanently reduced and somewhat distorted level. In general, the nearer the period of most rapid growth, the smaller will be the insult required to produce a given ultimate derangement in the adult. It is well known that the adult brain is remarkably resistant to changes in its weight, even in cases of severe starvation, provided that it has developed normally to a mature size before starvation begins. Malnutrition appears to affect those growth processes that are contemporaneous with it, as well as some that follow it; in other words, it does not usually perturb or terminate processes that occur prior to the insult. Though there is no overt "destruction" of structures that are already in place, the functions of these may be temporarily altered and could show various degrees of "recovery" later on as a result of dietary rehabilitation. Given that there are transient windows of special vulnerability related to precise periods of cell division, it is essential to distinguish between direct destruction of cells early in development and simply changing their proliferation rates. In either case, any later processes that depend on the earlier completion of events that have been altered will themselves be secondarily altered. One of the ways in which malnutrition insult exerts its effects is to impose limitations on the complexity of neuronal circuits by discoordinating the maturational events that depend on time-related interactions.

It is important to reiterate that the pathology of malnutrition insult does not involve deformations of the brain or even focal tissue destruction, but rather various irrecoverable distortions of developmental patterns. These include cellular arrangement patterns and alterations in normal age-related sequences of brain development. We need also to consider malnutrition as one aspect of a deprived environment. Clearly, malnourished animals are also understimulated animals and do not adequately interact with their environment.

It might also be well to point out that the reason we appear to have so many studies of the effects of postnatal malnutrition is, in part, due to Dobbing's persistent emphasis on the so-called brain growth spurt period. It is long past due, based on more recent cellular and molecular analyses of the effect of malnutrition, to give special attention to the effects of prenatal malnutrition insults, given the many vital brain developmental processes impinged upon during this crucial time of development. Thus, it is not the remarkable weight changes that define the brain growth spurt that are of greatest significance, but rather the early formation and organizational periods related to the birth and migration of brain cells, since these events are absolutely essential to the resulting organization of the brain into functional circuit complexes.

Finally, we would like to stress that human malnutrition has biological, psychological, and sociological aspects. Because of these, predispositions and behavioral practices that are associated with malnutrition tend to be passed from generation to generation. The extent to which such effects become perpetuated and even cumulative in their effects over generations requires a combined educational, economic, behavioral, and nutritional rehabilitation, probably lasting beyond a single generation.

ACKNOWLEDGMENTS. This research was supported by NIH grants HD-22539 and HD-23338. The authors wish to thank Dr. Joseph Altman for many comments and suggestions.

# REFERENCES

Altman, J., 1970, Postnatal neurogenesis and the problem of neural plasticity, in: *Developmental Neurobiology* (W. Himwich, ed.), C.C. Thomas, Springfield, IL, pp. 197–237.

Altman, J., 1986, An animal model of minimal brain dysfunction, in: *Learning Disabilities and Prenatal Risk* (M. Lewis, ed.), University of Illinois Press, Urbana and Chicago, pp. 241–304.

Altman, J., 1987, Morphological and behavioral markers of environmentally induced retardation of brain development: An animal model, *Environ. Health Persp.* 74:153–168.

Altman, J., and Bayer, S.A., 1990a, Mosaic organization of the hippocampal neuroepithelium and the multiple germinal sources of dentate granule cells, *J. Comp. Neurol.* 301:325–342.

Altman, J., and Bayer, S.A., 1990b, Prolonged sojourn of developing pyramidal cells in the intermediate zone of the hippocampus and their settling in the stratum pyramidale, *J. Comp. Neurol.* 301:343–364.

Altman, J., and Bayer, S.A., 1990c, Migration and distribution of two populations of hippocampal granule cell precursors during the perinatal and postnatal periods, *J. Comp. Neurol.* 301:365–381.

Austin, K.B., Bronzino, J.D., and Morgane, P.J., 1986, Prenatal protein malnutrition affects synaptic potentiation in the dentate gyrus of rats in adulthood, *Dev. Brain Res.* 29:267–273.

Austin, K.B., Bronzino, J.D., and Morgane, P.J., 1989, Paired-pulse facilitation and inhibition in the dentate gyrus is dependent on behavioral state, *Exp. Brain Res.* 77:594–604.

Austin, K.B., Beiswanger, C., Bronzino, J.D., Austin-LaFrance, R.J., Galler, J.R., and Morgane, P.J., 1992, Prenatal protein malnutrition alters behavioral state modulation of inhibition and facilitation in the dentate gyrus, *Brain Res. Bull.* 28:245–255.

Austin-LaFrance, R.J., Tonkiss, J., Galler, J.R., Bronzino, J.D., and Morgane, P.J., 1991, Prenatal protein malnutrition and hippocampal function: Spatial learning and long-term potentiation, in: *21st Ann Soc. Neurosci. Abstr.*, p. 663.

Balázs, R., Lewis, P.D., and Patel, A.J., 1975, Effects of metabolic factors on brain development, in: *Growth and Development of the Brain* (M.A.B. Brazier, ed.), Raven Press, New York, pp. 83–115.

Balázs, R., Patel, A.J., and Lewis, P.D., 1977, Metabolic influences on cell proliferation in the brain, in: *Biochemical Correlates of Brain Structure and Function* (A.N. Davison, ed.), Academic Press, London, pp. 43–83.

Balázs, R., Lewis, P.D., and Patel, A.J., 1979, Nutritional deficiencies and brain development, in: *Human Growth, Vol. 3, Neurobiology and Nutrition* (F. Falkner and J. Tanner, eds.), Plenum Press, New York, pp. 415–480.

Barnes, R.H., 1976, Dual role of environmental deprivation and malnutrition in retarding intellectual development, *Am. J. Clin. Nutr.* 29:912–917.

Basco, E., Hajos, F., and Fulop, Z., 1977, Proliferation of Bergmann glia in the developing rat cerebellum, *Anat. Embryol.* 151:219–222.

Bass, N.H., Netsky, M.G., and Young, E., 1970, Effect of neonatal malnutrition on developing cerebrum. I. Microchemical and histologic study of cellular differentiation in the rat, *Arch. Neurol.* 23:289–302.

Bennett, T.L., 1975, The electrical activity of the hippocampus and processes of attention, in: *The Hippocampus*, Vol. 2, (R.L. Isaacson and K.H. Pribram, eds.), Plenum Press, New York, pp. 71–100.

Bilkey, D.K., and Goddard, G.V., 1987, Septohippocampal and commissural pathways antagonistically control inhibitory interneurons in the dentate gyrus, *Brain Res.*, 405:320–325.

Black, A.H., 1975, Hippocampal electrical activity and behavior, in: *The Hippocampus*, Vol. 2, (R.L. Isaacson and K.H. Pribram, eds.), Plenum Press, New York, pp. 129–168.

Bronzino, J.D., Austin, K.B., Siok, C.S., Cordova, C., and Morgane, P.J., 1983, Spectral analysis of neocortical and hippocampal EEG following protein malnutrition, *Electroencephalog. Clin. Neurophysiol.* 55:699–709.

Bronzino, J.D., Austin-LaFrance, R.J., Siok, C.J., and Morgane, P.J., 1986, Effect of protein malnutrition on hippocampal kindling: Electrographic and behavioral measures, *Brain Res.* 384:348–354.

Bronzino, J.D., Austin-LaFrance, R.J., and Morgane, P.J., 1990, Effects of prenatal protein malnutrition on perforant path kindling in the rat, *Brain Res.* 515:45–50.

Bronzino, J.D., Austin-LaFrance, R.J., Morgane, P.J., and Galler, J.R., 1991a, Effects of prenatal protein malnutrition on kindling-induced alterations in dentate granule cell excitability. I. Synaptic transmission measures, *Exp. Neurol.* 112:206–215.

Bronzino, J.D., Austin-LaFrance, R.J., Morgane, P.J., and Galler, J.R., 1991b, Effects of prenatal protein malnutrition on kindling-induced alterations in dentate granule cell excitability. II. Paired-pulse measures, *Exp. Neurol.* 112:216–223.

Campbell, L.F., and Bedi, K.S., 1989, The effects of undernutrition in early life on spatial learning, *Physiol. Behav.* 45:883–890.

Castro, C.A., and Rudy, J.W., 1987, Early-life malnutrition selectively retards the development of distal- but not proximal-cue navigation, *Devp. Psychobiol.* 20:521–537.

Castro, C.A., Tracy, M., and Rudy, J.W., 1989, Early-life undernutrition impairs the development of the learning and short-term memory processes mediating performance in a conditional-spatial discrimination task, *Behav. Brain Res.* 32:255–264.

Chase, H.P., Lindsley, W.F.B., and O'Brien, D., 1969, Undernutrition and cerebellar development, *Nature* 221:554–555.

Chase, H.P., Dabiere, C.S., Welch, N.N., and O'Brien, D., 1971, Intrauterine undernutrition and brain development, *Pediatrics* 47:491–500.

Choi, B.H., and Lapham, L.W., 1978, Radial glia in the human fetal cerebrum: A combined Golgi immunofluorescent and electron microscopic study, *Brain Res.* 148:295–311.

Chow, B.F., 1974, Effect of maternal dietary protein on anthropometric and behavioral development of the offspring, *Adv. Exp. Med. Biol.*, 49:183–219.

Cintra, L., Díaz-Cintra, S., Kemper, T., and Morgane, P.J., 1982, Nucleus locus coeruleus: A morphometric Golgi study in rats of three age groups, *Brain Res.* 247:17–28.

Cintra, L., Díaz-Cintra, S., Galvan, A., Kemper, T., and Morgane, P.J., 1990, Effects of protein undernutrition on the dentate gyrus in rats of three age groups, *Brain Res.* 532:271–277.

Collins, R.C., 1987, Neurotoxins and the selective vulnerability of the brain, in: *Neurotoxins and their Pharmacological Implications*, Peter Jenn Press, New York, pp. 1–17.

Colombo, P., 1982, The critical period concept: Research, methodology, and theoretical issues, *Psychol. Bull.* 91:269–275.
Coursin, D.B., 1975, Malnutrition, brain development, and behavior: Anatomic, biochemical, and electrophysiological constructs, in: *Growth and Development of the Brain* (M.A.B. Brazier, ed.), Raven Press, New York, pp. 289–305.
Cragg, B.G., 1972, The development of cortical synapses during starvation in the rat, *Brain,* 95:143–150.
Culley, W.J., and Lineberger, R.D., 1968, Effect of undernutrition on the size and composition of the rat brain, *J. Nutr.* 96:375–381.
Dahl, D., and Winson, J., 1985, Action of norepinephrine in the dentate gyrus. I. Stimulation of locus coeruleus, *Exp. Brain Res.,* 59:491–496.
Davison, A.N., and Dobbing, J., 1968, The developing brain, in: *Applied Neurochemistry* (A.N. Davison and J. Dobbing, eds.), F.A. Davis, Philadelphia, pp. 253–286.
Díaz-Cintra, S., Cintra, L., Kemper, T., Resnick, O., and Morgane, P.J., 1981a, Nucleus raphé dorsalis: A morphometric Golgi study in rats of three age groups, *Brain Res.* 207:1–16.
Díaz-Cintra, S., Cintra, L., Kemper, T., Resnick, O., and Morgane, P.J., 1981b, The effects of protein deprivation on the nucleus raphé dorsalis: A morphometric Golgi study in rats of three age groups, *Brain Res.* 221:243–255.
Díaz-Cintra, S., Cintra, L., Kemper, T., Resnick, O., and Morgane, P.J., 1984, The effects of protein deprivation on the nucleus locus coeruleus: A morphometric Golgi study in rats of three age groups, *Brain Res.* 304:242–253.
Díaz-Cintra, S., Cintra, L., Galvan, A., Kemper, T., and Morgane, P.J., 1991, Effects of prenatal protein malnutrition on the postnatal development of granule cells in the fascia dentata, *J. Comp. Neurol.* **310**:356–364.
Dobbing, J., 1968a, Effects of experimental undernutrition on development of the nervous system, in: *Malnutrition, Learning and Behavior* (N. Scrimshaw and J. Gordon, eds.), MIT Press, Cambridge, MA, pp. 181–202.
Dobbing, J., 1968b, Vulnerable periods in developing brain, in: *Applied Neurochemistry* (A.N. Davison and J. Dobbing, eds.), F.A. Davis, Philadelphia, pp. 287–316.
Dobbing, J., 1970, Undernutrition and the developing brain: The relevance of animal models to the human problem, *Am. J. Dis. Child.* 20:411–415.
Dobbing, J., 1971, Undernutrition and the developing brain: The use of animal models to elucidate the human problem, in: *Advances in Experimental Medicine and Biology, Vol. 13, Chemistry and Brain Development* (R. Paoletti and A. Davison, eds.), Plenum Press, New York, pp. 399–412.
Dobbing, J., 1972, Vulnerable periods of brain development, in: *Lipids, Malnutrition and the Developing Brain,* CIBA Foundation Symposium, Elsevier, Amsterdam, pp. 9–29.
Dobbing, J., 1984, Infant nutrition and later achievement, *Nutr. Rev.* 42:1–7.
Dobbing, J., 1985, Maternal nutrition in pregnancy and later achievement of offspring: A personal interpretation, *Early Hum. Dev.* 12:1–8.
Dobbing, J., 1990, Early nutrition and later achievement, *Proc. Nutr. Soc.* 49:103–118.
Fisher, S.E., 1988, Selective fetal malnutrition: The fetal alcohol syndrome, *J. Am. Coll. Nutr.* 7:101–106.
Fish, I., and Winick, M., 1969, Effect of malnutrition on regional growth and development of the developing rat brain, *Exp. Neurol.* 25:534–540.
Fleischer, S.F., and Turkewitz, G., 1984, The use of animals for understanding the effects of malnutrition on human behavior: Models vs. a comparative approach, in: *Human Nutrition, Vol. 5, Nutrition and Behavior* (J.R. Galler, ed.), Plenum Press, New York, pp. 37–61.
Frankova, S., 1974, Interaction between early malnutrition and stimulation in animals, in: *Early Malnutrition and Mental Development* (J. Cravioto, L. Hambraeus, and B. Vahlquist, eds.), XII Symp. Swedish Nutrition Found., Almquist and Wiksell, Uppsala, pp. 202–209.
Freund, T.F., and Antal, M., 1988, GABA-containing neurons in the septum control inhibitory interneurons in the hippocampus, *Nature* 336:170–173.
Freund, T.F., Gulyás, A.I., Acsády, L., Görcs, T., and Tóth, K., 1990, Serotonergic control of the hippocampus via local inhibitory interneurons. *Proc. Natl. Acad. Sci. USA* 87:8501–8505.
Frotscher, M., and Leranth, C., Catecholaminergic innervation of pyramidal and GABA-ergic non-pyramidal neurons in the rat hippocampus, *Histochemistry,* 88:313–319, 1988.
Galler, J.R., 1984, The behavioral consequences of malnutrition in early life, in: *Nutrition and Behavior* (J.R. Galler, ed.), Plenum Press, New York, pp. 63–118.
Galler, J.R., and Kanis, K.B., 1987, Animals models of malnutrition applied to brain research, in: *Current Topics in Nutrition and Disease, Vol. 16, Basic and Clinical Aspects of Nutrition and Brain Development,* Alan R. Liss, New York, pp. 57–73.
Galler, J.R., and Turkewitz, G., 1977, Motor competence in rats of different stocks reared in large and small litters, *Physiol. Behav.* 19:696–699.
Galler, J.R., Ricciuti, H.N., Crawford, M.A., and Kucharski, L.T., 1984, The role of the mother–infant interaction in nutritional disorders, in: *Nutrition and Behavior* (J.R. Galler, ed.), Plenum Press, New York, pp. 269–304.
Goodlett, C.R., Valentino, M.L., Morgane, P.J., and Resnick, O., 1986, Spatial cue utilization in chronically malnourished rats: Task-specific learning deficits, *Dev. Psychobiol.* 19:1–15.
Gramsbergen, A., 1974, The effect of undernutrition on the development of the EEG in rats, in: *Ontogenesis of the Brain* (L. Jilek and S. Trojan, eds.), Universitas Carolinas Pragensis, Prague, pp. 181–191.
Gramsbergen, A., 1976, The development of the EEG in the rat, *Dev. Psychobiol.* 9:501–515.
Gray, J.A., and McNaughton, N., 1983, Comparison between the behavioral effects of septal and hippocampal lesions: A review, *Neurosci. Biobehav. Rev.,* 7:119–188.

Guthrie, H.A., 1968, Severe undernutrition in early infancy and behavior in rehabilitated albino rats, *Physiol. Behav.* 3:619–623.

Halas, E.S., and Sandstead, H.H., 1980, Malnutrition and behavior: The performance versus learning problem revisited, *J. Nutr.* 110:1858–1864.

Halas, E.S., Burger, P.A., and Sandstead, H.H., 1980, Food motivation of rehabilitated malnourished rats: Implications for learning studies, *Anim. Learn. Behav.* 8:152–158.

Hall, R.D., 1983, Is hippocampal function in the adult rat impaired by early protein or protein-calorie deficiencies? *Dev. Psychobiol.* 16:395–411.

Herschkowitz, H., and Rossi, E., 1972, Critical periods in brain development, in: *Lipids, Malnutrition and the Developing Brain*, CIBA Foundation Symposium, Elsevier, Amsterdam, pp. 107–119.

Jordan, T.C., Howells, K.F., and Piggott, S.M., 1979, Effects of early undernutrition on motor coordination in the adult rat, *Behav. Neural Biol.*, 25:126–132.

Jordan, T.C., Cane, S.E., and Howells, K.F., 1981, Deficits in spatial memory performance induced by early undernutrition, *Dev. Psychobiol.* 14:317–325.

Jordan, T.C., Howells, K.F., McNaughton, N., and Heatlie, P., 1982, Effects of early undernutrition on hippocampal development and function, *Res. Exp. Med.* 180:201–207.

Katz, H.B., and Davies, C.A., 1983, The separate and combined effects of early undernutrition and environmental complexity at different ages on cerebral measures in rats, *Dev. Psychobiol.* 16:47–58.

Lewis, P.D., Baláz, R., Patel, A.J., and Johnson, A.L., 1975, The effect of undernutrition in early life on cell generation in the rat brain, *Brain Res.* 83:235–247.

Lewis, P.D., Patel, A.J., and Balázs, R., 1979, Effects of undernutrition on cell generation in the rat hippocampus, *Brain Res.* 168:186–189.

Lynch, A., Smart, J.L., and Dobbing, J., 1975, Motor coordination and cerebellar size in adult rats undernourished in early life, *Brain Res.* 83:249–259.

Monmaur, P., Depoortere, H., and M'Harzi, M., 1981, $\alpha$-adrenoceptive influences on hippocampal theta rhythm in the rat, *Behav. Neural Biol.* 33:129–132.

Morgan, B.L., and Naismith, D.J., 1982, The effect of early postnatal undernutrition on the growth and development of the rat brain, *Br. J. Nutr.* 48:15–23.

Morgane, P.J., Miller, M., Kemper, T., Stern, W.C., Forbes, W.B., Hall, R., Bronzino, J.D., Kissane, J., Hawrlewicz, E., and Resnick, O., 1978, The effects of protein malnutrition on the developing central nervous system in the rat, *Neurosci. Biobehav. Rev.* 2:137–230.

Morgane, P.J., Resnick, O., Stern, W.C., Forbes, W.B., Bronzino, J.D., Miller, M., Leahy, J.P., Hawrelewicz, E., and Kissane, J., 1979, Maternal protein malnutrition and the developing central nervous system, in: *Malnutrition, Environment and Behavior: New Perspectives* (D. Levitsky, ed.), Cornell University Press, Ithaca, NY, pp. 94–122.

Morgane, P.J., Austin, K.B., Siok, C.J., LaFrance, R.J., and Bronzino, J.D., 1985, Power spectral analysis of hippocampal and cortical EEG activity following severe prenatal protein malnutrition in the rat, *Dev. Brain Res.* 22:211–218.

Morgane, P.J., Austin, K.B., Palmer, S.J., Austin-LaFrance, R.J., and Bronzino, J.D., 1990, Prenatal protein malnutrition results in the loss of behavior-mediated theta frequency shifting, in: *20th Ann. Soc. Neurosci. Abstr.*, p. 35.

Morris, R.G.M., Garrud, P., Rawlins, J.N.P., and O'Keefe, J., 1982, Place navigation impaired in rats with hippocampal lesions, *Nature* 297:681–683.

Morris, R.G.M., Hagen, J.J., and Rawlins, J.N.P., 1986, Allocentric spatial learning by hippocampectomized rats: A further test of the "spatial mapping" and "working memory" theories of hippocampal function, *Q. J. Exp. Psychol.* 388:365–369.

Noback, C.R., and Eisenman, L.M., 1981, Some effects of protein-calorie undernutrition on the developing central nervous of the rat, *Anat. Rec.* 201:67–73.

O'Keefe, J., and Nadel, L., 1978, *The Hippocampus as a Cognitive Map*, Clarendon Press, Oxford.

Olton, D.S., 1983, Memory functions of the hippocampus, in: *Neurobiology of the Hippocampus* (W. Seifert, ed.), Academic Press, London, pp. 335–373.

Olton, D.S., and Feustle, W.A., 1981, Hippocampal function required for nonspatial working memory, *Exp. Brain Res.* 41:380–384.

Olton, D.S., Becker, J.T., and Handelmann, G.E., 1979, Hippocampus, space and memory, *Behav. Brain Sci.* 2:313–365.

Oppenheim, R.W., 1991, Cell death during development of the nervous system, *Ann. Rev. Neurosci.* 14:453–501.

Rakic, P., 1975, Cell migration and neuronal ectopias in the brain, in: *Birth Defects: Original Article Series*, Vol. 11 (D. Bergsma, ed.), Alan R. Liss, New York, pp. 95–129.

Ribak, C.E., and Seress, L., 1983, Five types of basket cell in the hippocampal dentate gyrus: A combined Golgi and electron microscopic study, *J. Neurocytol.* 12:577–596.

Rodier, P.M., 1976, Critical periods for behavioral anomalies in mice, *Environ. Health Perspect.* 18:79–83.

Rodier, P.M., 1977, Correlations between prenatally-induced alterations in CNS cell populations and postnatal function, *Teratology* 16:235–246.

Rodier, P.M., 1980, Chronology of neuron development: Animal studies and their clinical implications, *Dev. Med. Child Neurol.* 22:525–545.

Rodier, P.M., 1988, Structural-functional relationships in experimentally induced brain damage, in: *Progress in Brain Research*, Vol. 73 (G.J. Boer, M.G.P. Feenstra, M. Mirmiran, and F. Van Haaren, eds.), Elsevier Science Publishers, Amsterdam, pp. 335–348.

Rodier, P.M., Reynolds, S.S., and Roberts, W.N., 1979, Behavioral consequences of interference with CNS development in the early fetal period, *Teratology* 19:327–336.

Rosso, P., 1984, Nutrition during pregnancy: Myths and realities, in: *Concurrent Concepts in Nutrition, Vol. 13: Nutrition in the 20th Century* (M. Winick, ed.), John Wiley, New York, pp. 47–70.

Rosso, P., 1987, Maternal and fetal growth: Implications for subsequent mental competence, in: *Current Topics in Nutrition and Disease, Vol. 16: Basic and Clinical Aspects of Nutrition and Brain Development* (D.K. Rassin, ed.), Alan R. Liss, New York, pp. 339–357.

Rudy, J.W., and Castro, C.A., 1990, Undernutrition during the brain growth period of the rat significantly delays development of processes mediating Pavlovian trace conditioning, *Behav. Neural Biol.* 53:307–320.

Sacher, G.A., and Staffeldt, E.F., 1974, Relation of gestation time to brain weight for placental mammals: Implications for the theory of vertebrate growth, *Am. Natural.* 108:593–615.

Schmaltz, L.W., and Isaacson, R.L., 1966, Retention of a DRL-20 Schedule by hippocampectomized and partially neodecorticate rats. *J. Comp. Physiol. Psychol.* 62:128–132.

Schulte, F.J., Schrempf, G., and Hinze, G., 1972, Maternal toxemia, fetal malnutrition, and motor behavior of the newborn, *Pediatrics* 48:871–882.

Schwerdtfeger, W.K., 1986, Afferent fibers from the septum terminate on gamma-aminobutyric acid (GABA-) interneurons and granule cells in the area dentata of the rat, *Experientia* 42:392–394.

Scott, J.P., 1979, Critical periods in organizational processes, in: *Human Growth: Neurobiology and Nutrition, Vol. 3* (F. Falkner and J. Tanner, eds.), Plenum Press, New York, pp. 223–241.

Seress, L., 1977, The postnatal development of rat dentate gyrus and the effect of early thyroid hormone treatment, *Anat. Embryol.* 151:335–339.

Shimada, M., and Morikawa, Y., 1978, Effect of early experimental undernutrition on brain development, *Asian Med. J.* 21:88–97.

Shimada, M., Yamano, T., Nakamura, T., Morikawa, Y., and Kusunoki, T., 1977, Effect of maternal malnutrition on matrix cell proliferation in the cerebrum of mouse embryo: An autoradiographic study, *Pediatr. Res.* 11:728–731.

Shoemaker, W.J., and Bloom, F.E., 1977, Effect of undernutrition on brain morphology, in: *Nutrition and the Brain, Vol. 2* (R.J. Wurtman and J.J. Wurtman, eds.), Raven Press, New York, pp. 147–192.

Slob, A.K., Snow, C.E., and de Natris-Mathot, E., 1973, Absence of behavioral deficits following neonatal undernutrition in the rat, *Dev. Psychobiol.* 6:177–186.

Smart, J.L., 1977, Early life malnutrition and later life ability: A critical analysis, in: *Genetics, Environment and Intelligence*, (A. Oliverio, ed.), Elsevier/North Holland Biomedical Press, Amsterdam, pp. 215–235.

Smart, J.L., 1987, The need for and the relevance of animal studies of early undernutrition, in: *Early Nutrition and Later Achievement* (J Dobbing, ed.) Academic Press, London, pp. 50–85.

Smart, J.L., 1990, Vulnerability of developing brain to undernutrition, *Ups. J. Med. Sci.* 48:21–41, 1990.

Smart, J.L., and Bedi, K.S., 1982, Early life undernutrition in rats, 3. Motor performance in adulthood, *Br. J. Nutr.* 47:439–444.

Smart, J.L., Dobbing, J., Adlard, B.P.F., Lynch, A., and Sands, J., 1973, Vulnerability of developing brain: Relative effects of growth restriction during the fetal suckling periods on behavior and brain composition of adult rats, *J. Nutr.* 103:1327–1338.

Stanfield, B.B., and Cowan, W.M., 1988, The development of the hippocampal region, in: *Cerebral Cortex, Vol. 7, Development and Maturation of Cerebral Cortex* (A. Peters and E.G. Jones, eds.), Plenum Press, New York, pp. 91–131.

Swarz, J.R., and Oster-Granite, M.L., 1978, Presence of radial glia in foetal mouse cerebellum, *J. Neurocytol.* 7:301–312.

Teyler, T.J., and Discenna, P., 1984, Long-term potentiation as a candidate mnemonic device, *Brain Res. Rev.* 7:15–28.

Thompson, R., Huestis, P.W., Crinella, F.M., and Yu, J., 1986, The neuroanatomy of mental retardation in the white rat, *Neurosci. Biobehav. Rev.* 10:317–338.

Thompson, R., Huestis, P.W., Crinella, F.M., and Yu, J., 1987, Further lesion studies on the neuroanatomy of mental retardation in the white rat, *Neurosci. Biobehav. Rev.* 11:415–440.

Tonkiss, J., and Galler, J.R., 1990, Prenatal protein malnutrition and working memory performance in adult rats, *Behav. Brain Res.* 40:95–107.

Tonkiss, J., Galler, J.R., Formica, R.N., Shukitt-Hale, B., and Timm, R.R., 1990a, Fetal protein malnutrition impairs acquisition of a DRL task in adult rats, *Physiol. Behav.* 48:73–77.

Tonkiss, J., Shukitt-Hale, B., Formica, R.N., Rocco, F.J., and Galler, J.R., 1990b, Prenatal protein malnutrition alters response to reward in adult rats, *Physiol. Behav.* 48:675–680.

Tonkiss, J., Galler, J.R., Shukitt-Hale, B., and Rocco, F.J., 1991, Prenatal protein malnutrition impairs visual discrimination learning in adult rats, *Psychobiology* **19**:247–250.

Vanderwolf, C.H., and Leung, L.-W.S., 1983, Hippocampal rhythmical slow activity: A brief history and the effects of entorhinal lesions and phencyclidine, in: *Neurobiology of the Hippocampus* (W. Seifert, ed.), Academic Press, London, pp. 175–302.

Wallingford, J.C., Shrader, R.E., and Zeman, F.J., 1980, Effect of maternal protein-calorie malnutrition on fetal cerebellar neurogenesis, *J. Nutr.* 110:543–551.

Wasterlain, C.G., Hattori, H., Yang, C., Schwartz, P.H., Fujikawa, D.G., Morin, A.M., and Dwyer, B.E., 1990, Selective vulnerability of neuronal subpopulations during ontogeny reflects discrete molecular events associated with normal brain development, in: *Neonatal Seizures* (C.G. Wasterlain and P. Vert, eds.), Raven Press, New York, pp. 69–81.

Winick, M., 1969, Food, time and cellular growth of the brain, *N.Y. State J. Med.* 69:302–304.
Winick, M., and Noble, A., 1966, Cellular response in rats during malnutrition at various ages, *J. Nutr.* 89:300–306.
Winson, J., 1975, The theta mode of hippocampal function, in: *The Hippocampus,* Vol. 2 (R.L. Isaacson and K.H. Pribram, eds.), Plenum Press, New York, pp. 169–184.
Winson, J., 1986, Behaviorally dependent neuronal gating in the hippocampus, in: *The Hippocampus,* Vol. 4 (R. Isaacson and K. Pribram, eds.), Plenum Press, New York, pp. 77–91.
Winson, J., and Abzug, C., 1978, Neuronal transmission through hippocampal pathways dependent on behavior, *J. Neurophysiol.* 41:716–732.
Zamenhof, S., and van Marthens, E., 1978, Nutritional influences on prenatal brain development, in: *Studies on the Development of Behavior and the Nervous System, Vol. 4, Early Influences* (G. Gottlieb, ed.), Academic Press, New York, pp. 149–186.
Zamenhof, S., van Marthens, E., and Margolis, F.L., 1968, DNA (cell number) and protein in neonatal brain: Alteration by maternal dietary protein restriction, *Science* 160:322–323.
Zamenhof, S., van Marthens, E., and Grauel, L., 1971, DNA (cell number) and protein in neonatal rat brain: Alteration by timing maternal dietary protein restriction, *J. Nutr.* 101:1265–1270.

Chapter 2

# Prolonged Dietary Restriction and Its Effects on Dopamine Systems of the Brain

*Frank M. Scalzo*

## 1. INTRODUCTION

This chapter examines the role that nutritional factors can potentially play in reducing vulnerability to the adverse effects of toxicant exposure on dopamine systems of the brain. Unlike most of the chapters in this volume, this chapter is about a deficiency, not a contaminant or endogenous toxin found in food. In this case, the insult is a lack of food itself. The putative beneficial effects of reduced dietary intake on the dopamine systems of the brain will be examined, and implications for predicting vulnerability to toxicant exposure will be discussed.

It has been known for over half a century that caloric restriction, which is a reduction in the amount of dietary energy intake by approximately 50%, without essential nutrient deficiency, prolongs the average life span of rodents (Fig. 1) (McCay *et al.*, 1935; Ross, 1961; Weindruch *et al.*, 1986; Weindruch and Walford, 1988). Since then, it has been demonstrated that such caloric restriction elicits diverse biochemical changes (Feuers *et al.*, 1989; Koizumi *et al.*, 1987; Laganiere and Yu, 1989; Leakey *et al.*, 1989a, 1989b; Masoro, 1990; Ross, 1969; Weindruch and Walford, 1988), reduces the incidence of pituitary and other tumors (Tannenbaum, 1940, 1942a, 1942b; Visscher *et al.*, 1942; Weindruch and Walford, 1988), delays puberty and reproductive senescence (Holehan and

---

*Frank M. Scalzo* • Department of Pediatrics, University of Arkansas for Medical Sciences and Arkansas Children's Hospital, Little Rock, Arkansas 72205.
*The Vulnerable Brain and Environmental Risks, Volume 1: Malnutrition and Hazard Assessment,* edited by Robert L. Isaacson and Karl F. Jensen. Plenum Press, New York, 1992.

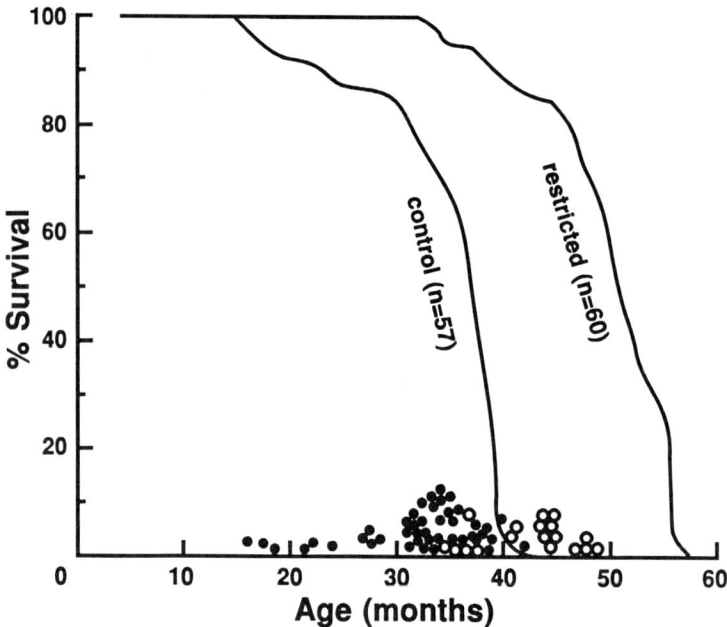

**FIGURE 1.** Longevity and tumor incidence in female mice from long-lived C3B10Rf$_1$ hybrid strain fed either a control or restricted diet. The filled circles show the age of death for tumor-bearing mice fed the control diet; open circles represent restricted mice. From Weindruch (1989), with permission.

Merry, 1985; Koizumi et al., 1989), and enhances immune function (Fernandes et al., 1976; Gerbase-Delima et al., 1975; Mann, 1978; Weindruch et al., 1979, 1986), learning and motor performance (Harrison and Archer, 1987; Idrobo et al., 1987; Ingram et al., 1987). Yet, the public and, until recently, the scientific community, have not been enamored of this phenomenon, perhaps due largely to the lack of clinical data. As more is learned about the benefits of prolonged decreases in food intake (without malnutrition), research on dietary restriction may be on the verge of major advances, with the potential to improve the health and well-being of the world's population.

Support for dietary restriction research is provided in part by a collaboration between the National Institute on Aging (NIA) and the National Center for Toxicological Research (NCTR). In an effort to reduce variation between laboratories in animal models, animal husbandry, diets, and experimental procedures, the NIA together with the NCTR have developed an animal colony of aged mice and rats. Four mouse genotypes (C57BL/6NNia, DBA/2NNia, B6D2F1, B6C3F1) and three rat genotypes (Fischer-344, Brown Norway, F344 × BNF1) are being maintained at the NCTR on ad lib and 60% caloric-restricted diets (Sprott, 1988). This 10-year initiative, which was begun in 1988, provides a unique opportunity in aging, diet, and toxicity research to control many sources of variation that often make the interpretation of data between (and sometimes within) laboratories difficult.

**TABLE 1.** Delayed Development of Tumors in Mildly Underfed Mice

| Tumor | Incidence (%) | | Age of occurrence (months) | |
|---|---|---|---|---|
| | Ad lib | Restricted | Ad lib | Restricted |
| Pituitary adenoma | 33 | 8 | 25 | 31 |
| Mammary | 14 | 6 | 25 | 29 |
| Lymphosarcoma | 11 | 10 | 20 | 27 |
| RCS—Type A | 4 | 3 | 26 | 33 |
| RCS—Type B | 7 | 2 | 23 | 26 |
| Lung—single adenoma | 21 | 13 | 23 | 27 |
| Lung—multiple adenoma | 6 | 3 | 23 | 29 |
| Lung—adenocarcinoma | 11 | 15 | 24 | 28 |

From Weindruch (1989), with permission.

## 2. GENERAL BENEFITS OF DIETARY RESTRICTION

Much research on dietary restriction has focused on tumors (Table 1) and biochemical toxicology. Several reports describe dietary restriction effects on the development of tumors (Weindruch, 1989), liver function (Cutler, 1981; Feuers et al., 1989; Laganiere and Yu, 1989; Leakey et al., 1989a, 1989b) and the endocrine system (Holehan and Merry, 1985; Koizumi et al., 1990; Merry and Holehan, 1979; Stewart et al., 1988). A comprehensive study by Duffy et al. (1989) on the physiology of Fischer-344 rats during chronic caloric restriction demonstrates circadian patterns of body temperature, activity, metabolism, and feeding behavior that are different from ad-libitum-fed animals. One striking finding is that average body temperature is significantly lower in restricted rats, with a reduction in body temperature occurring for a short interval during the transition stage between dark and light. This temperature reduction may reflect decreased energy metabolism, but it is not clear whether this is a consequence of or is caused by caloric restriction.

During chronic caloric restriction, the energy requirements of the brain must continue to be supported. The above findings suggest that the brain, endocrine, and immune systems compensate for energy restriction by maintaining homeostasis, perhaps in a way similar to hibernation or torpor. The mechanisms of this compensation are poorly understood, and thus far only a few studies have begun to address the effects of diet restriction on brain and behavior. These studies usually have been conducted within the context of aging research, with the primary focus on understanding the aging process and the determination of beneficial effects of chronic dietary restriction on longevity and quality of life. The interaction of diet with neurotoxicant exposure has received even less attention. With increased understanding of non-nervous system changes in physiology during dietary restriction and the identification of biomarkers for aging- and toxicant-induced neurobehavioral deficits (see Ingram, 1988a; Landfield, 1988; Mooradian, 1990 for a discussion of biomarkers of aging), study of behavior and the central nervous system during dietary restriction will be more accessible to investigation.

## 3. METHODOLOGY

Before discussing data on dietary restriction and the brain it is important to define the terminology used in these studies. Subtle differences in phrasing can have very different meanings for feeding regimens in dietary restriction studies.

### 3.1. Terminology

*Food restriction* refers to reducing the amount of all or most specific nutrients as well as a reduction in calories (Masoro, 1988). Severe food restriction results in essential nutrient deficiencies. Under these conditions, one or more essential nutrients (e.g., protein) are lacking and, depending on the degree of restriction, undernourishment or malnourishment occurs. Much valuable information about the brain has been gained from studies on undernutrition and malnutrition. Malnutrition is the result of inadequate levels of nutrient supply, in contrast to the controlled reduction in caloric intake (without essential nutrient deficiencies) used in caloric-restriction studies. For a discussion of undernutrition effects on the nervous system and behavior, see Chapters 1 and 3. It is important to make the distinction between food restriction and caloric restriction, because animals undergoing caloric restriction are not malnourished. It is the reduced intake of calories, in the absence of malnutrition, which appears to produce beneficial effects in chronic caloric-restriction studies. For consistency, the term *caloric restriction* will be used for the remainder of this chapter and refers to a specified reduction in caloric intake (e.g., to 60% of ad libitum intake) that does not cause malnutrition.

### 3.2. Methods of Caloric Restriction

There are at least two methods currently used for implementing a caloric-restriction feeding regimen. These are by a daily reduction in calorie intake or by using the every other day (EOD) method of feeding. Daily reduction in food intake was first used by McKay to increase longevity (McCay *et al.*, 1935). This same basic approach is used by the NCTR in raising animals for the NIA. Rats and mice are raised from birth in a specific pathogen-free environment, maintained on a 12 hr/12 hr light/dark cycle under ad libitum food conditions until the animals are assigned to a diet condition. At maturity (14 weeks of age), animals are either fed under ad libitum conditions or under conditions of caloric restriction. Restricted animals are fed a predetermined amount of food (e.g., a 25-g mouse would receive approximately one 3.5-g food pellet a day), supplemented with the full recommended daily requirement of vitamins and minerals, at a specified time each day, to maintain the restricted animals at 60% of the ad libitum body weight (Duffy *et al.*, 1989). Young (18 months) and old (30 months) animals raised under this regimen are visibly smaller and have a healthier appearance (e.g., are well groomed and have healthy coats) compared to the ad libitum animals.

Another feeding regime used in the study of aging and diet effects on the brain, the EOD method, involves a different feeding procedure. Under this regimen, animals are allowed access to diet for 24 hr every other day. Food is placed in hoppers on alternate mornings and the hoppers, and any remaining food, are removed from the cages the next morning (London et al., 1985). This regimen has been initiated at different ages. For example, in one study, EOD feeding was initiated at 6–10 weeks, 25 weeks, or 40 weeks of age (Goodrick et al., 1990). This regimen results in the EOD animals receiving approximately 70% of the calories that the ad libitum control group consumes (Goodrick et al., 1982; London et al., 1985).

Differences in feeding regimens raise important questions of validity in comparing data from the two methods of caloric restriction. Animals raised under both regimens live longer and have fewer tumors. However, animals fed on a daily restriction schedule can only consume the predetermined amount of food (e.g., one pellet), while animals under the EOD regimen can consume more than one pellet. The two groups are therefore likely to have different physiological response profiles during feeding and fasting. The bases for this assertion are data on circadian rhythms for body temperature and activity in daily restricted animals (Duffy et al., 1989). It is possible that 48-hr rhythms develop in the EOD model for these same parameters. This would have important implications for many behavioral and biochemical endpoints typically investigated in neurotoxicity studies. For example, in the daily restriction regimen for restricted Fischer-344 rats fed during lights-on, total activity peaks approximately 5 hr after lights-on (feeding time) and is at its lowest at approximately 1 hr before lights-on (Duffy et al., 1989), while in light-fed restricted B6C3F1 mice, plasma corticosterone levels peak at lights-off and are at their lowest approximately 5 hr later (Holson et al., 1991). These rhythms appear to be linked to the light cycle, which is also predictive of diet delivery (Duffy et al., 1989).

## 3.3. Caloric Restriction, Aging, and Toxicology

The convincing results from longevity and tumor studies, which clearly demonstrate the beneficial effects of dietary restriction, compel neurotoxicologists to examine the potential for dietary restriction to decrease vulnerability to neurotoxicants throughout the life span. Recent work on the neurobehavioral effects of dietary restriction is contradictory (see Section 4.4). These studies suggest that the brain may or may not enjoy the beneficial effects of chronic dietary restriction.

Because the brain, together with the endocrine and immune systems, acts to control and integrate all body functions, it is likely that during aging (and probably during toxicant exposure) malfunctions in these systems lead to declines in body function and to a reduced ability to maintain body homeostasis (Holehan and Merry, 1985; Meites et al., 1987, 1990; Merry and Holehan, 1979). However, intensive studies of diet restriction and these interactions have yet to be published. This author is aware of only one published study that has investigated the interaction of caloric restriction with a known neurotoxicant (see Section 5).

## 4. BIOMARKERS FOR NEUROTOXICITY

Caloric restriction effects on brain and behavior have been reported primarily in the context of aging studies. Thus, in order to determine the potential for caloric restriction to protect against toxicant-induced deficits in the dopamine system, it is first necessary to discuss the reported beneficial effects of caloric restriction on age-related deficits in the dopamine system. Declines in dopamine function with aging have been widely studied (Joseph and Roth, 1988, 1989; Lieberman and Abou-Nader, 1986; Morgan and Finch, 1988; Roth, 1988; Strong, 1988), but only recently have there been a number of studies investigating the effects of caloric restriction on aging and the dopamine system.

### 4.1. Neurochemical Assessment of Aged Animals

The most consistent finding in investigations of neurochemical changes in the dopamine system during aging has been a reduction in striatal D2 dopamine receptor binding that is related to a decrease in $B_{max}$. Results from early studies with D2 ligands have been corroborated by more recent studies that have found similar reduction in D2 binding with more specific D2 ligands (Table 2). Data from primate studies is limited but also corroborate findings in rodents where decreases in D2 binding appear to be related to the rate of aging and the maximal life span (Lai *et al.*, 1987). For reviews on aging and alterations in the dopamine neurochemistry see Burchinsky (1984), Joseph and Roth (1988, 1989), Meites (1990), Morgan and Finch (1988), Randall (1980), Roth (1988), Roth and Joseph (1988), and Strong (1988).

Randall *et al.* (1980) reviewed aging effects in the nigrostriatal system, suggesting that age-related changes in the nigrostriatal pathway appear to be coordinated between pre- and postsynaptic components. Postsynaptic deficits may be more severe and earlier to occur than presynaptic losses in the nigrostriatal pathway itself. For example, dopamine receptor binding and dopamine-activated adenyl cyclase decrease at an earlier age and to a greater extent than do the presynaptic markers of the dopamine neurons themselves. Aging C57BL/6J mice do not exhibit behavioral or biochemical supersensitivity following chronic haloperidol treatment, which resulted in both phenomena in young- and middle-aged mice.

During aging there is an increase in lipofuscin deposits in brain as well as other tissues (Strehler, 1977). Such deposits in substantia nigra may be related to age-related cell death. However, given that relatively high levels of dopamine depletion (50%) are necessary to produce behavioral deficits, a neurotoxic insult coupled with a preexisting "silent lesion" might produce more severe neurotoxicity, which is expressed as a behavioral deficit. It is possible that caloric restriction may protect against naturally occurring degenerative processes that predispose the brain to enhanced neurotoxicity, even at low levels of exposure that might have no effect in younger animals. It has been difficult to characterize behavioral deficits caused by dysfunction of the dopamine system in rodents that model these levels of lesions presumed to occur gradually over time. Characterizing this behavioral decline would greatly aid the demonstration of beneficial effects of caloric restriction prior to massive neurochemical and behavioral deficits.

### 4.2. Effects of Chronic Caloric Restriction on Neurochemistry in Aged Animals

There are few studies that examine the role of diet restriction in preventing decreases in dopamine function during aging (Table 3). EOD restriction has been shown to delay the loss in rat striatal D2 receptors observed during aging (Levin *et al.*, 1981; London *et al.*,

TABLE 2. Summary of Aging Effects on Dopamine Neurochemistry

| Strain | Brain region | Biomarker | Aging change | Reference |
|---|---|---|---|---|
| **Rat** | | | | |
| Sprague-Dawley | Striatum | DA levels | → | Strong et al., 1982 |
| Sprague-Dawley | Striatum | D2 ($^3$H-spiperone) | → | O'Boyle and Waddington, 1984 |
| Sprague-Dawley | Striatum | D1 ($^3$H-piflutixol) | nc | O'Boyle and Waddington, 1984 |
| Long-Evans | Striatum | DA levels | → | Simpkins, 1984 |
| Wistar | Striatum | D1 ($^3$H-piflutixol) | → | Henry et al., 1986 |
| Wistar | Striatum | D2 ($^3$H-spiperone) | → | Henry et al., 1986 |
| Wistar | Striatum | DA stimulated adenylate cyclase | → | Henry et al., 1986 |
| Fischer-344 | CPU | D2 ($^3$H-spiroperidol) | → | Joyce et al., 1986 |
| Sprague-Dawley | Striatum | Na$^+$ $^3$H-cocaine binding | → | Missale et al., 1986 |
| Sprague-Dawley | FC | Na$^+$ $^3$H-cocaine binding | nc | Missale et al., 1986 |
| Sprague-Dawley | Striatum | $^3$H-dopamine uptake, Km | ← | Missale et al., 1986 |
| Wistar | Striatum | D1, D2 recovery following EEDQ | → | Henry et al., 1987 |
| Sprague-Dawley | Striatum | D1 ($^3$H-SCH-23390) | → | Giorgi et al., 1987 |
| Fischer-344 | Striatum | $^3$H-DA release | nc | McIntosh and Westfall, 1987 |
| Fischer-344 | Striatum | DA levels | → | Govoni et al., 1988 |
| Wistar | Striatum | Muscarinic control of DA autoreceptors | → | Joseph et al., 1988 |
| Wistar | Striatum, CX, HPT | D2 ($^3$H-spiroperidol) | → | Petkov et al., 1988 |
| Wistar | Striatum, CX | DA levels | → | Petkov et al., 1988 |
| Wistar | Striatum, CX | MAO-A | ← | Petkov et al., 1988 |
| Sprague-Dawley | Striatum, HPC | HVA | → | Godefroy et al., 1989 |
| Sprague-Dawley | HPC | DA levels | → | Godefroy et al., 1989 |
| Sprague-Dawley | CX | DA levels | ← | Godefroy et al., 1989 |
| Wistar | Striatum | D2 ($^3$H-spiperone) | → | Han et al., 1989 |
| Wistar | Striatum | D1 ($^3$H-SCH-23390) | → | Hyttel, 1989 |
| Wistar | Striatum | D2 ($^3$H-spiperone) | → | Hyttel, 1989 |
| Wistar | Pituitary | Sensitivity to estradiol reduction in DA receptors | → | Kochman et al., 1989 |

(continued)

TABLE 2. (Continued)

| Strain | Brain region | Biomarker | Aging change | Reference |
|---|---|---|---|---|
| Holtzman albino | Striatum | DA release | → | Dluzen et al., 1989 |
| Wistar | Striatum | DA release (K$^+$) | nc | Stamford, 1989 |
| Wistar | SN | DA, HVA, DOPAC levels | → | Venero et al., 1989 |
| Long-Evans | Striatum | ChAct | → | Gallagher et al., 1990 |
| Wistar | SN | DA levels | → | Gozlan et al., 1990 |
| Wistar | SN | DOPAC/DA ratio | ← | Gozlan et al., 1990 |
| Wistar | SN | D2 ($^3$H-spiperone) | → | Gozlan et al., 1990 |
| Wistar | Neostriatum | Enhancement of DA release (K$^+$) | | Joseph et al., 1990 |
| Sprague-Dawley | Striatum | DA release (K$^+$) | → | Laping et al., 1990 |
| Fischer-344 | VCPU | DA, HVA, DOPA, DOPAC levels | → | Marshall and Rosenstein, 1990 |
| Sprague-Dawley | CPU, OT, NAC | D1 ($^3$H-SCH-23390) | → | Morelli et al., 1990 |
| Sprague-Dawley | CPU, OT, NAC | D2 ($^3$H-sulpiride) | → | Morelli et al., 1990 |
| Wistar | PFC | DA | ← | Venero et al., 1990 |
| Wistar | PFC | MAO-A/MAO-B ratio | → | Venero et al., 1990 |
| Sprague-Dawley | FC | D1 cAMP coupling | → | Amenta et al., 1990 |
| Sprague-Dawley | FC | D2 cAMP inhibition | ← | Amenta et al., 1990 |

| Mouse | | | | |
|---|---|---|---|---|
| C57BL/6J | Striatum | DA levels | → | Finch, 1973 |
| C57BL/6J, C3HeB/FeJ | Striatum | D1/D2 ($^3$H-ADTN) | → | Severson and Finch, 1980 |
| C57BL/6J | Striatum, HPT | D2 ($^3$H-spiroperidol) | → | Severson and Finch, 1980 |
| C57BL/6J | Olfactory bulb | D2 ($^3$H-spiroperidol) | nc | Severson and Finch, 1980 |
| C3HeB/FeJ | Striatum | D2 ($^3$H-spiroperidol) | → | Severson and Finch, 1980 |
| C57BL/6J | Striatum | D2 ($^3$H-spiperone) | → | Severson and Randall, 1985 |
| C57BL, BALB/c | Striatum | DA levels | nc | Ebel et al., 1987 |
| BALB/c | Striatum | DOPA levels | → | Ebel et al., 1987 |
| C57BL, BALB | Striatum | DOPAC, HVA | → | Ebel et al., 1987 |
| BALB/c | Striatum | DA release | ← | Freeman and Gibson, 1987 |
| C57BL/6J | Striatum | D2 ($^3$H-spiperone) | nc | Leprohon-Greenwood and Cinader, 1987 |
| A/J, SJL/J, C3/HeJ, DBA/1J | Striatum | D2 ($^3$H-spiperone) | → | Leprohon-Greenwood and Cinader, 1987 |
| C57BL/6N | SN | Number of DA neurons | nc | McNeill et al., 1988 |
| C57BL6 | Striatum | D1 ($^3$H-piflutixol) | → | Henry et al., 1986 |
| C57BL6 | Striatum | D2 ($^3$H-spiperone) | → | Henry et al., 1986 |

CPU = caudate putamen; CX = cortex; FC = frontal cortex; HPC = hippocampus; HPT = hypothalamus; NAC = nucleus accumbens; OT = olfactory tubercles; PFC = prefrontal cortex; SN = substantia nigra; VCPU = ventral caudate putamen; nc = no change.

**TABLE 3.** Summary of Caloric-Restriction Effects on Aging-Induced Alterations in Dopamine Neurochemistry

| Strain | Restriction method | Brain region | Biomarker | Restriction effect compared to age-matched ad lib control | Reference |
|---|---|---|---|---|---|
| *Rat* | | | | | |
| Wistar | EOD | Striatum | ³H-ADTN | ↑ | Levin *et al.*, 1981 |
| Wistar | EOD | Striatum | D2 ³H-spiperone | ↑ | Roth *et al.*, 1984 |
| Wistar | EOD | Striatum | Muscarinic ³H-QNB binding | ↑ | London *et al.*, 1985 |
| Fischer-344 | Daily | Caudate | DA levels | ↓ | Kolta *et al.*, 1989 |
| Fischer-344 | Daily | Caudate | DOPAC, HVA levels | nc | Kolta *et al.*, 1989 |
| Fischer-344 | Daily | HPT | DA levels | ↓ | Kolta *et al.*, 1989 |
| Fischer-344 | Daily | HPT | DOPAC, HVA levels | nc | Kolta *et al.*, 1989 |
| *Mouse* | | | | | |
| B6C3F1 | Daily | Caudate | D1 (³H-SCH-23390) | nc | Holson *et al.*, 1991 |
|  |  |  | D2 (³H-spiroperidol) | nc | Holson *et al.*, 1991 |
| B6C3F1 | Daily | HPT | DA, HVA, DOPAC levels | nc | Holson *et al.*, 1991 |

HPT = hypothalamus; nc = no change.

1985; Meites, 1990; Roth and Joseph, 1988; Roth *et al.*, 1984, 1986), although in B6C3F1 mice no such effect of 60% daily caloric restriction was observed in striatal D2 or hippocampal muscarinic binding, both of which showed a decline with age that was similar under both diet conditions (Table 4). However, the results from the latter study were obtained from single point assays, and it may be necessary to examine binding characteristics over several ligand concentrations. Intensive studies on dopamine receptor binding in daily caloric-restricted animals have yet to be reported.

An ongoing study in rhesus and squirrel monkeys investigating dietary manipulations on several endpoints should shed more light on the effects of caloric restriction on dopamine neurochemistry (Ingram *et al.*, 1990). In this study, monkeys are fed ad libitum or 70% of the ad lib diet, with 50% of the diet made available two times each day. Thus far, only preliminary data have been published describing animal husbandry techniques, diet formulations, food intake, and blood chemistry (Ingram *et al.*, 1990).

### 4.3. Behavioral Assessment of Aged Animals

It is not clear what role alterations in the dopamine system play in age-related behavioral deficits. Based on what is known about neurochemical deficits in the dopamine system during aging, one can predict what functional deficits might occur. These would likely be deficits in locomotor activity and sensorimotor activity based on reported deficits in striatal dopamine neurochemistry (Gallagher and Burwell, 1989; Ingram, 1988b; Joseph and Roth, 1988; Morgan and Finch, 1988).

**TABLE 4.** Dopaminergic and Muscarinic Receptor Binding in B6C3F1 Mice

| | Age (months) | | | | | |
|---|---|---|---|---|---|---|
| | 7 | | 18 | | 30 | |
| Diet | AL | RES | AL | RES | AL | RES |
| Hippocampus | | | | | | |
| $^3$[H]-QNB[a] | 1361 | 1309 | 1333 | 1276 | 1190[b,c] | 1113[b,c] |
| | ±44 | ±53 | ±63 | ±35 | ±26 | ±40 |
| Caudate | | | | | | |
| $^3$[H]-QNB[a] | 1136 | 1199 | 1149 | 1067 | 1134 | 1107 |
| | ±49 | ±61 | ±85 | ±985 | ±40 | ±68 |
| $^3$[H]-SCH-23390[a] | 111.2 | 111.0 | 104.1 | 114.2 | 125.8 | 133.9 |
| | ±3.5 | ±2.5 | ±5.4 | ±7.2 | ±12.2 | ±12.5 |
| $^3$[H]-spiroperidol[a] | 189.8 | 211.0 | 107.3[b] | 110.2[b] | 103.3[b] | 92.3[b] |
| | ±4.2 | ±7.7 | ±7.9 | ±5.4 | ±9.5 | ±10.6 |

· AL = ad lib; RES = 60% calorie restricted.
[a]Mean fmoles/mg protein ± SEM.
[b]Significantly different from 7-month group, $p \leq .05$.
[c]Significantly different from 18-month group, $p \leq .05$.
From Holson et al. (1991), with permission.

Behavioral assessment during aging in rodents has taken many approaches, including motor behavior, learning, and memory (Gallagher and Burwell, 1989; Ingram, 1988c; Morgan and Finch, 1988). Each task is designed to assess the integrity of specific brain systems, where neurochemical deficits may be manifest as functional deficits. Ingram and colleagues (Ingram, 1988a, 1988b; Spangler et al., 1989) have conducted several studies on motor performance, and learning and memory in several rat and mice strains, and have shown a robust age-related impairment in acquisition in the Stone maze in outbred, inbred, and hybrid rat and mice strains (Fig. 2). Interactions of the cholinergic system thus appear to play a key role in the observed deficits shown by pharmacological and lesion studies. Gallagher and colleagues (Gallagher et al., 1990) have shown that the analysis of choline acetyltransferase (ChAT) in the basal forebrain and striatum appear to be the best predictors of spatial learning impairment in Long-Evans rats.

Joseph et al. (1989) examined the effects of chronic estrogen and modified ovine prolactin on inclined screen performance during aging and found that administration of either substance was effective in improving both inclined screen performance and increasing striatal D2 receptor concentrations. However, the improvements in inclined screen performance were observed prior to any increases in striatal D2 concentrations.

Molloy and Waddington (1988) investigated the effects of D1 and D2 agonist challenges in young (4 months) and old (22 months) Sprague-Dawley rats and found that stereotypic behavior induced by 0.5 mg/kg apomorphine was increased and prolonged in old rats (which have reduced D2 but not D1 dopamine receptors), suggesting a pharmacokinetic effect rather than a receptor-mediated effect. Stereotypic behavior induced by the D2 agonist RU-24213 was not different in young vs. old rats. Thus, the well-documented decrease in striatal D2 dopamine receptors does not appear to produce significant behavioral alterations in response to these drug challenges. This may be related to the observation that large lesions in the striatal dopamine system are needed to produce severe behavioral alterations.

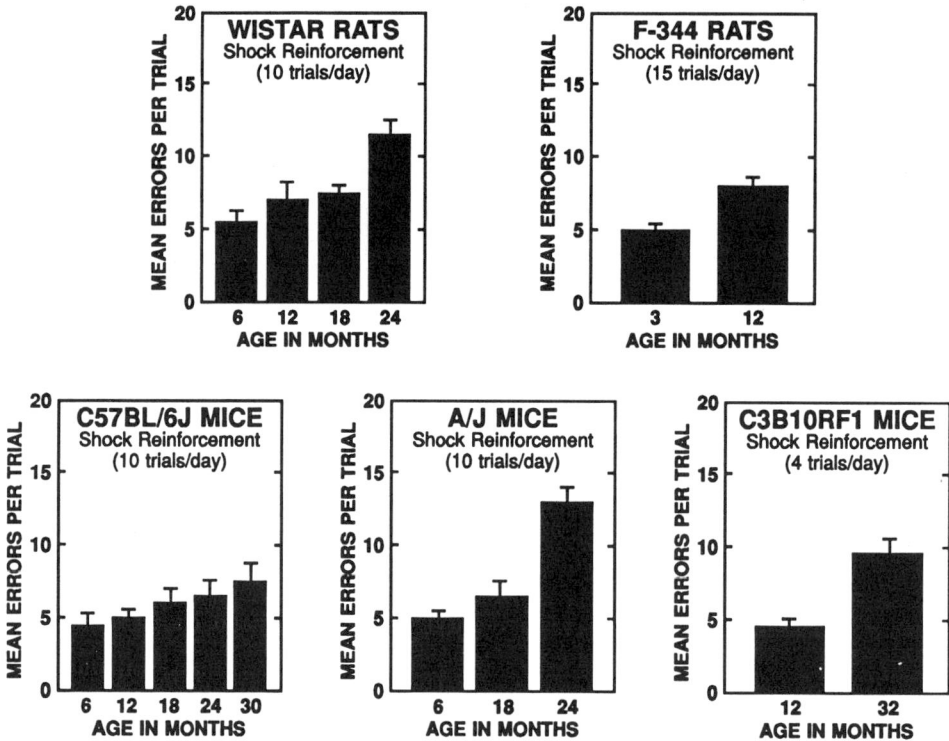

**FIGURE 2.** Age comparisons of mean (+SEM) errors per trial made by male Wistar rats, male F-344 rats, male C57BL/6J mice, male A/J mice, and female C3B10RF$_1$ mice during acquisition training in the Stone maze (n's = 6–10). From Ingram (1988), with permission.

Stoessl et al. (1989) found that spontaneous locomotor activity and motor coordination decreased with aging in Sprague-Dawley rats, as did responsiveness to low doses (10–50 μg/kg) of apomorphine. They suggest that aging is associated with decreased responsiveness to stimulation of dopamine autoreceptors, resulting from the loss of dopaminergic nerve terminals. They also observed a decrease in functional response to the D2 agonist (+)-4-propyl-9-hydroxynaphthoxazine, suggesting a decrease in postsynaptic D2 receptors, which would agree with observations from receptor binding studies.

It is clear that behavioral deficits do occur with aging, but the role of the dopamine system in these deficits is not well understood. This makes the assessment of the potential beneficial effects of caloric restriction on behaviors mediated by the dopamine system a difficult task compared to neurochemical studies, which have focused primarily on receptor binding properties in the striatum.

### 4.4. Effects of Chronic Caloric Restriction on Behavior of Aged Animals

While the documentation of age-related deficits in behavior is convincing, the ability of caloric restriction to ameliorate these deficits is still an enigma. Ingram and colleagues

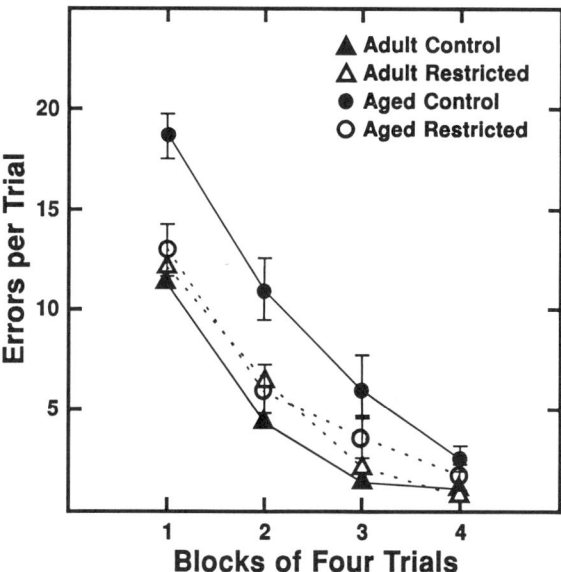

**FIGURE 3.** Age and diet comparisons of mean (+SEM) errors per trial for female C3B10RF$_1$ mice in a 14-unit T-maze. From Ingram *et al.* (1987), with permission.

(Ingram *et al.*, 1987) have shown that in female C3B10RF1 mice age-related declines in motor coordination (rotorod test) and learning (complex maze) were prevented by EOD caloric restriction (Fig. 3). In addition, caloric restriction increased locomotor activity in a running wheel cage among middle-aged (11–15 months) and aged (31–35 months) mice but did not affect exploratory activity in a novel arena.

Stewart *et al.* (1989) studied ad lib and 60% caloric-restricted Fischer-344 rats at three ages—8, 16, and 24 months—on spatial memory tasks (eight-arm radial maze and the Morris water maze) and found that life-long food restriction appeared to delay the impairments of age but does not prevent them. However, Bond *et al.* (1989) examined male Wistar rats in a radial-arm maze and found that dietary restriction does not protect rats from the memory loss observed in aged animals.

In male CD-COBS rats studied at 4, 12, and 24 months of age, Pitsikas *et al.* (1990) found that rats fed a hypocaloric diet that resulted in body weights that were 67% of ad lib did not have the cognitive deficits (i.e., delayed learning and impaired memory utilization) that ad lib animals exhibited in the Morris water maze.

Holson *et al.* (1991) have shown performance deficits in old ad lib and 60% caloric-restricted Brown Norway rats, tested with water as a reward, that are remarkably similar to those observed in trimethyltin- (TMT) treated rats. In these studies, older rats (14 and 23 months old) could find the goal box but experienced great difficulty in finding their way back to the start region. However, at no age did diet have an effect on maze performance; thus chronic caloric restriction neither retarded nor accelerated the memory loss observed in older rats (Fig. 4).

Idrobo *et al.* (1987) have shown that in C57BL/6 mice dietary restriction improved performance on radial maze learning. This improvement was associated with a significant reduction in lipofuscin pigment deposition in the hippocampus and frontal cortex.

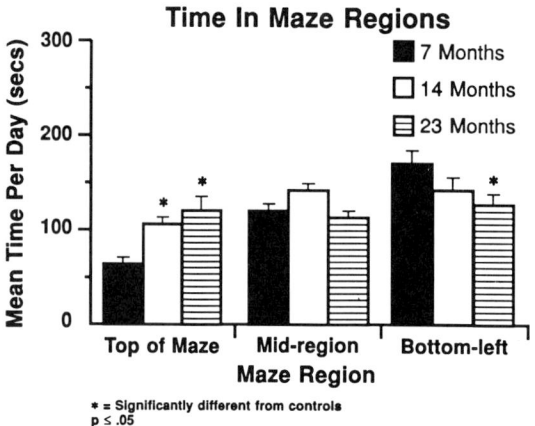

**FIGURE 4.** Maze performance in 7-, 14-, and 23-month-old ad lib and restricted Brown Norway rats (data collapsed over diet condition; n = 10–12/group). From Holson et al. (1991), with permission.

## 5. INTERACTION OF CHRONIC CALORIC RESTRICTION WITH TRIMETHYLTIN TOXICITY IN AGED ANIMALS

Because chronic caloric restriction has beneficial effects on health and longevity, it is possible that vulnerability to toxicants may be reduced following chronic caloric restriction. Because of the general beneficial effects of chronic caloric restriction, the brain may be more resistant to insults (e.g., retains plasticity) and less susceptible to the adverse effects of neurotoxicants. Thus, the critical experimental hypothesis for chronic caloric restriction in relation to this volume is as follows: *Chronic caloric restriction decreases vulnerability to neurotoxicity.*

All of the data discussed thus far have focused on the putative beneficial effects of chronic caloric restriction on longevity, behavior, and the dopamine system. To date, the aforementioned hypothesis has not been adequately tested regarding any neurotoxicant discussed in this volume.

One approach to testing this hypothesis is to assess neurotoxicity after exposure to a neurotoxicant in animals that have been raised either ad libitum or under chronic caloric restriction. While this approach may first appear rather straightforward, there are significant methodological and data-interpretation problems. These include differences in sensory detection thresholds, physical size, and potential differences in the metabolism and pharmacokinetics of the neurotoxicant (especially regarding the larger fat compartment in ad libitum animals, which could alter the pharmacokinetics of both lipophilic and lipophobic substances). The assessment of behavior in caloric-restriction studies is also complicated by circadian patterns of activity and other variables (Duffy et al., 1989). Because restricted animals always appear to be interested in consuming food and will work harder to get food, the choice of reinforcer (e.g., food or water) and motivational factors (e.g., to feed or not to feed before behavioral testing) are critical. Restricted animals are also more active than ad libitum animals (Duffy et al., 1989), and this activity may reflect some kind of practice or learning effect, which in turn prevents the deterioration seen in more sedentary aging ad libitum rodents. The selection of appropriate control groups is also a problem. Issues such as baseline locomotor ability, body weight, age, and the overall health of aged controls are all important factors to consider. For example,

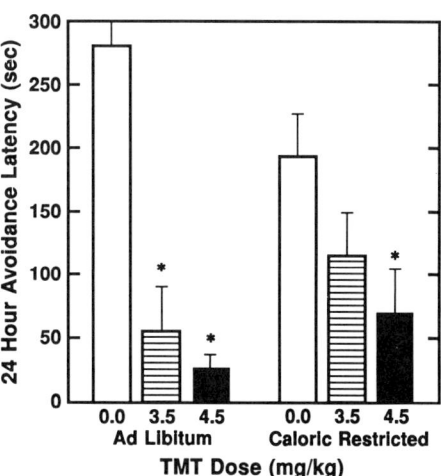

FIGURE 5. Response latencies on passive avoidance test presented as functions of TMT dose and diet. TMT-treated group means that are significantly different ($p < .05$) from the saline-treated controls of the same diet condition are marked by an asterisk. The latencies (mean sec ± SEM) for the rats to reenter the darkened test box containing the electrified shock grid for the training-trial box 24 hr after the training trial are presented here. In no case was there a significant difference between diet conditions at a single level of the TMT dose. The TMT effects on escape and 24-hr retention were significant at both doses in ad lib fed rats, while they were significant only at the high dose in caloric-restricted rats. From Matthews and Scallet (1991), with permission.

Hicks et al. (1980) observed that longer latencies to initiation and longer durations of amphetamine induce gnawing behavior in C57BL/6J mice that appeared to be caused by differences in the pharmacokinetics of amphetamine between young and old mice. This type of pharmacokinetic problem is significant in the determination of the beneficial effects of caloric restriction on the dopamine system, because the pharmacokinetics of many compounds used to probe the central nervous system are either poorly understood or have not been examined at all in caloric-restricted animals or during aging.

In a recent attempt to examine the potential interaction of caloric restriction with neurotoxicity, Matthews and Scallet (1991) investigated the effects of aging and diet on TMT neurotoxicity. Three doses of TMT (0, 3.5, or 4.5 mg/kg) were administered to separate groups of 17-month-old Fischer-344 rats raised ad libitum or on a 60% calorie-restricted diet. Animals were then tested in a passive avoidance test. There was no effect of caloric restriction on escape latencies during training or on the 24- or 48-hr retention tests. There was a significant TMT treatment effect on escape latencies and on 24- (Fig. 5) and 48-hr retention tests, but there were no significant TMT by diet interactions. The TMT effect on escape latencies was primarily on the ad-libitum-fed rats, since individual mean comparisons indicated that only the ad libitum latencies of TMT-treated rats were significantly greater than their saline-treated control. Similarly, in the retention tests, although the TMT by diet interactions were not significant, ad libitum rats exhibited larger changes in latency scores compared to their saline-treated controls than did the caloric-restriction groups. It is also interesting to note that in the 24-hr retention test, caloric-restricted animals exhibited a trend toward impaired performance on the passive avoidance test relative to the ad lib controls. This raises the possibility that there may be some detrimental effects of prolonged caloric restriction at the level (60% of ad lib) utilized in this study.

The results from this study raise important questions regarding experimental design and data interpretation. For example, recent evidence suggests that pain sensitivity may be altered during aging (Tucker, 1989). This difference in sensitivity may interact with behavioral testing in a shock paradigm and may also be affected by TMT treatment.

Based on available data, it is difficult to draw any sound conclusions about the potential beneficial effects of caloric restriction on vulnerability to neurotoxicants. Only through careful experimental design and the development of a baseline database for specific behaviors used in neurotoxicological assessment will efforts be successful in determining if caloric restriction protects against or exacerbates neurotoxicant insults.

## 6. DOPAMINE AGONISTS, AGING, AND NEUROTOXICITY

The focus of this chapter thus far has been on the potential for diet manipulations to reduce vulnerability to dopaminergic deficits during aging or following toxicant exposure. Although it is not clear what the links are between caloric restriction and toxicant or aging vulnerability in the dopamine system, there are a few reports worthy of mention that raise some interesting possibilities about the role of the dopamine system in reducing vulnerability to insults and in extending life span.

Results from at least two laboratories strongly support the notion that life span can be increased with the administration of L-deprenyl (Knoll, 1988; Knoll *et al.*, 1989; Milgram *et al.*, 1990) (Table 5). L-deprenyl is a monoamine oxidase B inhibitor and is widely used as an adjunct to therapy for Parkinson's disease. It has been hypothesized that L-deprenyl protects against neurotoxic byproducts of MAO-mediated metabolism (Cohen *et al.*, 1984) and may play a protective role against some neurotoxicants (Cohen *et al.*, 1984; Fuller *et al.*, 1988; Langston *et al.*, 1983).

Another report provides evidence that mice chronically treated with L-dopa have significantly longer life spans (Cotzias *et al.*, 1974). Similarly, rats chronically treated with ibopamine, a catecholaminergic drug, were less likely to have tumors than age-matched controls, and although life span was not measured, it appeared that ibopamine-treated rats had significantly less malignant lesions than controls, suggesting a potentially positive effect of treatment on survival (Walker *et al.*, 1988).

**TABLE 5.** Life Span of Rats Treated with Saline (n = 66) and (-)-Deprenyl (n = 66)

| Classification of the groups according to sexual performance before treatment | No. of animals | Average life span (weeks) | |
|---|---|---|---|
| | | Saline treated | (-)Deprenyl treated |
| Noncopulators | 23 | 142.74 ± 0.38 A | 187.90 ± 3.27 D |
| Mounting rats | 21 | 146.95 ± 0.42 B | 191.95 ± 3.59 E |
| Sluggish rats | 22 | 152.00 ± 0.92 C | 214.05 ± 3.07 F |
| Total | 66 | 147.05 ± 0.56 G | 197.98 ± 2.36 H |

Significances according to the Student's *t*-test for two means:

| | | | | |
|---|---|---|---|---|
| A:B | $p < 0.001$ | | C:F | $p < 0.001$ |
| A:C | $p < 0.001$ | | D:E | $p > 0.05$ |
| B:C | $p < 0.001$ | | D:F | $p < 0.001$ |
| A:D | $p < 0.001$ | | E:F | $p < 0.001$ |
| B:E | $p < 0.001$ | | G:H | $p < 0.001$ |

From Knoll (1988), with permission.

## 7. CHRONIC CALORIC-RESTRICTION EFFECTS AND IMPLICATIONS FOR TOXICITY TESTING

One of the immediate practical gains to be made with caloric-restriction technology is in the area of safety assessment. At present, standard toxicity testing is conducted on both an acute and chronic basis. Typically, chronic studies involve exposure to a given test compound for approximately 2 years. A given rate of mortality is expected in both the control and experimental groups, but in light of the beneficial effects of caloric restriction, there are potential confounds in chronic toxicity data that can make accurate interpretations difficult.

Many test chemicals, as a result of toxicity, reduce food intake. If food intake is reduced moderately in a chronic toxicity study, the results of the study are potentially confounded by this unintentional dietary restriction. Treatment groups that are consuming less food are in effect being raised under a diet-restriction regimen (although they may also be malnourished). However, assuming that nutrient intake is not severely reduced, and if indeed diet restriction has beneficial effects, then one would predict less toxicity in this treatment group compared to a "non-diet-restricted" group (e.g., a group being treated at a lower test dose but consuming more diet). Furthermore, if the control group is fed ad libitum, this would exaggerate potential group differences, since the control group would likely develop tumors and other endpoints of toxicity at the normally expected rate. If the control group is pair-fed with the treatment group (to control for diet effects), the control group now potentially becomes a diet-restricted group, thus producing the potential of having fewer toxic effects (because of the putative beneficial effects of dietary restriction) than a control group fed ad libitum. This potential confound may be important in designing chronic toxicity studies in which a toxicant-induced reduction in food intake occurs, thereby necessitating the inclusion of more than a pair-fed control group. However, pair-feeding is also known to produce effects that are not well understood and, depending on the method employed, pair-feeding may in fact drive behavioral (e.g., animals become more active around feeding time) and biochemical rhythms.

Another potential problem in chronic toxicity testing is that caloric restriction might appear to be an effective remedy for the loss of subjects from 2-year studies. While extending the life span in chronic toxicity testing through dietary restriction is an attractive means to reduce normal tumorigenesis and mortality, it creates major problems in data interpretation. For example, in a rat strain such as Sprague-Dawley, which is commonly used in toxicity testing, the expected life span is approximately 24 months. A compound observed to be neurotoxic in ad-libitum-fed rats after chronic exposure might not produce the same degree of toxicity in caloric-restricted rats. Under restricted conditions, maximum achievable life span would increase and the potential beneficial effects of caloric restriction might protect against the neurotoxic effects that were previously observed in the 2-year chronic study of ad-libitum-fed rats.

## 8. SUMMARY AND CONCLUSIONS

It is clear that chronic caloric restriction has beneficial effects on the quality of life and longevity in rodents. However, the mechanisms of how this occurs are poorly understood. As more data are collected on these mechanisms it seems likely that efforts to understand how caloric restriction affects brain and behavior will be improved.

Caloric restriction appears to yield beneficial effects under relatively severe levels of restriction. This severity may be an impediment in conducting clinical research on the potential benefits of caloric restriction in humans. Perhaps if the degree of caloric restriction presumed to be required to produce beneficial effects in humans was not so severe, humans might be more likely to change life-styles and take advantage of this relatively simple approach to potentially longer, healthier lives. Through these same changes perhaps resistance to neurotoxicants and many other pathologies could be enhanced.

As our understanding of nutrition improves, a clearer picture should emerge regarding the role of various diet components (e.g., fatty acids) in caloric restriction. This might then allow for implementation of a comprehensive health plan for humans to change unhealthy eating habits, improve diets, and potentially live longer, healthier lives. As more is learned about diet, brain, hormonal, and immune interactions, the next decade is sure to bring many exciting findings in the area of prolonged dietary restriction effects on brain and behavior.

ACKNOWLEDGMENTS. Part of this work was supported by an appointment to the Oak Ridge Associated Universities Postgraduate Research Program at the National Center for Toxicological Research, administered by Oak Ridge Associated Universities through an interagency agreement between the U.S. Department of Energy and the U.S. Food and Drug Administration.

## REFERENCES

Amenta, F., Cavallotti, C., Collier, W.L., De Michele, M., and Ricci, A., 1990, Age-related changes of dopamine sensitive cyclic AMP generation in the rat frontal cortex, *Mech. Ageing Dev.* 54:63–73.

Bond, N.W., Everitt, A.V., and Walton, J., 1989, Effects of dietary restriction on radial-arm maze performance and flavor memory in aged rats, *Neurobiol. Aging* 10:27–30.

Burchinsky, S.G., 1984, Neurotransmitter receptors in the central nervous system and aging: Pharmacological aspect, *Exp. Gerontol.* 19:227–239.

Cohen, G., Pasik, B., Cohen, B., Leist, C., Mytilineous, C., and Yahr, M.D., 1984, Pargyline and deprenyl prevent the neurotoxicity of 1-methyl-4-phenyl-1,2,3,6-tetrahydropyridine (MPTP) in monkeys, *Eur. J. Pharmacol.* 106:209–210.

Cotzias, G.C., Miller, S.T., Nicholson, A.R., Jr., Matson, W.H., and Tang, L.C., 1974, Prolongation of the life-span in mice adapted to large amounts of L-dopa, *Proc. Natl. Acad. Sci. USA* 71:2466–2469.

Cutler, R.G., 1981, Life-span extension, in: *Aging: Biology and Behavior* (J.L. McGaugh and S.B. Kiesler, eds.), Academic Press, New York. pp. 31–76.

Dluzen, D.E., McDermott, J.L., and Ramirez, V.D., 1989, The effect of l-DOPA upon in vitro dopamine release from the corpus striatum of young and old male rats, *Exp. Neurol.* 106:259–264.

Duffy, P.H., Feuers, R.J., Leakey, J.A., Nakamura, K.D., Turturro, A., and Hart, R.W., 1989, Effect of chronic caloric restriction on physiological variables related to energy metabolism in the male Fischer 344 rat, *Mech. Ageing Dev.* 48:117–133.

Ebel, A., Strosser, M.T., and Kempf, E., 1987, Genotypic differences in central neurotransmitter responses to aging in mice, *Neurobiol. Aging* 8:417–427.

Fernandes, G., Yunis, E.J., and Good, R.A., 1976, Influence of diet on survival of mice, *Proc. Natl. Acad. Sci. USA* 73:1279–1283.

Feuers, R.J., Duffy, P.H., Leakey, J.A., Turturro, A., Mittelstaedt, R.A., and Hart, R.W., 1989, Effect of chronic caloric restriction on hepatic enzymes of intermediary metabolism in the male Fischer 344 rat, *Mech. Ageing Dev.* 48:179–189.

Finch, C.E., 1973, Catecholamine metabolism in the brains of aging male mice, *Brain Res.* 52:261–276.

Freeman, G.B., and Gibson, G.E., 1987, Selective alteration of mouse brain neurotransmitter release with age, *Neurobiol. Aging* 8:147–152.

Fuller, R.W., Hemricke-Luecke, S., and Perry, K.W., 1988, Deprenyl antagonizes acute lethality of 1-methyl-4-phenyl-1,2,3,6-tetrahydropyridine in mice, *J. Pharmacol. Exp. Ther.* 247:531–535.

Gallagher, M., and Burwell, R.D., 1989, Relationship of age-related decline across several behavioral domains, *Neurobiol. Aging* 10:691–708.

Gallagher, M., Burwell, R.D., Kodsi, M.H., McKinney, M., Southerland, S., Vella-Rountree, L., and Lewis, M.H., 1990, Markers for biogenic amines in the aged rat brain: Relationship to decline in spatial learning ability, *Neurobiol. Aging* 11:507–514.

Gerbase-Delima, M., Liu, R.K., Cheney, R., Mickey, R., and Walford, R.L., 1975, Immune function and survival in a long-lived mouse strain subjected to undernutrition, *Gerontology* 21:184–202.

Giorgi, O., Calderini, G., Toffano, G., and Biggio, G., 1987, D-1 dopamine receptors labelled with 3H-SCH 23390: Decrease in the striatum of aged rats, *Neurobiol. Aging* 8:51–54.

Godefroy, F., Bassant, M.H., Weil-Fugazza, J., and Lamour, Y., 1989, Age-related changes in dopaminergic and serotonergic indices in the rat forebrain, *Neurobiol. Aging* 10:187–190.

Goodrick, C., Ingram, D.K., Reynolds, M.A., Freeman, J.R., and Cider, N.L., 1982, Effects of intermittent feeding upon growth and lifespan in rats, *Gerontology* 28:233–241.

Goodrick, C.L., Ingram, D.K., Reynolds, M.A., Freeman, J.R., and Cider, N., 1990, Effects of intermittent feeding upon body weight and lifespan in inbred mice: Interaction of genotype and age, *Mech. Ageing Dev.* 55:69–87.

Govoni, S., Rius, R.A., Battaini, F., Magnoni, M.S., Lucchi, L., and Trabucchi, M., 1988, The central dopaminergic system: Susceptibility to risk factors for accelerated aging, *Gerontology* 34:29–34.

Gozlan, H., Daval, G., Verge, D., Spampinata, U., Fattaccini, C.M., Gallissot, M.C., El Mestikawy, S., and Hamon, M., 1990, Aging associated changes in serotonergic and dopaminergic pre- and postsynaptic neurochemical markers in the rat brain, *Neurobiol. Aging* 11:437–449.

Han, Z., Kuyatt, B.L., Kochman, K.A., DeSouza, E.B., and Roth, G.S., 1989, Effect of aging on concentrations of D2-receptor-containing neurons in the rat striatum, *Brain Res.* 498:299–307.

Harrison, D.E., and Archer, J.R., 1987, Genetic differences in effects of food restriction on aging mice, *J. Nutr.* 117:376–382.

Henry, J.M., Filburn, C.R., Joseph, J.A., and Roth, G.S., 1986, Effect of aging on striatal dopamine receptor subtypes in Wistar rats, *Neurobiol. Aging* 7:357–361.

Henry, J.M., Joseph, J.A., Kochman, K., and Roth, G.S., 1987, Effect of aging on striatal dopamine receptor subtype recovery following N-ethoxycarbonyl-2-ethoxy-1,2-dihydroquinoline blockade and relation to motor function in Wistar rats, *Brain Res.* 418:334–342.

Hicks, P., Strong, R., Schoolar, J.C., and Samorajski, T., 1980, Aging alters amphetamine-induced stereotyped gnawing and neostriatal elimination of amphetamine in mice, *Life Sci.* 27:715–722.

Holehan, A.N., and Merry, B.J., 1985, The control of puberty in the dietary restricted female rat, *Mech. Ageing Dev.* 32:179–191.

Holson, R.R., Duffy, P., Ali, S.F., and Scalzo, F.M., 1991, Aging, dietary restriction and glucocorticoids: A critical review of the "Glucocorticoid Hypothesis," in: *The Biological Effects of Dietary Restriction* (L. Fishbein, ed.), International Life Sciences Institute, Washington, D.C. pp. 123–139.

Hyttel, J., 1989, Parallel decreases in the density of dopamine D1 and D2 receptors in corpus striatum of rats from 3 to 25 months of age, *Pharmacol. Toxicol.* 64:55–57.

Idrobo, F., Nandy, K., Mostofsky, D.I., Blatt, L., and Nandy, L., 1987, Dietary restriction: Effects on radial maze learning and lipofuscin pigment deposition in the hippocampus and frontal cortex, *Arch. Gerontol. Geriatr.* 6:355–362.

Ingram, D.K., 1988a, Key questions in developing biomarkers of aging, *Exp. Gerontol.* 23:429–434.

Ingram, D.K., 1988b, Motor performance variability during aging in rodents. Assessment of reliability and validity of individual differences, *Ann. N.Y. Acad. Sci.* 515:70–96.

Ingram, D.K., 1988c, Complex maze learning in rodents as a model of age-related memory impairment, *Neurobiol. Aging* 9:475–485.

Ingram, D.K., Weindruch, R., Spangler, E.L., Freeman, J.R., and Walford, R.L., 1987, Dietary restriction benefits learning and motor performance of aged mice, *J. Gerontol.* 42:78–81.

Ingram, D.K., Cutler, R.G., Weindruch, R., Renquist, D.M., Knapka, J.J., April, M., Belcher, C.T., Clark, M.A., Hatcherson, C.D., Marriott, B.M., and Roth, G.S., 1990, Dietary restriction and agingL the initiation of a primate study, *J. Gerontal.* 45:b148–b163.

Joseph, J.A., and Roth, G.S., 1988, Altered striatal dopaminergic and cholinergic reciprocal inhibitory control and motor behavioral decrements in senescence, *Ann. N.Y. Acad. Sci.* 521:110–122.

Joseph, J.A., and Roth, G.S., 1989, Upregulation of striatal dopamine receptors and improvement of motor performance in senescence, *Exp. Cell Res.* 180:234–242.

Joseph, J.A., Dalton, T.K., and Hunt, W.A., 1988, Age-related decrements in the muscarinic enhancement of $K^+$-evoked release of endogenous striatal dopamine: An indicator of altered cholinergic-dopaminergic reciprocal inhibitory control in senescence, *Brain Res.* 454:140–148.

Joseph, J.A., Kochman, K., and Roth, G.S., 1989, Reduction of motor behavioural deficits in senescence via chronic prolactin or estrogen administration: Time course and putative mechanisms of action, *Brain Res.* 505:195–202.

Joseph, J.A., Kowatch, M.A., Maki, T., and Roth, G.S., 1990, Selective cross-activation/inhibition of second messenger systems and the reduction of age-related deficits in the muscarinic control of dopamine release from perifused rat striata, *Brain Res.* 537:40–48.

Joyce, J.N., Loeschen, S.K., Sapp, D.W., and Marshall, J.F., 1986, Age-related regional loss of caudate-putamen dopamine receptors revealed by quantitative autoradiography, *Brain Res.* 378:158–163.

Knoll, J., 1988, The striatal dopamine dependency of life span in male rats. Longevity study with (-)deprenyl, *Mech. Ageing Dev.* 46:237–262.
Knoll, J., Dallo, J., and Yen, T.T., 1989, Striatal dopamine, sexual activity and lifespan. Longevity of rats treated with (-)deprenyl, *Life Sci.* 45:525–531.
Kochman, K., Joseph, J.A., Blackman, M.R., Stagg, C.A., and Roth, G.S., 1989, Impaired down-regulation of pituitary dopamine receptors by estradiol in aged rats, *Proc. Soc. Exp. Biol. Med.* 92:23–26.
Koizumi, A., Weindruch, R., and Walford, R.L., 1987, Influences of dietary restriction and age on liver enzyme activities and lipid peroxidation, *J. Nutr.* 117:361–367.
Koizumi, A., Masuda, H., Wada, Y., Tsukada, M., Kawamura, K., Kamiyama, S., and Walford, R.L., 1989, Caloric restriction perturbs the pituitary-ovarian axis and inhibits mouse mammary tumor virus production in a high-spontaneous-mammary-tumor-incidence mouse strain (C3H/SHN), *Mech. Ageing Dev.* 49:93–104.
Koizumi, A., Wada, Y., Tsukada, M., Kamiyama, S., and Weindruch, R., 1990, Effects of energy restriction on mouse mammary tumor virus mRNA levels in mammary glands and uterus and on uterine endometrial hyperplasia and pituitary histology in C3H/SHN F1 mice, *J. Nutr.* 120:1401–1411.
Kolta, M.G., Holson, R., Duffy, P., and Hart, R.W., 1989, Effect of long-term caloric restriction on brain monoamines in aging male and female Fischer 344 rats, *Mech. Ageing Dev.* 48:191–198.
Laganiere, S., and Yu, B.P., 1989, Effect of chronic food restriction in aging rats II. Liver cytosolic antioxidants and related enzymes, *Mech. Ageing Dev.* 48:221–230.
Lai, H., Bowden, D.M., and Horita, A., 1987, Age-related decreases in dopamine receptors in the caudate nucleus and putamen of the Rhesus monkey (*Macaca mulatta*), *Neurobiol. Aging* 8:45–49.
Landfield, P.W., 1988, Commentary on biomarkers of aging in the nervous system, *Exp. Gerontol.* 23:413–416.
Langston, J.W., Ballard, J.W., Tetrud, J.W., and Irwin, I., 1983, Chronic Parkinsonism in humans due to a product of meperidine analog synthesis, *Science* 219:979–980.
Laping, N.J., Dluzen, D.E., and Ramirez, V.D., 1990, Aging alters opiate inhibition of potassium ($K^+$)-stimulated dopamine release from the corpus striatum of male rats, *Neurobiol. Aging* 11:395–399.
Leakey, J.E.A., Cunny, H.C., Bazare, J., Jr., Webb, P.J., Lipscomb, J.C., Slikker, W., Jr., Feuers, R.J., Duffy, P.H., and Hart, R.W., 1989a, Effects of aging and caloric restriction on hepatic drug metabolizing enzymes in the Fischer 344 rat. I: The cytochrome P-450 dependent monooxygenase system, *Mech. Ageing Dev.* 48:145–155.
Leakey, J.E.A., Cunny, H.C., Bazare, J., Jr., Webb, P.J., Lipscomb, J.C., Slikker, W., Jr., Feuers, R.J., Duffy, P.H., and Hart, R.W., 1989b, Effects of aging and caloric restriction on hepatic drug metabolizing enzymes in the Fischer 344 rat. II: Effects on conjugating enzymes, *Mech. Ageing Dev.* 48:157–166.
Leprohon-Greenwood, C.E., and Cinader, B., 1987, Variations in age-related decline in striatal D2-dopamine receptors in a variety of mouse strains, *Mech. Ageing Dev.* 38:199–206.
Levin, P., Janda, J.K., Joseph, J.A., Ingram, D.K., and Roth, G.S., 1981, Dietary restriction retards the age-associated loss of rat striatal dopaminergic receptors, *Science* 214:561–562.
Lieberman, H.R., and Abou-Nader, T.M., 1986, Possible dietary strategies to reduce cognitive deficits in old age, in: *Progress in Brain Research* (D.F. Swaab, E. Fliers, M. Mirmiran, W.A. Van Gool, and F. Van Haaren, eds.), Elsevier Science, Amsterdam, pp. 461–471.
London, E.D., Waller, S.B., Ellis, A.T., and Ingram, D.K., 1985, Effects of intermittent feeding on neurochemical markers in aging rat brain, *Neurobiol. Aging* 6:199–204.
Mann, P.L., 1978, The effect of various dietary restricted regimes on some immunological parameters of mice, *Growth* 42:87–103.
Marshall, J.F., and Rosenstein, A.J., 1990, Age-related decline in rat striatal dopamine metabolism is regionally homogeneous, *Neurobiol. Aging* 11:131–137.
Masoro, E.J., 1988, Food restriction in rodents: An evaluation of its role in the study of aging, *J. Gerontol.* 43:b59–b64.
Masoro, E.J., 1990, Assessment of nutritional components in prolongation of life and health by diet, *Proc. Soc. Exp. Biol. Med.* 93:31–34.
Matthews, J.C., and Scallet, A.C., 1991, Nutrition, neurotoxicants, and age-related neurodegeneration, *Neurotoxicology* 12(3):547–558.
McCay, C.M., Crowell, M.F., and Maynard, L.A., 1935, The effect of retarded growth upon the length of life span and upon the ultimate body size, *J. Nutr.* 10:63–79.
McIntosh, H.H., and Westfall, T.C., 1987, Influence of aging on catecholamine levels, accumulation, and release in F-344 rats, *Neurobiol. Aging* 8:233–239.
McNeill, T.H., Koek, L.L., Brown, S.A., and Rafols, J.A., 1988, Age-related changes in the nigrostriatal system, *Ann. N.Y. Acad. Sci.* 515:239–248.
Meites, J., 1990, Aging: Hypothalamic catecholamines, neuroendocrine-immune interactions, and dietary restriction, *Proc. Soc. Exp. Biol. Med.* 195:304–311.
Meites, J., Goya, R., and Takahashi, S., 1987, Why the neuroendocrine system is important in aging processes, *Exp. Gerontol.* 22:1–15.
Merry, B.J., and Holehan, A.M., 1979, Onset of puberty and duration of fertility in rats fed a restricted diet, *J. Reprod. Fertil.* 57:253–259.
Milgram, N.W., Racine, R.J., Nellis, P., Mendonca, A., and Ivy, G.O., 1990, Maintenance on l-deprenyl prolongs life in aged male rats, *Life Sci.* 47:415–420.

Missale, C., Govoni, S., Pasinetti, G., Assini, C., Spana, P.F., Battaini, F., and Trabucchi, M., 1986, Age-dependent changes in the mechanisms regulating dopamine uptake in the central nervous system, *J. Gerontol.* 41:136–139.

Molloy, A.G., and Waddington, J.L., 1988, Behavioural responses to the selective d1-dopamine receptor agonist R-SK&F 38393 and the selective d2-agonist RU 24213 in young compared with aged rats, *Br. J. Pharmacol.* 95:335–342.

Mooradian, A.D., 1990, Biomarkers of aging: Do we know what to look for? *J. Gerontol.* 45:183–186.

Morelli, M., Mennini, T., Cagnotto, A., Toffano, G., and DiChiara, G., 1990, Quantitative autoradiographical analysis of the age-related modulation of central dopamine D1 and D2 receptors, *Neuroscience* 36:403–410.

Morgan, D.G., and Finch, C.E., 1988, Dopaminergic changes in the basal ganglia. A generalized phenomenon of aging in mammals, *Ann. N.Y. Acad. Sci.* 515:145–160.

O'Boyle, K.M., and Waddington, J.L., 1984, Loss of rat striatal dopamine receptors with ageing is selective for D-2 but not D-1 sites: Association with increased non-specific binding of the D-1 ligand $^3$[H]piflutixol, *Eur. J. Pharmacol.* 105:171–174.

Petkov, V.D., Petkov, V.V., and Stancheva, S.L., 1988, Age-related changes in brain neurotransmission, *Gerontology* 34:14–21.

Pitsikas, N., Carli, M., Fidecka, S., and Algeri, S., 1990, Effect of life-long hypocaloric diet on age-related changes in motor and cognitive behavior in a rat population, *Neurobiol. Aging* 11:417–423.

Randall, P.K., 1980, Functional aging of the nigro-striatal system, *Peptides* 1 (Suppl. 1):177–184.

Ross, M.H., 1961, Length of life and nutrition in the rat, *J. Nutr.* 75:197–210.

Ross, M.H., 1969, Aging, nutrition and hepatic enzyme activity patterns in the rat, *J. Nutr.* 97:565–601.

Roth, G.S., 1988, Age changes in adrenergic and dopaminergic signal transduction mechanisms: Parallels and contrasts, *Neurobiol. Aging* 9:63–64.

Roth, G.S., and Joseph, J.A., 1988, Peculiarities of the effect of hormones and transmitters during aging: Modulation of changes in dopaminergic action, *Gerontology* 34:22–28.

Roth, G.S., Ingram, D.K., and Joseph, J.A., 1984, Delayed loss of striatal dopamine receptors during aging of dietarily restricted rats, *Brain Res.* 300:27–32.

Roth, G.S., Henry, J.M., and Joseph, J.A., 1986, The striatal dopaminergic system as a model for modulation of altered neurotransmitter action during aging: Effects of dietary and neuroendocrine manipulations, in: *Progress in Brain Research, Vol. 70* (D.F. Swaab, E. Fliers, M. Mirmiran, W.A. Van Gool, and F. Van Haaren, eds.), Elsevier Science, Amsterdam, pp. 473–484.

Severson, J.A., and Finch, C.E., 1980, Reduced dopaminergic binding during aging in the rodent striatum, *Brain Res.* 192:147–162.

Severson, J.A., and Randall, P.K., 1985, D-2 dopamine receptors in aging mouse striatum: Determination of high- and low-affinity agonist binding sites, *J. Pharmacol. Exp. Ther.* 233:361–368.

Simpkins, J.W., 1984, Regional changes in monoamine metabolism in the aging constant estrous rat, *Neurobiol. Aging* 5:309–313.

Spangler, E.L., Chachich, M.E., Curtis, N.J., and Ingram, D.K., 1989, Age-related impairment in complex maze learning in rats: Relationship to neophobia and cholinergic antagonism, *Neurobiol. Aging* 10:133–141.

Sprott, R.L., 1988, Age-related variability, *Ann. N.Y. Acad. Sci.* 515:121–123.

Stamford, J.A., 1989, Development and ageing of the rat nigrostriatal dopamine system studied with fast cyclic voltammetry, *J. Neurochem.* 52:1582–1589.

Stewart, J., Meaney, M.J., Aitken, D., Jenson, L., and Kalant, N., 1988, The effects of acute and life-long food restriction on basal and stress-induced serum corticosterone levels in young and aged rats, *Endocrinology* 123:1934–1941.

Stewart, J., Mitchell, J., and Kalant, N., 1989, The effects of life-long food restriction on spatial memory in young and aged Fischer 344 rats measured in the eight-arm radial and the Morris water mazes, *Neurobiol. Aging* 10:669–675.

Stoessl, A.J., Martin-Iverson, M.T., Barth, T.M., Dourish, C.T., and Iversen, S.D., 1989, Effects of aging on the behavioural responses to dopamine agonists: Decreased yawning and locomotion, but increased stereotypy, *Brain Res.* 495:20–30.

Strehler, B.L., 1977, *Time, Cells, and Aging,* 2nd ed., Academic Press, New York.

Strong, R., 1988, Regionally selective manifestations of neostriatal aging, *Ann. N.Y. Acad. Sci.* 515:161–177.

Strong, R., Samorajski, T., and Gottesfeld, Z., 1982, Regional mapping of neostriatal neurotransmitter systems as a function of aging, *J. Neurochem.* 39:831–836.

Tannenbaum, A., 1940, The initiation and growth of tumors: Introduction. I. Effects of underfeeding, *Am. J. Cancer* 38:335–350.

Tannenbaum, A., 1942a, The genesis and growth of tumors. II. Effects of caloric restriction per se, *Cancer Res.* 2:460–475.

Tannenbaum, A., 1942b, The genesis and growth of tumors. III. Effects of a high fat diet, *Cancer Res.* 2:468–475.

Tucker, M.A., 1989, Age-associated change in pain threshold measured by transcutaneous neuronal electrical stimulation, *Age Ageing* 18:241–246.

Venero, J.L., Machado, A., and Cano, J., 1989, Changes in monoamines and their metabolite levels in substantia nigra of aged rats, *Mech. Ageing Dev.* 49:227–233.

Venero, J.L., Machado, A., and Cano, J., 1990, Determination of levels of biogenic amines and their metabolites and both forms of monoamine oxidase in prefrontal cortex of aged rats, *Mech. Ageing Dev.* 56:253–263.

Visscher, M.S., Ball, Z.B., Barnes, R.H., and Siverstonr, I., 1942, The influence of caloric restriction upon the incidence of spontaneous mammary carcinoma in mice, *Surgery* 11:48–55.

Walker, R.F., Weidman, C.A., and Wheeldon, E.B., 1988, Reduced disease in aged rats treated chronically with ibopamine, a catecholaminergic drug, *Neurobiol. Aging* 9:291–301.

Weindruch, R., 1989, Dietary restriction, tumors, and aging in rodents, *J. Gerontol.* 44:67–71.
Weindruch, R., and Walford, R.L., 1988, *The Retardation of Aging and Disease by Dietary Restriction*, Charles C. Thomas, Springfield, IL.
Weindruch, R., Kristie, J.A., Cheney, R., and Walford, R.L., 1979, Influence of controlled dietary restriction on immunologic function and aging, *Fed. Proc.* 38:2007–2016.
Weindruch, R., Walford, R.L., Fligiel, S., and Guthrie, O., 1986, The retardation of aging in mice by dietary restriction: Longevity, cancer, immunity and lifetime energy intake, *J. Nutr.* 116:641–654.

Chapter 3

# Dietary Factors That Influence the Neural Substrates of Memory

*Gary L. Wenk*

## 1. INTRODUCTION

Drugs that alter brain function and influence cognitive function often interact with specific neurotransmitter systems and their receptors. These drugs may function by impairing or enhancing the production, storage, and/or release of specific neurotransmitter molecules that are formed from nutrients in the diet. Under certain circumstances, the dietary nutrients themselves may be viewed as drugs that can significantly influence behavior (Essman, 1987; Kruesi and Rapoport, 1986). An important difference between drugs and nutrients may be the nature of the dose-response curve that defines their effects on cognitive function and behavior. For example, it is important to consider the range over which the dose-response curve is horizontal, i.e., when the effects are constant across a variety of doses. This region of the dose-response curve will be much greater for dietary nutrients than for most drugs. Furthermore, if specific dietary nutrients are manipulated over an entire dose range, as is often done with drugs, virtually all nutrients are likely to produce a change in behavior. Finally, one must consider that the cognitive effects of specific dietary nutrients, such as glucose, proteins, or fats, may be either quite immediate or very delayed following ingestion, and selected nutrients may affect different behaviors in specific individuals differentially (Boal *et al.,* 1988).

This chapter will introduce specific examples of how dietary constituents influence cognitive function, with special emphasis on learning and memory, as determined by timing behavior and performance in mazes that require spatial memory abilities.

---

*Gary L. Wenk* • Division of Neural Systems, Memory and Aging, University of Arizona, Tucson, Arizona 85724.
*The Vulnerable Brain and Environmental Risks, Volume 1: Malnutrition and Hazard Assessment,* edited by Robert L. Isaacson and Karl F. Jensen. Plenum Press, New York, 1992.

## 2. BEHAVIORAL EFFECTS OF SPECIFIC DIETARY NUTRIENTS

### 2.1. Dietary Proteins

The dietary amino acids tryptophan and tyrosine produce the neurotransmitter molecules serotonin and dopamine, norepinephrine, and epinephrine, respectively. Dietary amino acids also serve as precursors to the formation of the neuropeptides, such as the hypothalamic neuroendocrine transmitters and endogenous opiates. The production and release of many of these neurotransmitters are subject to precursor control, e.g., increased dietary levels of tryptophan increases the production and release of serotonin (Moir and Eccleston, 1968; Wurtman et al., 1981; although see Teff et al., 1989). Many of these neurotransmitters have been shown to influence cognitive function, particularly learning and memory.

Elevated levels of the amino acid proline has been shown to significantly impair memory in chicks (Cherkin and Van Harreveld, 1978). The amnestic effects of proline may be related to its ability to antagonize the synaptic actions of endogenous glutamate (Van Harreveld and Fifkova, 1974).

Endogenous opiates derived de novo from dietary amino acids clearly influence brain mechanisms that underlie learning and memory (Kapp and Gallagher, 1979). For example, when endogenous opiates or analogs are administered, performance in learning and memory tasks is impaired (Bostock et al., 1988; Introini et al., 1985; Linden and Martinez, 1986; Zhang et al., 1987). In contrast, opiate receptor antagonists, such as naloxone, improve both acquisition and retention performance in avoidance tasks and in the radial-arm maze (Gallagher, 1982; Gallagher and Kapp, 1978; Messing et al., 1979). When naloxone was given to monkeys that had been previously trained in a delayed nonmatching-to-sample task with trial-unique objects, 80% of the monkeys demonstrated a significant increase in the number of objects that were correctly recognized (Aigner and Mishkin, 1988).

In addition, the neuropeptide neurotransmitter vasopressin can facilitate neural processes associated with learning and memory in normal young (Koob et al., 1986; Kovacs et al., 1979; Le Moal et al., 1981; Meck et al., 1986; Sahgal and Wright, 1983) and aged animals and humans. Vasopressin may function via specific receptors in the brain. When injected directly into the brain it enhanced performance in an inhibitory avoidance task (Koob et al., 1986, and see Wenk, 1989a for a discussion of vasopressin's mechanism of action). Impaired utilization of dietary amino acids by the brain might be expected to alter the production of these polypeptide neurotransmitters.

Some foods contain substances that resemble endogenous neuropeptides, and these may act to influence our mood and general feelings of well-being. For example, peptides with pharmacological activity similar to that of the endogenous opiates and morphine were discovered in pepsin hydrolysates of wheat gluten and casein. These peptides, called exorphins because of their exogenous origin and morphine-like activity, interact with opiate receptors and are resistant to pronase degradation. Similar compounds were also found in enzymatic digests of milk and milk products. If these compounds were to form naturally in the gastrointestinal tract, and in sufficient quantities, they might enter the brain (Hemmings, 1978), alter many opiate-related neurophysiological processes, and thereby alter mood and behavior. For example, the consumption of wheat gluten has been associated with specific mental disorders (Singh and Kay, 1976). Those individuals without an intact blood–brain barrier, such as newborns and a small population of the elderly, would be particularly susceptible to the effects of elevated levels of exogenous psychoactive dietary substances.

## 2.2. Dietary Fats

Dietary fats contribute to the formation of specific neurotransmitters and adrenal steroids, and are an essential component of neural membranes. Adrenal steroids are released during periods of stress and increased sympathetic activity. These steroids easily enter the brain and may influence cognitive function. Adrenalectomy abolishes the positive effects on performance in memory tasks produced by selected cognitive enhancers, such as amphetamine, vasopressin, and the nootropics (Mondadori and Petschke, 1987; for review, see Wenk, 1989a). Pharmacological antagonism of aldosterone receptors was able to block the enhancement related to nootropic therapy (Mondadori et al., 1990). The nootropics are a new class of agents that have been investigated for their ability to enhance the performance of humans and laboratory animals (Nicholson, 1990). The mechanism of their action is unknown (Wenk, 1989a), although they may influence the function of acetylcholinergic and GABAergic neurons. The findings outlined above are consistent with the hypothesis that dietary fats may indirectly influence cognitive function by their role as precursors for peripheral hormonal systems.

Furthermore, when diets are modified to contain higher levels of polyunsaturated fats (up to 20%), e.g., with soybean oil, performance in a spatial learning task in a water maze is improved as compared to a diet with saturated fats (Coscina et al., 1986). The mechanism that underlies this benefit in learning and memory is unknown.

Dietary omega-3 fatty acids are important for brain chemistry. They form the largest lipid component of the cerebral cortex and can only be derived from the diet. Omega-3 fatty acids, in the form of linolenic acid, are found in many land plants as well as in phytoplankton and algae. The precise effects of omega-3 deficiency on brain function are unknown, although there may be a significant impairment in visual acuity and function of the retina (Connor and Neuringer, 1988).

Dietary fats are also involved in the biosynthesis of lecithin and its constituent choline for the production of phosphatidylserine and other constituents of the neural membrane, such as the cerebrosides and gangliosides. Choline, as phosphatidylcholine, is found in a variety of foods, including eggs, liver, soybeans, wheat germ, and peanuts. Most fruits and vegetables contain very low levels of choline.

The dietary administration of choline or choline-containing compounds can increase the synthesis of acetylcholine in the brain, particularly when cholinergic neurons are already active (Cohen and Wurtman, 1976; Jenden et al., 1982; Wecker, 1986). Enhanced cholinergic function has been closely linked to improved learning and memory abilities in humans and laboratory animals (Drachman et al., 1982; for review see Wenk and Olton, 1989). Pretreatment with choline chloride can partially reverse the scopolamine-induced impairment in a verbal learning task (Mohs et al., 1981). This improved behavioral performance may be related to increased formation of acetylcholine. However, increased formation of acetylcholine may not always lead to increased release of acetylcholine or increased activity in the cholinergic system (Eckernas et al., 1977). Therefore, the precise mechanism that underlies the therapeutic benefit of choline therapy is undetermined.

Furthermore, choline therapy has not been effective when there is evidence of cholinergic cell loss, such as associated with aging or Alzheimer's Disease (Wenk and Olton, 1989).

## 2.3. Dietary Carbohydrates

Carbohydrates act as a precursor to the formation of many different neurotransmitter compounds (McIlwain and Bachelard, 1985). Under normal conditions the brain depends on an adequate supply of glucose for energy and as the major source of carbon for the production of a wide variety of neuronal components and many essential neurotransmitters, including the inhibitory neurotransmitters glycine and gamma-aminobutyric acid, and the excitatory amino acid neurotransmitters glutamate and aspartate. Glucose is also used to produce triose phosphates for the ultimate production of membrane lipids and prostaglandins.

Dietary carbohydrates increase the release of insulin and may elevate the levels of tryptophan in the brain, thereby increasing serotonin production. Dietary carbohydrates also increase the level of blood glucose and lead to elevated glucose uptake by the brain. Increased levels of glucose can have dramatic effects on behavior. For example, glucose has been shown to significantly enhance memory in both rodents and humans (Gold, 1986; Gold et al., 1986; for review and hypothesis of its action, see Wenk, 1989a) by its influence on the acetylcholinergic neurotransmitter system. Glucose is a precursor to the formation of acetylcholine, and its availability may influence the synthesis and release of acetylcholine (Messier et al., 1990).

Cholinergic function can be antagonized by injections of scopolamine. Scopolamine treatment impairs learning and memory, and impaired cholinergic function produced by drugs or selective brain lesions is related to deficits in the acquisition and retention of new information. Peripheral glucose injections significantly attenuated the scopolamine-induced amnesia and enhanced the action of the cholinergic agonist physostigmine (Gold and Stone, 1988). These findings are all consistent with the hypothesis that glucose administration enhances memory by its effects on the acetylcholinergic system.

Deficits in the ability of normal aged animals to regulate glucose levels in the blood are associated with deficits in learning and memory (Gold and Stone, 1988). Furthermore, deficits in learning and memory are correlated with impaired glucose utilization by the brain. These findings have important implications for elderly patients with impaired liver or pancreatic function, and suggest a possible relationship between impaired glucose regulation and changes in specific cognitive abilities observed with normal human aging.

Impaired cholinergic function is correlated with memory deficits in aged humans (Drachman et al., 1982). The recent results of experimental studies of glucose supplementation therapy suggest that glucose or carbohydrate dietary supplementation may be a reasonable therapy to enhance the moderately impaired cholinergic function that may accompany normal aging (Hall et al., 1989). Furthermore, abnormal glucose metabolism may be a primary abnormality in early-onset dementia of the Alzheimer's type (Hoyer et al., 1988) and may underlie the initial symptoms of the amnesia observed in these patients (Wenk, 1989b).

In contrast to the effects observed in these animal studies, very large doses of carbohydrates can reduce alertness, increase fatigue and sleepiness, and increase self-reports of depression in human subjects (Lieberman et al., 1986). This change in mood has been related to changes in tryptophan metabolism and serotonergic function. However, glucose may also suppress the firing rate of dopaminergic cells in the midbrain (Saller and Chiodo, 1980) and thereby alter mood in a manner similar to the classical antipsychotics.

The association between nutritional status and cognitive abilities extends beyond the importance of carbohydrates to include many other dietary nutrients as well (Essman, 1987; Goodwin et al., 1983), including specific vitamins and minerals, which may in turn influence glucose utilization.

In summary, increased carbohydrate consumption (as glucose) can modulate the function of at least four separate neurotransmitter systems and thereby significantly influence behavior: (1) The production and release of serotonin is increased because tryptophan uptake into the brain is increased by glucose; (2) the production and release of dopamine and norepinephrine are decreased because tyrosine uptake into the brain is decreased by glucose (see discussion below or behavioral timing studies); and (3) The formation of acetylcholine is increased because glucose can act as a precursor to the production of acetyl coenzyme-A.

Taken together, the data from these studies are consistent with the hypothesis that peripheral glucose regulation, and its ultimate utilization by the brain, plays a critical role in cognitive function; furthermore, enhancement of glucose regulation or utilization might enhance the neural processes that underlie cognitive function. Alternatively, there is some evidence that increased blood glucose levels might also influence the brain via the liver (Sawchenko and Friedman, 1979).

## 2.4. Caffeine and Benzodiazepines in Food

Caffeine is found naturally in many foods sources, e.g., tea, coffee, and cocoa. When given to normal individuals caffeine enhanced both their mood and cognitive abilities. A single dose of caffeine given to healthy adult subjects improved self-reports of general well-being and enhanced performance in two tasks, auditory vigilance and visual reaction time (Lieberman et al., 1987). Caffeine also improved the performance of young healthy subjects on a battery of psychomotor tests (Swift and Tiplady, 1988). These subjects also reported an improved feeling of well-being and that they were more alert, calmer, and more interested in the experiment.

Detectable levels (up to 0.5 ng per gram of tissue) of the antianxiety agents diazepam and desmethyldiazepam (and a few other benzodiazepine analogs that are not currently used for the treatment of anxiety) have been discovered in wheat grain, potato tuber, brown lentils, yellow soybeans, rice, maize corn, cherries, egg whites, and mushrooms (Klotz, 1991). Diazepam and the other benzodiazepine drugs can produce amnesia and impair cognitive function in both laboratory animals and humans (Gilbert et al., 1989; Lister et al., 1985). Germination significantly increased the levels of the various benzodiazepine analogs in wheat grains and potato tubers. The brains of many different species that consume these foods have been investigated for the presence of "endogenous" levels of similar benzodiazepines. These studies have found significant whole-brain levels that ranged from 600 ng/g (wet weight) for bovines to 3 ng/g for rats and from 0.17 to 0.34 ng/g for humans. It is unknown whether pharmacological levels of these benzodiazepines could be achieved by "natural" dietary sources. For example, it would require the ingestion of approximately 11 tons of potatoes to attain the whole-brain level of benzodiazepines that is typically achieved following a standard pharmacological treatment regimen in humans. However, under certain circumstances the brain might be able to selectively concentrate these compounds in specific brain regions. The "natural" presence of these compounds in the diet may provide a counterbalance to endogenous anxiety-inducing compounds found in the brain, including diazepam-binding inhibitor protein and the beta-carbolines (Klotz, 1991). It is possible that humans and other animals may actually regulate their own level of anxiety by the choice of specific foods.

## 3. EFFECTS OF SPECIFIC NUTRIENTS ON TIMING BEHAVIOR

### 3.1. The Timing Behavior Task

The importance of the ability to accurately estimate the passage of time cannot be overemphasized. Time estimates are critical for organizing any complex sequence of movements through the environment, for determining the recency of a visit to a known food source, for estimating the speed of movement of a predator or prey, and for numerous other behaviors that are critical to an animal's survival. Laboratory animals and humans are capable of accurately estimating the passage of time, and this ability can be altered by similar manipulations, such as dietary nutrients and drugs, e.g., hallucinogens and alcohol.

Operant procedures can examine the cognitive mechanisms involved in the timing of events of a relative short duration. Rats are first trained on a standard fixed interval (FI) schedule of reinforcement in which food is delivered for the first bar press after a certain interval of time from the beginning of an auditory or visual stimulus. Peak trials test the remembered time of reinforcement. Each peak trial begins with the standard FI signal. However, no food is provided for a bar press, and the signal continues for approximately twice as long as in the usual FI trial. Control rats have a symmetrical peak of responding, with the maximal rate occurring at the time when reinforcement is ordinarily available in the FI schedule. The *peak time* is defined as the time of the maximum rate of response.

### 3.2. The Role of Acetylcholine

Pharmacological manipulation of the acetylcholinergic neural system shifted the peak time (Meck and Church, 1987a). Enhancement of cholinergic function (e.g., physostigmine) produced a leftward shift in peak time, while antagonism of cholinergic function (e.g., atropine) produced a rightward shift in peak time. Similar to cholinergic antagonism, the destruction of the basal forebrain cholinergic system, including the nucleus basalis magnocellularis of rats, produced a rightward shift in the peak time (Meck *et al.*, 1987).

Dietary nutrients, such as lecithin, carbohydrates, and proteins, can also modify timing behavior (Meck and Church, 1987b). Lecithin increased plasma and brain choline levels, increased acetylcholine synthesis, and shifted the peak time leftward. This shift remained leftward with additional testing, and remained shifted for two testing sessions after the lecithin consumption was discontinued. Lecithin shifted the peak time in the same direction as treatment with pharmacological agents that enhance cholinergic function (e.g., physostigmine).

Carbohydrates shifted the peak time rightward, in the same direction as treatment with pharmacological agents that inhibit cholinergic function (e.g., scopolamine), but it returned to normal with additional consumption and testing. The peak time rebounded leftward when the carbohydrate supplementation was discontinued. This rightward shift suggests that increasing carbohydrate intake may decrease cholinergic function and impair temporal memory.

Protein, e.g., from the casein in milk, increased the uptake of tyrosine into the brain, increased the synthesis of the catecholamine neurotransmitters, reduced the uptake of tryptophan into the brain, and may have reduced the synthesis of serotonin. Increased dietary proteins shifted the peak time leftward, but it returned to normal with additional testing. When protein consumption was discontinued, the peak time rebounded rightward (Meck and Church, 1987).

The pattern of results obtained in these studies following protein consumption was the same as that following carbohydrate consumption, although the direction was opposite. This opposite pattern may be related to the enhanced production of competing neurotransmitter systems. For example, carbohydrate consumption enhanced serotonin production and release, while protein consumption enhanced catecholamine production and release. These two neurotransmitter systems appear to have different and competing influences on timing behavior. These changes in timing behavior produced by consumption of specific nutrients can be interpreted in terms of selective precursor effects on the synthesis of specific neurotransmitters substances.

Together, these studies are consistent with the hypothesis that the cholinergic system plays a vital role in the control of timing behavior in rats. Glucose may also have effects on this behavior that are independent of its effects on tryptophan uptake into the brain. These possible actions have already been discussed.

## 4. SUMMARY

Dietary nutrients are essential to supply the energy and to provide the precursors of materials that our brain requires for normal function. Some nutrients can be considered as drugs that can be given for their effects on specific neurotransmitter systems in the brain. Some can act as precursors or cofactors for the production of specific neurotransmitters and neuromodulators within the brain. A variety of cognitive processes can be influenced by dietary supplementation of specific amino acids that are precursors to the noradrenergic, dopaminergic, and serotonergic neurotransmitter systems. Glucose can significantly influence the brain uptake of many of these amino-acid precursors and can itself act as a precursor for the production of acetylcholine, a neurotransmitter that plays an important role in learning and memory. Glucose is also the primary source for energy metabolism within the brain. Therefore, the regulation of glucose by the body and the uptake and utilization of glucose by the brain can significantly influence brain function in many ways. Impaired glucose regulation, such as that associated with normal or abnormal aging, may lead to dysfunction of cholinergic and many noncholinergic neural systems within the brain. This impaired function can be expressed in many ways, e.g., a shift in timing behavior or a deficit in learning and memory. Someday, a drug or specific dietary nutrient that enhances the ability of the brain to utilize glucose may be used to reverse many age-related cognitive impairments and/or enhance learning and memory.

ACKNOWLEDGMENTS. The preparation of this chapter was supported in part by a grant from the National Science Foundation (BNS 89-14941). I thank Drs. David Olton, Paul Gold, and William Stone for helpful discussions related to the preparation of this chapter, and Jane Stieritz Wenk for typing the original manuscript.

# REFERENCES

Aigner, T.G., and Mishkin, M., 1988, Improved recognition memory in monkeys following naloxone administration, *Psychopharmacology* 94:21–23.

Aigner, T.G., Mitchell, S.J., Aggleton, J.P., De long, M.R., Struble, R.G., Price, D.L., Wenk, G.L., and Mishkin, M., 1987, Effects of scopolamine and physostigmine on recognition memory in monkeys with ibotenic-acid lesions of the nucleus basalis of Meynert, *Psychopharmacology* 92:292–300.

Boal, A.S., Young, S.N., Sutherland, M., Ervin, F.R., and Coppinger, R., 1988, The effect of breakfast on social behavior and brain amine metabolism in vervet monkeys, *Pharmacol. Biochem. Behav.* 29:115–123.

Cherkin, A., and Van Harreveld, A., 1978, L-proline and related compounds. Correlation of structure, amnesic potency and anti-spreading depression potency, *Brain Res.* 156:265–273.

Connor, W.E., and Neuringer, M., 1988, Importance of dietary omega-3 fatty acids in retinal function and brain chemistry, in: *Nutritional Modulation of Neural Function* (J.E. Morley, M.B. Sterman, and J.H. Walsh, eds.), Academic Press, New York, pp. 191–201.

De Weid, D., and Gispen, W.H., 1977, Behavioral effects of peptides, in: *Peptides in Neurobiology* (H. Ganier, ed.), Plenum Press, New York, pp. 397–448.

Drachman, D.A., Glosser, G., Fleming, P., and Longenecker, G., 1982, Memory decline in the aged: Treatment with lecithin and physostigmine, *Neurology* 32:944–590.

Essman, W.B., 1987, *Nutrients and Brain Function*, S. Karger, New York.

Gallagher, M., 1982, Naloxone enhancement of memory processes: Effects of other opiate antagonists, *Behav. Neural Biol.* 35:375–382.

Gallagher, M., and Kapp, B.A., 1978, Manipulation of opiate activity in the amygdala alters memory processes, *Life Sci.* 23:1974–1978.

Gallagher, M., King, R.A., and Young, N.B., 1983, Opiate antagonists improve spatial memory, *Science* 221:975–976.

Gibson, G.E., and Blass, J.P., 1976, Impaired synthesis of acetylcholine in brain accompanying mild hypoxia and hypoglycemia, *J. Neurochem.* 27:37–42.

Gilbert, D.B., Patterson, T.A., and Rose, S.P.R., 1989, Midazolam induces amnesia in a simple, one-trial, maze-learning task in young chicks, *Pharmacol. Biochem. Behav.* 34:439–442.

Gold, P.E., 1986, Glucose modulation of memory storage processing, *Behav. Neural Biol.* 45:342–349.

Gold, P.E., and Stone, W.S., 1988, Neuroendocrine effects on memory in aged rodents and humans, *Neurobiol. Aging* 9:709–717.

Gold, P.E., Vogt, J., and Hall, J.L., 1986, Posttraining glucose effects on memory: Behavioral and pharmacological characteristics, *Behav. Neural Biol.* 46:145–155.

Goodwin, J.S., Goodwin, J.M., and Garry, P.J., 1983, Association between nutritional status and cognitive functioning in a healthy elderly population. *JAMA*. 249:2917–2921.

Hall, J.L., Gonder-Frederick, L.A., Chewning, W.W., Silveira, J., and Gold, P.E., 1989, Glucose enhancement of performance on memory tests in young and aged humans, *Neuropsychologia* 9:1129–1138.

Hemmings, W.A., 1978, The entry into the brain of large molecules derived from dietary protein, *Proc. R. Soc. Lond.* 200:175–192.

Hoyer, S., Oesterreich, K., and Wager, O., 1988, Glucose metabolism as the site of the primary abnormality in early onset dementia of Alzheimer's type? *J. Neurol.* 235:143–148.

Introini-Collison, I.B., and McGaugh, J.L., 1988, Modulation of memory by post-training epinephrine: Involvement of cholinergic mechanisms, *Psychopharmacology* 94:379–385.

Introini-Collison, I.B., and McGaugh, J.L., and Baratti, C.M., 1985, Pharmacological evidence of a central effect of naltrexone, morphine, and beta-endorphin and a peripheral effect of Met- and Leu-enkephalin on retention of an inhibitory response in mice, *Behav. Neural Biol.* 44:434–446.

Jenden, D.J., Weiler, M.H., and Gundersen, C.B., 1982, Choline availability and acetylcholine synthesis, in: *Alzheimer's Disease: A Report of Progress*, Aging, Vol. 19 (S. Corkin, K.L. Davis, J.H. Growdon, E. Usdin, and R.J. Wurtman, eds.), Raven Press, New York, pp. 315–326.

Klotz, U., 1991, Occurrence of "natural" benzodiazepines, *Life Sci.* 48:209–215.

Koob, G.F., Dantzer, R., Bluthe, R-M., Le Brun, C., Bloom, F.E., and Le Moal, M., 1986, Central injections of arginine vasopressin prolong extinction of active avoidance, *Peptides* 7:213–218.

Kovacs, G.L., Bohus, B., and Versteeg, D.H.G., 1979, Facilitation of memory consolidation by vasopressin: Mediation by terminals of the dorsal noradrenergic bundle? *Brain Res.* 172:73–85.

Kruesi, M.J.P., and Rapoport, J.L., 1986, Diet and human behavior: How much do they affect each other? *Ann. Rev. Nutr.* 6:113–130.

Le Moal, M., Koog, G.F., Koda, L.Y., Bloom, F.E., Manning, M., Sawyer, W.H., and Rivier, J., 1981, Vasopressor receptor antagonist prevents behavioral effects of vasopressin, *Nature* 291:491–493.

Lieberman, H.R., Wurtman, J.J., and Chew, B., 1986, Changes in mood after carbohydrate consumption amoung obese individuals, *Am. J. Clin. Nutr.* 44:772–778.

Lister, R.G., 1985, The amnesic action of benzodiazepines in man, *Neurosci. Biobehav. Rev.* 9:87–94.

McIlwain, H., and Bachelard, H.S., 1985, *Biochemistry and the Central Nervous System*, Churchill, London.

Meck, W.H., and Church, R.M., 1987a, Cholinergic modulation of the content of temporal memory, *Behav. Neurosci.* 101:457–464.

Meck, W.H., and Church, R.M., 1987b, Nutrients that modify the speed of internal clock and memory storage processes, *Behav. Neurosci.* 101:465–475.

Meck, W.H., Church, R.M., and Wenk, G.L., 1986, Arginine vasopressin inoculates against age-related increases in sodium-dependent high affinity choline uptake and discrepancies in the content of temporal memory, *Eur. J. Pharmacol.* 130:327–331.

Meck, W.H., Church, R.M., Wenk, G.L., and Olton, D.S., 1987, Nucleus basalis magnocellularis and medial septal area lesions differentially impair temporal memory, *J. Neurosci.* 7:3505–3511.

Messier, C., Durkin, T., Mrabet, O., and Destrade, C., 1990, Memory-improving action of glucose: Indirect evidence for a facilitation of hippocampal acetylcholine synthesis, *Behav. Brain Res.* 39:135–143.

Messing, R.B., Jensen, R.A., Martinez, J.L., Jr., Speihler, V.R., Vasquez, B.J., Soumireu-Mourat, B., Liang, K.C., and McGaugh, J.L., 1979, Naloxone enhancement of memory, *Behav. Neural Biol.* 27:266–275.

Moir, A.T.B., and Eccleston, D., 1968, The effects of precursor loading in the cerebral metabolism of 5-hydroxyindoles, *J. Neurochem.* 15:1093–1108.

Mondadori, C., and Petschke, F., 1987, Do piracetam-like compounds act centrally via peripheral mechanisms? *Brain Res.* 435:310–314.

Mondadori, C., Bhatnagar, A., Borkowski, J., and Hausler, A., 1990, Involvement of a steroidal component in the mechanism of action of piracetam-like nootropics, *Brain Res.* 506:101–108.

Nicholson, C.D., 1990, Pharmacology of nootropics and metabolically active compounds in relation to their use in dementia, *Psychopharmacology* 101:147–159.

Sahgal, A., and Wright, C., 1983, A comparison of the effects of vasopressin and oxytocin with amphetamine and chlordiazepoxide on passive avoidance behavior in rats, *Psychopharmacology* 80:88–92.

Saller, C.F., and Chiodo, L.A., 1980, Glucose suppresses basal firing and haloperidol-induced increases in the firing rate of central dopaminergic neurons, *Science* 210:1269–1271.

Sawchenko, P.E., and Friedman, M.I., 1979, Sensory functions of the liver—a review, *Am. J. Physiol.* 236:R5–R20.

Singh, M.M., and Kay, S.R., 1976, Wheat gluten as a pathogenic factor in schizophrenia, *Science* 191:401–404.

Swift, C.G., and Tiplady, B., 1988, The effects of age on the response to caffeine, *Psychopharmacology* 94:29–31.

Teff, K.L., Young, S.N., Marchand, L., and Botez, M.I., 1989, Acute effect of protein and carbohydrate breakfasts on human cerebrospinal fluid monoamine precursor and metabolite levels, *J. Neurochem.* 52:235–241.

Van Harreveld, A., and Fifkova, E., 1974, Involvement of glutamate in memory formation, *Brain Res.* 81:455–467.

Wecker, L., 1989, Neurochemical effects of choline supplementation, *Can. J. Physiol. Pharmacol.* 64:329–333.

Wenk, G.L., 1989a, An hypothesis on the role of glucose in the mechanisms of action of cognitive enhancers, *Psychopharmacology* 99:431–438.

Wenk, G.L., 1989b, Nutrition, cognition and memory, in: *Topics in Geriatric Rehabilitation: Nutrition and Rehabilitation*, Vol. 5, No. 1 (R.B. Weg, ed.), Aspen Publishers, Frederick, MD, pp. 79–87.

Wenk, G.L., and Olton, D.S., 1989, Cognitive enhancers: Potential strategies and experimental results, *Prog. Neuropsychopharmacol. Biol. Psychiatry* 13:S117–139.

Wurtman, R.J., Hefti, F., and Melamed, E., Precursor control of neurotransmitter synthesis. *Pharmacol. Rev.* 32:315–335.

Zhang, S., McGaugh, J.L., Juler, R.G., and Introini-Collision, I.B., 1987, Naloxone and [Met$^5$]enkephaline effects on retention: Attenuation by adrenal denervation, *Eur. J. Pharmacol.* 138:37–44.

Chapter 4

# Neurotoxins in Herbs and Food Plants

*Ryan J. Huxtable*

## 1. INTRODUCTION

The modern flora has evolved in the face of continual assault from mammals, which are ultimately dependent on the plant kingdom. In addition to the physical defenses of spine, barb, thorn, and other devices, plants have developed complex systems of chemical defenses, varying enormously from genus to genus and family to family. The chemicals used, however, are classifiable under a relatively small number of structural headings, such as acetogenins, sugars, and modified amino acids. Most common plant secondary metabolites, including alkaloids, glycosides, steroids, and terpenes, can be subsumed under these headings. These substances deter because of their taste or because of their noxious or fatal effects on animals consuming them.

Plant predators, in turn, have evolved systems of defenses against plant chemicals. However, plants and those using them coexist in an uneasy balance of chemical power. In evolution, absolute tactical success is absolute strategic failure. If herbivores became too efficient in combating the chemical defenses of plants, numerous species in both kingdoms would become extinct. Conversely, if plants suppressed predation, the extinction of the animal kingdom would be rapidly followed by the impoverishment of the plant kingdom, as successful species colonized space and other resources.

Man protects himself from plant toxicity by relying on a relatively small number of highly selected cultivars for the bulk of his nutritional needs. Cultivars are plant varieties not occurring naturally, but derived culturally by selective breeding. These include corn (*Zea* spp.), wheat (*Triticum* spp.), rice (*Oryza sativa*), barley (*Hordeum* spp.), potatoes (*Solanum* spp.), and beans (*Phaseolus* spp.). Even so, many cultivars are

---

*Ryan J. Huxtable* • Department of Pharmacology, College of Medicine, University of Arizona, Tucson, Arizona 85724.
*The Vulnerable Brain and Environmental Risks, Volume 1: Malnutrition and Hazard Assessment,* edited by Robert L. Isaacson and Karl F. Jensen. Plenum Press, New York, 1992.

or can be highly toxic, and have to be stored or prepared with certain precautions. Thus, cassava (*Manihot esculenta*), used by millions of people in the tropical and subtropical worlds, must undergo a lengthy preparation to remove the cyanogenic glycoside, linamarin. Beans have to be aggressively boiled to inactivate their phytohemagglutinins (lectins) (Liener, 1983), and potatoes and tomatoes have to be harvested and stored appropriately to keep the levels of steroidal alkaloids in the safe range (Dalvi and Bowie, 1983; Jadhav *et al.*, 1981; Sharma and Salunkhe, 1989). Lectins, in fact, are present in numerous food plants, including fruits, spices, nuts, and cereals. Rye, although no longer extensively used, was for centuries a mainstay for the underclasses of Europe. A parasitic infestation of rye was responsible for the massive outbreaks of St. Anthony's fire, or ergotism, which alternated with the plague in punctuating the population growth of the continent.

Paradoxically, other plants are consumed in vast amounts because of their effects on the central nervous system. Such plants include coffee (*Coffea* spp.), tea (*Camellia sinensis*), marijuana (*Cannabis* spp.), maté (*Ilex paraguayensis*), and cocoa (*Theobroma cacao*). Such human use has spread vast plantations of these plants in areas remote from their native ranges and has ensured that, whatever else of Nature's botanical cornucopia may vanish forever in man's heedless pillage of natural resources, these species will survive for as long as the farmer. Thus, in a roundabout way, the defensive chemicals evolved by these plants are successful in ensuring the survival of their biosynthesizers.

The history of plants is the history of medicine. Plant products affecting the nervous system are legion, and little more than a brief overview can be attempted here to discuss the types of compounds involved and to refer the reader to more specialized literature. In the main, discussion has been limited to ethnobotanically significant compounds; that is to say, neurotoxins from plants used as foods or plants used ethnopharmacologically. Even here, constraints of space necessitate picking through the topics like a jaded party-goer faced with another bowl of nuts.

## 2. MAMMALIAN DEFENSES AGAINST PLANT TOXINS

Xenobiotics are non-nutritive chemicals found but not formed in the body. They are frequently toxic. The first line of defense against ingested xenobiotics is to prevent or reduce absorption. The high acidity of the stomach, transport-limited processes of absorption, and breakdown by gut microflora all serve in their limited ways to filter out dietary toxins.

Following absorption of a potentially toxic xenobiotic, mammals typically rely on an integrated triad of processes for defense: oxidation, conjugation, and excretion. Hepatic oxidation occurs via enzymes such as the cytochrome $P_{450}$ mixed-function oxidases. These are inducible enzymes, their activity rising on chronic or subacute exposure to a substrate. Oxidation increases water solubility of the substrate. Solubility is increased further by conjugation with such endogenous substances as glutathione, sulfate, or glucuronate. The oxidized and conjugated xenobiotic is released into the bloodstream, to be excreted via the kidneys into the urine. Usually, on oxidation both the degree of binding to plasma proteins and the biological half-life of the xenobiotic are sharply decreased. Thus, caffeine is almost totally metabolized in adults (Cornish and Christman, 1957) but almost unmetabolized in premature babies. As a result, while the half-life of caffeine is

4.9 ± 1.8 hr in adults, in premature babies it is 102.9 ± 17.9 hr (Aldridge et al., 1979; Dews, 1984).

Most at risk for the expression of toxicity are the gastrointestinal tract and the liver, because these organs are exposed to the highest concentrations of xenobiotics. In consequence, these organs have developed specialized protective mechanisms. Both organs have high regenerative capacity, and the liver has mechanisms for enzymatic detoxification. Next at risk is the kidney, which tends to accumulate metabolized and unmetabolized xenobiotics for urinary excretion. In certain cases, hepatic conjugates can be further metabolized and bioactivated in the kidney, producing toxicity (Dekant et al. 1989; Koob and Dekant, 1991). The lung is another organ at risk, as substances released from the liver come into intimate contact in a relatively concentrated form with the capillary bed of the lung. Thus, in laboratory rodents, hepatic metabolites of the pyrrolizidine alkaloid, monocrotaline, produce pulmonary arterial hypertension (Huxtable, 1990a).

Despite its lack of regenerative capacity, in the main the central nervous system is well protected from xenobiotics. The increase in water solubility following hepatic oxidation militates against entry into the brain. For lipid-soluble substances, other compartments in the body compete with the brain. Substances with affinity for protein bind to plasma albumin. Additionally, the blood–brain barrier provides a further defense against the entry of xenobiotics. In all, a primary neurotoxic action is uncommon for plant xenobiotics, although substances can cause hepatic encephalopathy due to a derangement of nitrogen metabolism in the liver.

The Maginot line of the gastrointestinal tract can be bypassed, invalidating the hepatic defenses behind it. Certain substances, such as coniine, cocaine, nicotine, or tropane alkaloids such as scopolamine or atropine, are absorbed across mucous membranes, such as the vagina, nose, or mouth, while numerous others are absorbable by the lungs when inhaled as dust or smoke. This is often the preferred method of administration for centrally active substances, such as cocaine or nicotine, precisely because they avoid the first pass through the liver, ensuring that greater amounts rapidly reach the brain. Hamlet's father was fraternally murdered by means of a plant extract being poured into his ear as he slept. The plant has been tentatively identified as *Conium maculatum,* a source of coniine (Max, 1988a).

Despite their relative scarcity, plants with actions on the central nervous system have been avidly sought by many cultures. Such plants include those elaborating caffeine and the related methylxanthines; morphine; reserpine; the ungrammatically named psychedelics and hallucinogens, such as mescaline, tetrahydrocannabinol, lysergic acid, and psilocybin; and the terpenes present in absinthe and spices.

## 3. PLANT NEUROTOXINS

Neurotoxic plant chemicals can be classified in a number of ways. These include their pharmacological action (e.g., excitant, depressant, psychotomimetic, narcotic), their mechanism of action, the receptor systems they act on (e.g., muscarinergic, nicotinergic, dopaminergic, serotonergic, glutaminergic), or their botanical source. In this chapter, plant neurotoxins will be grouped according to their chemical structures. Three main groups of compounds will be considered—alkaloids, amino acids, and monoterpenoids—along with a fourth, miscellaneous group.

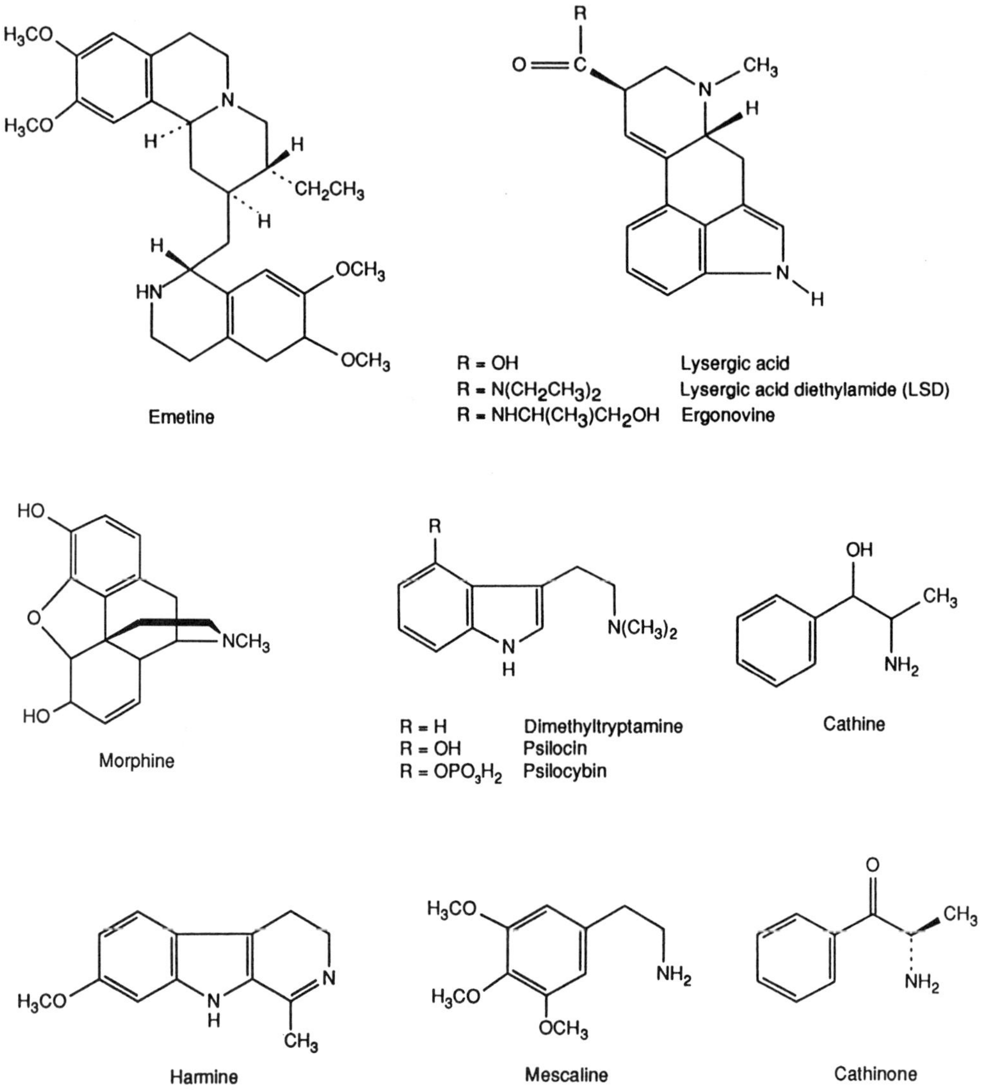

**FIGURE 1.** Neurotoxic alkaloids: Nonterpenoid alkaloids derived from aromatic amino acids.

Plant alkaloids are related, biogenetically and structurally, to mammalian neurotransmitters. With a few exceptions, they are basic derivatives of amino acids, typically formed by decarboxylation, which may be combined with other metabolic fragments. Thus, simple decarboxylation plus minor modifications yields mescaline (Fig. 1) from tyrosine, psilocybin and psilocin (Fig. 1) from tryptophan, and histamine from histidine. Combination of decarboxylated and deaminated aromatic amino acid fragments yields morphine (Figs. 1 and 5) or benzylisoquinoline alkaloids, such as papaverine. Other metabolic fragments include an acetate-derived mevalonate in the case of ergot alkaloids, such as ergonovine (Fig. 1), or a mevalonate-derived monoterpenoid $C_9$ or $C_{10}$ fragment in the case of the complex indole alkaloids, such as reserpine or strychnine (Fig. 2). Exceptions

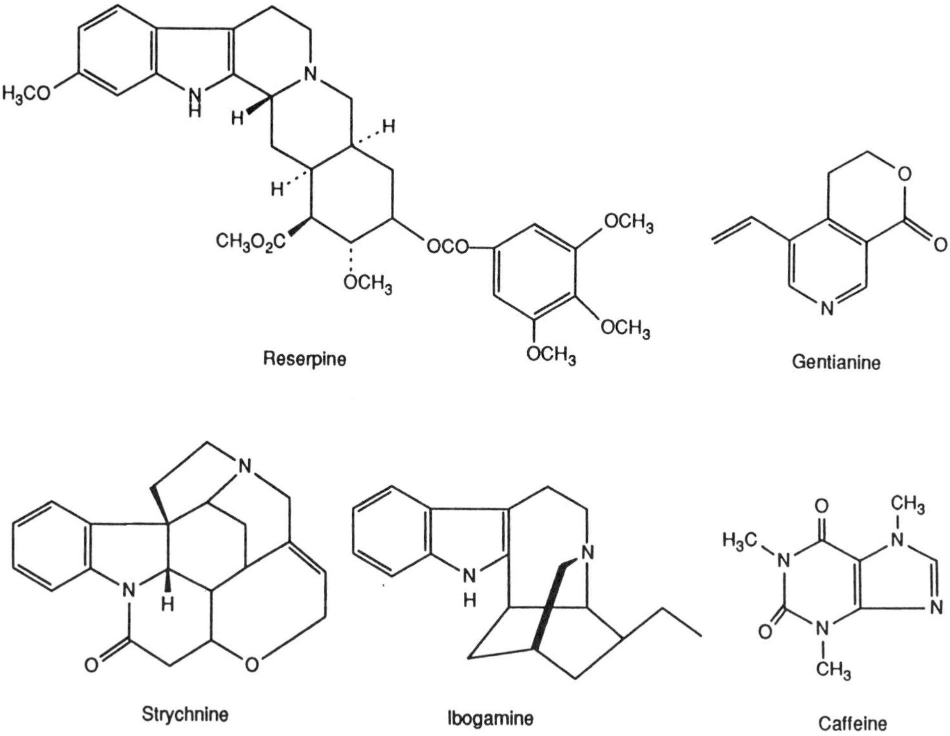

**FIGURE 2.** Neurotoxic monoterpenoid and purine alkaloids.

to this definition of an alkaloid include colchicine, which, although derived from tyrosine and phenylalanine, is a nonbasic N-acetyl compound, and the xanthines, caffeine (Fig. 2), theobromine, and theophylline, which are methylated derivatives of purine.

Almost without exception, alkaloids have pharmacological actions, largely due to the ability of the amine function to interact by charge transfer, proton transfer, hydrogen bonding, or ion bonding with numerous sites in the body. Actions on the central nervous system depend on the liposolubility of the alkaloid. This, in turn, is a function of the basicity. The greater the basicity of the alkaloid, the greater the proportion that is ionized at physiological pH and the lower the partition coefficient into lipid compartments such as the brain. Liposolubility also depends on the ratio of hydrophilic to hydrophobic groups on the molecule. Thus, phenolic groupings are more hydrophilic than the corresponding methyl ethers, while large aryl and alkyl substituents increase liposolubility.

Apart from their marked pharmacological effects, alkaloids tend to be bitter tasting. Foods containing them tend to be aversive. Exceptions include the monoamines, such as tyramine and serotonin, present in many foods, such as bananas, cheese, beer, chocolate, and fish, and contributing to the characteristic taste of these substances. Alkaloid-containing materials are, however, frequently taken as herbs or for their psychoactive effects.

Amino acids tend to be much more hydrophilic than alkaloids, partly because of their dipolar nature, and partly because of their lower molecular weights. In general, they contribute little to the taste or smell of the foods containing them. However, some, such as glycine and arginine, have distinctive tastes, while acidic amino acids tend to be flavor enhancers, accentuating the taste of foods in which they are present. Although plants contain many unusual amino acids that are non-nutritive to mammals, in the main these substances have little neurotoxicity. This is partly because concentrations are low in plants and partly because entry into the brain is limited by poor liposolubility. Important exceptions include the neuroexcitatory plant amino acids. These occur in certain plants, such as *Lathyrus, Sativa,* or *Cycas,* which are or were widely consumed, are neurotoxic in low concentrations, and enter the brain either in the circumventricular regions where blood vessels contain a fenestrated endothelium (i.e., the blood–brain barrier is not patent), or possibly by utilizing active transport systems for physiologically important amino acids.

The third group of neurotoxins to be considered is the monoterpenes. Terpenes derive from acetate via the intermediacy of mevalonate and isopentenyl pyrophosphate. Compounds such as tetrahydrocannabinol, one of the principal active components of marijuana, can be considered to be a modified monoterpene plus an olivetol fragment. Monoterpenes are responsible for the fragrance and taste of many pungent plants, such as the mints (*Mentha* spp.). They are highly liposoluble. If the liver fails to oxidize them sufficiently, they pass readily into the brain. They tend to be pharmacologically active, as the potency of their odors might indicate, and their smell derives from high-affinity activation of a chemoreceptor. Indeed, a qualitative relationship between olfaction or taste and central nervous system action is suggested by the culinary use of plants containing capsaicin (*Capsicum* spp.), the myrosinolates in the mustards (Cruciferae) and capers (Capparidaceae) (Kjaer, 1976, 1978), and sulfur compounds, such as those adding piquancy to materials ranging from coffee to mushrooms (Huxtable, 1986).

Overall, the importance of plant neurotoxins in the development of neuropharmacology cannot be overstated. The kainate and quisqualate subtypes of excitatory amino acid receptors and the muscarinic and nicotinic cholinergic receptors are all named for the plant chemicals that led to their discovery. Quisqualate is found in the seeds of the Chinese plant, *Quisqualis chinesis* (or *Q. indica*), while kainate comes from the red alga, *Digenia simplex* (Takemoto, 1978).

### 3.1. Neurotoxic Alkaloids

The major neurotoxic alkaloids encountered in foodstuffs and herbs are listed in Table 1. There has been a marked and continuing increase in the number of alkaloid-containing plants sold as teas, herbs, herbal remedies, food additives, and food supplements in North America. Of the 200 species Siegel (1976) reported as being sold as smoking mixtures and the 400 species being sold as teas or food supplements, many are alkaloidal. The species included *Corynanthe yohimbe* (yohimbine), *Cola* spp. (methylxanthines), *Lobelia inflata* (lobeline), *Argemone mexicana* (berberine), *Nicotiana* spp. (nicotine), *Ilex paraguayensis* (caffeine), *Ephedra* spp. (pseudoephedrine or ephedrine, depending on whether the plant derives from the New World or Old), *Passiflora incarnata* (harmine alkaloids), *Catharanthus roseus* (indoles), *Rauwolfia serpentina* (reserpine), and *Datura* spp. (tropane alkaloids). At least in the United States, these substances are largely unregulated. Not being sold as food or drugs, but as food additives, food supplements, or herbal remedies, they escape regulation by the Food and Drug Administration.

The class of plant compounds generating the most intense lay and professional interest is that known variously as hypnotics, psychotomimetics, psychedelics, psycho-

TABLE 1. Human Nonmedicinal Use of or Exposure to Neurotoxic Alkaloids

| Type | Alkaloid | Source[a] | Exposure | Geographic distribution | Neurotoxicity |
|---|---|---|---|---|---|
| I | Caffeine[b] | *Coffea* spp. | Beverages | Worldwide | Stimulant |
| | | *Cola nitida* | Condiment | West Indies, Brazil, Java, West Africa | |
| | | *Paulinia cupana* | Beverage | Brazil, Uruguay, Paraguay | |
| | | *Ilex paraguayensis* | Beverage | South America | |
| | | *Camellia sinesis* | Beverage | Worldwide | |
| | Theobromine | *Theobroma cacao* | Beverage, chocolate | Worldwide | Stimulant |
| II | Mescaline[c] | *Lophophora* spp. | Intoxicant | Mesoamerica (aboriginal) | Hallucinogen |
| | | *Trichocereus* spp. | | Developed world | |
| | Morphine[c] | *Papaver somniferum* | Intoxicant | Worldwide | Narcotic |
| | Cathine[c] | *Catha edulis* | Intoxicant | Arabia, East Africa, Europe | Stimulant |
| | Emetine[c] | *Cephaelis ipecacuanha* | Herb | South America (aboriginal) | Emetic |
| III | Ergonovine[c] | *Claviceps* spp. | Grain contamination | Europe | Delirium, hallucinogen |
| | Lysergic acid amide[c] | *Ipomea violacea* | Intoxicant | Mesoamerica (aboriginal) | Hallucinogen |
| | | *Rivea corymbosa* | | North America | |
| | Harmine[c] | *Banisteria caapi* | Intoxicant | South America (aboriginal) | Narcotic |

(*continued*)

TABLE 1. (Continued)

| Type | Alkaloid | Source[a] | Exposure | Geographic distribution | Neurotoxicity |
|---|---|---|---|---|---|
| | Dimethyl tryptamine[c] | *Piptadenia peregrina* | Snuff | America (aboriginal) | Hallucinogen |
| | | *Prestonia amazonica* | Intoxicant | Columbia, Peru | Hallucinogen |
| | Psilocybin[c] | *Psilocybe* spp. | Intoxicant | Mesoamerica (aboriginal) | Hallucinogen |
| IV | Reserpine[b] | *Rauwolfia serpentina* | Herb | India (Ayurvedic) | Tranquilizer |
| | Strychnine[b] | *Strychnos nuxvomica* | Herb | Indochina | Convulsant |
| | Ibogamine[b] | *Tabernanthe iboga* | Herb | West Africa | Stimulant |
| | 10-Methoxyibogamine | *Tabernanthe iboga* | Herb | West Africa | Hallucinogen |
| V | Trichodesmine | *Trichodesma incanum* | Grain contamination | Uzbekistan | Delirium |
| | Incanine | *Trichodesma incanum* | | | |
| | Nicotine[d] | *Nicotiana* | Tobacco | Worldwide | Adrenergic agonist |
| | Dioscorine[d] | *Dioscorea* spp. | Food | West Africa | Convulsant |
| | Cocaine[d] | *Erythroxylon coca* | Leaf, intoxicant | Andes (aboriginal), worldwide | Stimulant |
| | Atropine[d] | *Atropa belladonna* | Intoxicant, herb, contaminant | America, Europe | Psychotomimetic |
| | | *Datura* spp. | Intoxicant | | |
| VI | Lupinine[d] | *Lupinus alba* | Food | Mediterranean | Psychotomimetic Motoneuron disease |
| VII | Gentianine[b] | *Gentiana* spp. | Herbal tonic | Europe | Stimulant |

Biosynthetic or structural type: I: purine; II: phenylalanine and/or tyrosine; III: tryptophan: IV: monoterpenoid indole; V: ornithine; VI: lysine; VII: monoterpene.
[a] Alkaloids listed may be present in other plants; only plants of major ethnobotanic interest are given.
For structures, see [b]Fig. 2, [c]Fig. 1, and [d]Fig. 4.

dysleptics, hallucinogens, or pyschotropics (Emboden, 1979). This clutter of ill-defined terminology perhaps expresses the confusion of conflicting feelings such compounds generate. Do plants such as *Mandragora officinarum* or *Datura* represent "the insane root that takes the reason prisoner," as Banquo would have it, or do they provide a release from the cage of the body, with its imprisonment in space and time (Huxley, 1970)? But even Shakespeare is ambivalent, another of his characters concluding that, "We are such stuff as dreams are made on," and that life is merely an insubstantial pageant. The temptation to use these compounds to explore reality beyond the limits of the self has proven to be an irresistible allure to many (Dobkin de Rios, 1984; Emboden, 1979; Schultes and Hofmann, 1980). People of all cultures and times have taken advantage of the chemical ingenuity of plants to escape, temporarily, the travails of a fleshly existence.

Mind-altering or mind-expanding drugs variously alter self-consciousness, the sense of time and space, and the perception of the physical world. How such a definition varies from that of sleep is problematic. The relationship between consciousness (the state), the mind (the perceiving entity), and neurochemical alterations in the brain is opaque. One should not think that the discovery that hallucinogens or morphine bind to certain receptors in the brain and affect certain neurochemical processes somehow "explains" the effects of these chemicals on perception.

In most settings, "expanding the mind" impairs function. One function of consciousness is to triage or filter out the overwhelming and confusing mass of sensory input assailing us by the second. Writing an article takes a narrowed, focused consciousness. So does avoiding a predator or finding food. "Expanding the mind" safely can only occur in a structured, protected setting. It is not to be wondered at that most societies have drawn strict social or religious rules around the use of agents that alter perception.

### 3.1.1. Convulsants, Hallucinogens, and Psychotomimetics

Among the worst of toxins and the best of pharmacological agents is that plethora of peptide and nonpeptide tryptophan derivatives known as the ergot alkaloids. These are produced by a parasitic fungus, ergot (*Claviceps purpurea*), growing on rye (*Secale cereale*). The resultant contamination of the rye bread on which the peasantry of Europe subsisted for so many centuries was responsible for the terrible disease of ergotism, or St. Anthony's fire (Barger, 1931; Matossian, 1989; Schultes and Hofmann, 1980). Just one outbreak of ergotism in France in 994 AD killed 40,000 (Schultes and Hofmann, 1980). Ergot was never the problem in England it was on the continent, as rural workers in England never subsisted exclusively on rye (Barger, 1931).

Ergotism takes both a peripheral and a central form. The more common peripheral form involves alkaloid-induced vasoconstriction, leading to scintillating pain in the extremities, gangrene, and loss of limbs. The central form involves delirium, convulsions, and hallucinations.

The peripheral form, *ergotism gangrenosus*, is caused by the peptide alkaloids in ergot, while the central form, *ergotism convulsivus*, is caused by the nonpeptide lysergic acid amides. The natural variation in the ratio of these two classes of alkaloids is the probable reason for the variation in the clinical expression of ergotism. The forms were also differentiated geographically, presumably for the same reason, with the convulsive type being common east of the Rhine and the gangrenous type west of the Rhine.

Better public health measures and an increased liking for bread made from wheat rather than rye have attenuated the incidence of ergotism in the 20th century. Although largely a disease of the past, ergotism is not unknown in modern Europe. Major outbreaks occurred in Russia in 1926, in Ireland in 1929, and in France in 1953. In the Russian outbreak, over 11,000 people were affected in an area stretching from Kazan, 400 miles east of Moscow, to the Ural Mountains. Numerous deaths were reported (Barger, 1931). Outside of Europe, an outbreak occurred in 1979 in Ethiopia.

On the credit side, ergot has proven a veritable potpourri of valuable pharmacological agents (Goodman and Gilman *et al.*, 1990). Over two dozen alkaloids have been isolated. In the central nervous system, ergotamine acts as an α-adrenergic antagonist, while ergonovine and methylergonovine act as partial agonists or antagonist at serotonergic and dopaminergic receptors. These compounds are esters of lysergic acid (Fig. 1). Centrally acting alkaloids affect the vasomotor center, giving rise to the vasodilator, hypotensive, and bradycardiac effects of ergot. The psychotomimesis appears to be due to the hypothalamic actions.

Among the numerous hallucinogenic plants used by the Aztecs of Mesoamerica was one the seeds of which they named *ololiuqui*. For years the botanical identity of this plant was shrouded. In a 16th-century Aztec drawing made for the Spanish physician, Francisco Hernandez, *ololiuqui* resembled an *Ipomea*, or morning glory, species, but no hallucinogen had been found in a morning glory. By the dawn of the 20th century, the consensus was that *ololiuqui* was probably *Datura meteloides*, although in the Aztec drawings *ololiuqui* did not look solanaceous, and the effects of taking *ololiuqui* were not those to be expected for atropine, the psychoactive agent in *Datura*. The true *ololiuqui* was rediscovered for western science in 1939, growing in a Zapotec Indian garden in the Mexican state of Oaxaca (Schultes and Hofmann, 1980). Hidden from criticism, the use of the plant had survived the overthrow of the Aztec empire by 400 years, and had survived the successor Spanish empire. The plant was a morning glory, *Rivea corymbosa*.

The hallucinogens in *Rivea* are lysergic acid amides, similar to those present in ergot. It is a strange happenstance of biochemistry that species so botanically and geographically separated should make the same complex alkaloids. In both species, biogenesis involves the linking of an isoprene unit with tryptophan.

The chemist, A. Hofmann, discovered the hallucinogenic properties of lysergic acid diethylamide serendipitously, while purifying it (Swain, 1975). This compound is particularly effective as a serotonin antagonist. What on the one continent had been considered a visitation of the devil was on another seen as a visitation of the gods.

Another Mesoamerican species, *Ipomea violacea*, has been spread around the world as an ornamental. The seeds of the plant, also used by the Zapotecs as a hallucinogen, contain five times the level of lysergic acid amides as does *R. corymbosa*. The sight of *Ipomea* growing wild on the ruins of the Aztec temples at Teotihuacan instills a sense of *carpe diem*—the ruler and the ruled, all gone; in the words of the Elizabethan dramatist, James Shirley:

> *Sceptre and crown*
> *Must tumble down,*
> *And in the dust be equal made*
> *With the poor crooked scythe and spade*

Following the chemical analysis of these Mesoamerican plants, their use or abuse became popular among segments of the American population in the 1960s. Numerous cultivars were developed, with evocative names such as Heavenly Blue, Pearly Gates, and

Wedding Bells. In the 1990s, however, their use seems to have been largely replaced by the various cultivars of light beer.

Although all cultures had access to hallucinogens, the Aztecs were the most single-mindedly in their institutional pursuit of the visionary world revealed by such agents. The use of alcohol, however, was strictly banned, except for the old. A partial listing of Nahuatl words (the language of the Aztecs) for hallucinogenic plants shows the following: *coanenepilli (Passiflora jorullensis;* β-carboline-type alkaloids, such as harmine); *cochiztzapotl (Casimiroa edulis:* N-benzoyltyramine and other psychoactive compounds); *pipiltzintzintli (Salvia divinorum); coazhuitl (Rivea corymbosa); tlitliltzin (Ipomea violacea),* and *toloache (Datura* spp.). Three of the plants used by the Aztecs were considered so potent that they were elevated to godhood: the above-discussed *ololiuqui; peyotl* (the dried heads of the cactus *Lophophora williamsii* or *L. diffusa,* containing the hallucinogenic mescaline or simple tetrahydroisoquinolines such as pellotine); and *teonanacatl* (the word literally meaning "flesh of the God"—a *Psilocybe* mushroom containing psilocybin or 4-phospho-N,N-dimethyltryptamine). Psilocybin is dephosphorylated to yield the actual hallucinogen, psilocin (Fig. 1).

Hallucinogenic mushrooms have been revered in many cultures (and feared in as many others). Wasson has developed a theory of mycolatry, or mushroom worship, based on the pharmacological activities of the Mesoamerican *Psilocybe* and the old world *Amanita* species (Wasson, 1979, 1980). The obvious phallic symbolism of mushrooms is made explicit in much art of both the New and Old World.

The psychotropic mushroom, *Amanita muscaria,* has been equated with the *soma* of the old Ayurvedic scripts (Wasson, 1968). *Soma* conferred immortality on those consuming it. The active agent in *A. muscaria* is the GABA-mimetic, muscimole (Fig. 3) (Tyler, 1963). Muscimole is an artifact of isolation, being formed from ibotenic acid (Fig. 3). Others dispute the identification of *A. muscaria* as *soma.* Indeed, one could stock a fair-sized garden with species proposed as candidates over the years. Current front-runners include *Ephedra sinica,* source of ephedrine (McCaleb, 1990), and *Peganum harmala,* source of harmaline (Flattery and Schwartz, 1989; Jones, 1990). In modern times, Aldous Huxley reintroduced *soma* into his *Brave New World,* but there it tasted of strawberry ice cream, and those taking it toasted their own annihilation rather than immortalization.

The use of *peyotl* in a religious setting survives in the Native American Church and elsewhere (Anderson, 1980; Myerhoff, 1974). Mescal buttons, or the dried heads of the plants, are chewed. This is not to be confused with *Agave,* or an alcoholic drink made from *Agave,* both of which are also known as mescal. Mescaline is present in a number of other cacti, including the South American species, San Pedro, *Trichocereus pachanoi,* which is also an object of hallucinogenic use.

Other hallucinogenic plants used by various cultures include *Banisteriopsis, Lobelia, Tagetes,* and *Pegamum* (Emboden, 1979; Schultes and Hofmann, 1979). *Banisteriopsis caapi* is used in South America under a variety of regional names, including *caapi, ayahuasca, yajé,* and *cadána.* It contains β-carbolines. These substances act as monoamine oxidase inhibitors, potentiating the actions of both endogenous monoamines, such as epinephrine and norepinephrine, and exogenous monoamines, such as N,N-dimethyltryptamine. In a nice example of ethnopharmacology, users of *B. caapi* often add tryptamine-containing plants to the preparation, thereby taking advantage of the potentiating properties.

Tropane alkaloids such as atropine have both anticholinergic actions on the autonomic nervous system and central psychotomimetic actions. An intoxicated individual is

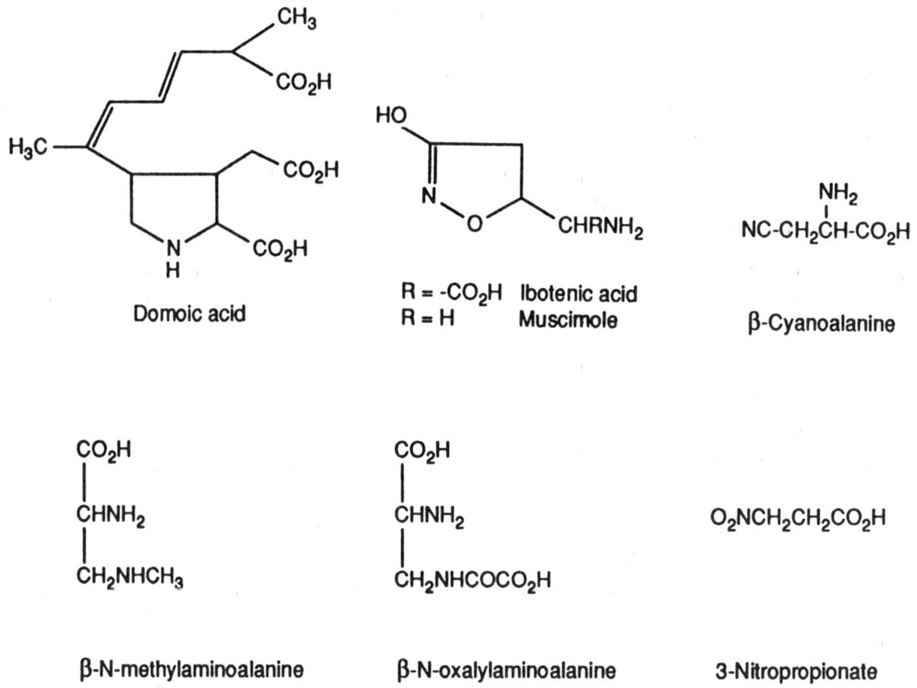

**FIGURE 3.** Muscimole and neurotoxic acids.

described in mnemonic phrases as hot as a hare, dry as a bone, blind as a bat, mad as a hatter, and red as a beet. Atropine itself is an artifact of isolation, being formed from the racemization of l-hyoscyamine.

The well-established ethnobotanic place of the these *Datura, Atropa,* and *Hyoscyamus* alkaloids is indicated by the species epithet for *A. belladonna*. The name, *bella donna,* or beautiful lady in Italian, stems from the cosmetic use of plant extracts to induce mydriasis, with the accompanying wide-eyed look considered so attractive in certain cultures. The obverse of the plant's pharmacological effects is given by the common English name, deadly nightshade, and by the genus name. Atropa was one of the three fates, the daughters of necessity. While Clotho spun the thread of life and Lachesis allotted each man's portion, Atropos cut the thread at the appointed time, her name deriving from the Greek for "not turning."

*Datura* poisoning is one of the more common plant intoxications in North America (e.g., Ulrich *et al.,* 1982). These plants are consumed as a result of commercial contamination of other plants (Awang and Kindack, 1989), or misidentification or lack of knowledge of their toxicity by persons collecting for themselves. *D. stramonium* is sold as an asthma medication, and poisonings have occurred as a result (Feenaghty, 1982). Many poisonings result from the intentional use of *Datura* for its psychotomimetic effect. Typically it is taken as a tea. *D. stramonium* is also smoked as a hallucinogen. Occasionally, accidental poisonings occur, as with a group on a desert survival course in southern California (Huxtable, 1990b). A couple in Canada were poisoned following the accidental addition of *Datura* seeds to hamburgers (Anonymous, 1984).

The convulsants, strychnine and brucine, come from the Indian tree, *Strychnos nuxvomica.* Strychnine blocks postsynaptic inhibition at glycinergic sites and is a valued tool in the study of amino acid neurotransmitter mechanisms. This highly complex alkaloid was first isolated in 1817, but its structure was not elucidated until 1946.

South American *Strychnos*, such as *S. toxifera*, are the source of the curare alkaloids, such as toxiferine I, used ethnobotanically as arrow poisons (the Greek word for which giving us our word, *toxic*) (Gardner and Sakiewicz, 1963). These are quaternary dimeric compounds that, unlike the tertiary alkaloids from *S. nuxvomica*, do not penetrate the central nervous system. Their major action is that of neuromuscular blockade at the nicotinic cholinergic receptor (McIntyre, 1972). Curare is a resinous extract of various plants from the Orinoco and Amazon basins. Depending on preparation and storage, it is classed as calabash, pot, gourd, or tube curare, the latter being packed into bamboo tubes. At one time, the alkaloid composition of these classes varied, although in this century this seems to be no longer true. d-Tubocurarine, isolated from tube curare, derives from *Chondrodendron tomentosum*. Quaternary alkaloids are present in all types of curare, and pot and calabash curare additionally contained tertiary alkaloids. These lack effect at the neuromuscular junction, but are central convulsants.

Yams (*Dioscorea* spp.) are solanaceous plants comprising a major food source in tropical countries. Worldwide production is about 20 million tons per annum (Jadhav *et al.*, 1981). In certain west African communities, yams may supply half the calories. Many wild species are highly toxic due to their content of isoquinuclidine alkaloids such as dioscorine (Fig. 4). This alkaloid, which has convulsant effects on the central nervous system, can be partially removed by soaking and leaching the yams in water.

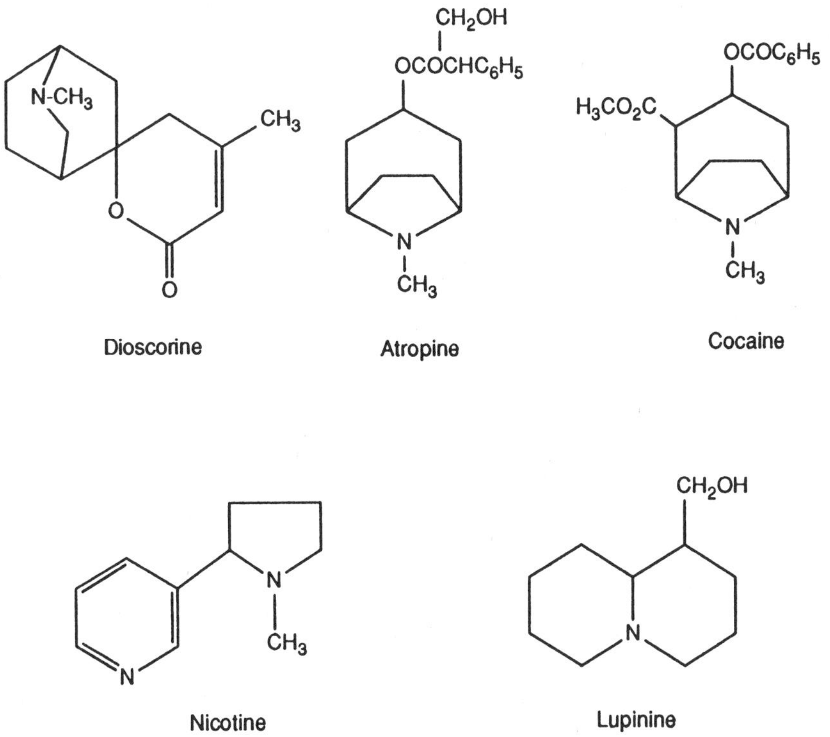

**FIGURE 4.** Some neurotoxic pyridine and piperidine alkaloids.

### 3.1.2. Stimulant or Euphoriant Alkaloids

Worldwide caffeine consumption has been estimated to be 70 mg per person each day, or some $1.1 \times 10^8$ kg per annum (120,000 tons) (Spiller, 1984; Max, 1986). This makes caffeine the most widely consumed neuroactive substance in the world. It has been considered to be a model drug of abuse (Holtzman, 1990). Caffeine is contained in tea, coffee, cocoa, chocolate, headache remedies, soft drinks, and a variety of regional herbs and drinks. Although caffeine is found in at least 63 plant species, 54% of the world's consumption derives from two *Coffea* species, *C. arabica* and *C. robusta,* and 43% from the tea plant, *Camellia sinensis* (Max, 1986). The caffeine in soft drinks is derived from the decaffeination of coffee, a pharmacological illustration of the principle that what you lose on the swings you gain on the roundabouts. The average daily intake for U.S. adults is 2.5 mg per kg body weight, and for Europeans 3.5 mg (Stavric, 1988a). The motivation for this enormous consumption is, of course, the central nervous system stimulation people get from caffeine. Theobromine, the major xanthine in chocolate, has only weak central actions, due to its low liposolubility (Stavric, 1988b). Although other activities can be demonstrated *in vitro*, the central actions of caffeine result largely from its antagonism of purinergic receptors.

Caffeine is addictive, the withdrawal syndrome involving headaches and lassitude. Apart from this, the methylxanthines have low toxicity in adults, numerous studies failing to sustain a relationship between caffeine consumption and the risk of cardiovascular disease (e.g., Grobbee *et al.,* 1990).

The form in which caffeine is consumed varies from country to country. Annual tea consumption ranges from 3.44 kg per person in Ireland to 0.02 kg per person in Thailand. Coffee consumption is highest in Finland, at 12.41 kg per person per year. In the United States, the corresponding figure is 4.68 kg. These numbers apply to 1981–1982 (Max, 1986). This represents a 54% drop since 1960, the difference being made up by the consumption of caffeine-containing soft drinks. In 1982, Americans drank 149 liters per person of such beverages.

Caffeine consumption is clearly within the pharmacological range. The minimum stimulant dose in humans falls between 85 and 250 mg. Average per capita daily consumption in the United Kingdom is around 165 mg, in the United States around 246 mg, and in Finland 465 mg. A considerable fraction of the populations of these countries, of course, consume much greater amounts. Thus, for the United States the upper decile is 7.0 mg/kg, or three times the mean daily intake (Dews, 1984).

Although this massive consumption of alkaloids seems relatively innocuous (Dalvi, 1986), humankind perhaps receiving more benefit than harm from "the reviving brew" or a fragrant cup of coffee, it may pose a developmental hazard. It is difficult to find a newborn baby who does not have caffeine in the blood. Even pregnant or nursing women who eschew coffee may be exposed to caffeine from a variety of other sources. Babies are exposed to caffeine both *in utero* and via the milk. Although the mean intake may be low [for the United States it is estimated to be 0.18 mg/kg for babies under the age of one (Dews, 1984)], a 16–20x longer half-life of excretion, due to the lack of liver metabolizing enzymes, means that even a low daily intake of caffeine can lead to an accumulating body burden (Aldridge *et al.,* 1979; Aranda *et al.,* 1979).

The developmental consequences of caffeine exposure is a generally unconsidered aspect of the wide use of this generally safe substance. Although developmental studies in humans are difficult because of the near impossibility of finding a control group of unexposed babies, the results of animal experiments give cause for alarm. Known developmental effects based on animal studies include increased circulating catecholamine levels in the fetus, decreased placental weight, lactate accumulation, and altered uterine perfusion. When nursing rats were given caffeine equivalent to a human consumption of approximately 3 cups of coffee a day (rats metabolize caffeine faster), protein concentration in the brains of their pups increased, while the levels of zinc and activities of zinc-dependent enzymes, such as alkaline phosphatase, decreased (Nakamoto et al., 1989). When caffeine exposure was combined with the additional stress of protein malnutrition, a different spectrum of changes obtained, including increases in the levels of DNA and cholesterol in the brain.

The first European to describe coffee drinking was Leonhard Rauwolf, for whom the genus *Rauwolfia* is named. In 1579, he observed the coffee habit in the Middle East. The drink quickly spread to Europe, spawning coffee shops, newspapers, and social interchange. The introduction of tea came later, one of the first mentions in England being Samuel Pepys' diary for September 25, 1660. It was not long before Pope was already describing a young lady with nothing to occupy her time but to

> . . . spill her solitary tea,
> Or o'er cold coffee trifle with the spoon.

The drinks have solaced many a European existence. The asthmatic novelist, Anthony Trollope, writes a few weeks before his death that, "Nothing seems to do me so much good as a cup of hot tea" (Trollope, 1983). Perhaps the most famous English tea drinker was Samuel Johnson, of whom Boswell muses, "I suppose no person ever enjoyed with more relish the infusion of that fragrant leaf." The artist, Sir Joshua Reynolds, alarmed on one occasion by the quantities Johnson was imbibing, reminded him that he had had 11 cups already. Johnson, annoyed, reprimanded him, "Sir, I do not count your glasses of wine. Why should you number my cups of tea?" and loudly called for a 12th cup.

A major plant of abuse in east Africa and certain Arab nations is khat, *Catha edulis*. Chewing the leaves and stems induces an amphetamine-like stimulation due to the presence of α-aminopropiophenone, also known as cathinone (Fig. 1). Cathinone oxidizes readily in wilted plants to norpseudoephedrine (Fig. 1), which is much less active (Brenneisen et al., 1986; Geisshüsler and Brenneisen, 1987). The appetite-suppressing effects of khat leads to a drug-induced anorexia in its users (Elmi, 1983). The khat habit is spreading to Europe with the immigration of formerly colonized peoples to the homelands of their colonizers.

Like atropine, cocaine is a tropane alkaloid, although its pharmacology differs. This well-known agent, from yet another South American plant, *Erythroxylon coca*, functions peripherally as a local anesthetic and centrally as a stimulant or euphoriant. Its actions are subjectively indistinguishable from the amphetamines, although its mechanism is different. Whereas cocaine blocks the reuptake of neuronally released dopamine and other monoamines, the amphetamines increase the release of monoamines from intraneuronal storage sites.

Given the entrepreneurial nature of American ingenuity, one can be assured that should supplies of South American cocaine be seriously interrupted, enterprising chemists will meet demand with the readily synthesized and almost infinitely variable amphetamines.

Cephaeline and emetine (Fig. 1) are emetic alkaloids from the Brazilian tree,

*Cephaelis ipecacuanha.* This plant was used ethnomedicinally, and ipecac has passed into common usage around the world as an emetic in cases of poisoning. The action of the alkaloids is centrally mediated, involving stimulation of the chemoceptor trigger zone in the area postrema of the medulla (Manno and Manno, 1977). Vomiting occurs within a few minutes of ingestion.

Motoneuron diseases precipitated by excitotoxic amino acids found in plants are discussed in Section 3.2. It has been reported that similar disease can be produced by ingestion of *Lupinus* seeds, probably *L. albus* (Agid et al., 1988). Such seeds are widely used for culinary purposes in Mediterranean countries, and their use is spreading to other countries. The toxicity of the quinolizine alkaloids such as lupinine (Fig. 4) in lupin has been well established. The toxicity of the seeds has been known since classical times. One method of preparation involves boiling to remove the bitterness (Sturtevant, 1919). In stock animals, excessive consumption of lupin leads to death from respiratory paralysis. Central nervous system involvement at lower levels of consumption is indicated by behavioral changes, including an affected animal standing with its head pressed against an object (Kingsbury, 1964). This is the first report, however, of primary neurotoxicity in a human associated with the consumption of lupin seeds (Agid et al., 1988).

### 3.1.3. Narcotics and Tranquilizers

Reserpine (Fig. 2), one of the first effective tranquilizers, comes from the Indian medicinal plant, *Rauwolfia serpentina*. Mahatma Gandhi supposedly used a tea made from the plant to help him in his periods of introspection and relaxation. Pharmacologically, reserpine causes prolonged depletion of neuronal norepinephrine and serotonin stores. As the storage vesicles are destroyed, the effects of reserpine are long lasting, recovery of neuronal function being dependent on *de novo* synthesis of storage sites.

The neurotoxic alkaloid that has wound the strangest and most revealing course through western history is doubtless morphine (Fig. 1). This compound is named for Morpheus, Ovid's name for the god of dreams, the name thereby revealing one of the most prominent subjective features of morphine intoxication. Morphine is isolated from the latex of the poppy, *Papaver somniferum*. The method of collecting the latex by incising the seed pod has remained unchanged for millennia. Opium is prepared from the dried latex. *P. somniferum* appears to be a cultivar of *P. setigerum,* although, like other species discussed in this chapter, it is a plant so domesticated, so cultivated, so selectively bred by man, that where it came from and what it came from are no longer easily discernable. No truly wild populations of *P. somniferum* are known. Individual plants can apparently be either diploid or polyploid, which again suggests that the "species" is a hybrid (Merlin, 1984). The modern pattern of distribution is related more to economics than to climate. Collecting opium is highly labor intensive, and so it is only produced in countries having a low cost of labor. Otherwise, the poppy grows happily, even in the environs of the northern city of Liverpool where the initial studies on its biosynthesis were carried out (Battersby et al., 1964).

The association of morphine and man is long standing, poppy seeds having been found in Neolithic sites in Europe dating to 5000 B.C. As the poppy is also the source of a valued oil, nutrition may possibly have been of more importance than the aspects of this varicolored flower that are so significant in modern times. However, the narcotic activity of opium was exploited early. The poppy is included in the prescriptions listed on a

Sumerian clay tablet in 2100 B.C. Opium was used by the Minoan, Ptolemaic, Assyrian, and Hellenic civilizations. Morphine has been detected in a Theban (Egyptian) funeral pot dating to about 1500 B.C. (Majno, 1977). Perhaps no substance has been more involved in man's search for a reality lying beyond reality, summarized in de Quincy's exultation, "Thou has the keys of paradise, O just, subtle and mighty opium" (de Quincey, 1948).

Although morphine was isolated in crude form by the Parisian apothecary, Derosne, in 1803–1804, the credit for isolating crystalline morphine belongs to Sertürner, who also named the alkaloid and showed that it produced sleep in dogs. Sertürner tried his new compound out on his friends, at 10 times a modern recommended dose, reminding one of the aphorism that "A man should choose his enemies more carefully than his friends, because he will have them longer." Although the structure of this complex alkaloid was not proven until 1952, Robert Robinson suggested the correct structure in 1923, based on biosynthetic considerations. Robinson realized that a morphine-type structure could be obtained by rotation through 90° of the 1-benzyl group of a tetrahydroisoquinoline such as reticuline followed by bond formation between the 2' position of the benzyl group and the 10 position of the isoquinoline ring (Fig. 5). Tetrahydroisoquinolines, in turn, could be formed from two molecules of tyrosine. The tyrosine-derived rings form the stem and one wing of the final, rigid T-shaped morphine molecule.

In addition to deducing the correct structure, Robinson also deduced a biosynthetic scheme, which transpired to be correct in the main, and unknowingly established the chemical relationship between the prosilient metabolite of the poppy and the structurally mundane peptides of the brain exhibiting a similar neuropharmacology. The first of these peptides was discovered by Hughes and Kosterlitz in 1975 (Hughes and Kosterlitz, 1975). Since then, many others have been isolated, acting at an increasing number of opioid receptors. The structural feature held in common by these various enkephalins, endorphins, and dynorphins is the presence of a tetrapeptide sequence, Try-Gly-Gly-Phe. Three opioid receptors are currently recognized, the $\mu$, $\delta$, and $\kappa$, each having its bevy of subtypes. Strangely, the pharmacology of morphine seems to be exerted largely via the $\mu$ receptor. Even more strangely, the function of these receptors is unclear, as the administration of naloxone, an antagonist at all three types, is unassociated with deleterious consequences in laboratory animals. Despite this, the brain generates cascades of these three classes of peptides via the actions of various peptidases, all exhibiting pharmacological activities at one or more of the opioid receptors (Hollt, 1986).

Evolution of higher animals was paralleled by the abridgement of considerable chemical ingenuity: Plants are better chemists than mammals. We, with our limited ability for postribosomal modification of proteins and peptides, achieve molecules with similar pharmacological activities to those of morphine by incorporating two unmodified aromatic amino acid residues into a polypeptide chain, spacing them with two glycine molecules to allow the aromatic rings to twist themselves into the appropriate T-shaped relationship needed to bind to the opiate receptors. Thus, from the pharmacological point of view, morphine is simply a modified dipeptide. The apparent lack of structural consonance between morphine and the endorphins and enkephalins of the central nervous system is a perceptual artifact induced by the limitations of representing three-dimensional structures on paper. In fact, both poppy and man achieve the same pharmacological end from the same starting materials. The difference resides in the sophistication and economy of the chemistry employed. Morphine can, therefore, serve as an important model for neuropharmacology and as a lesson that if problems in neuropharmacology are considered

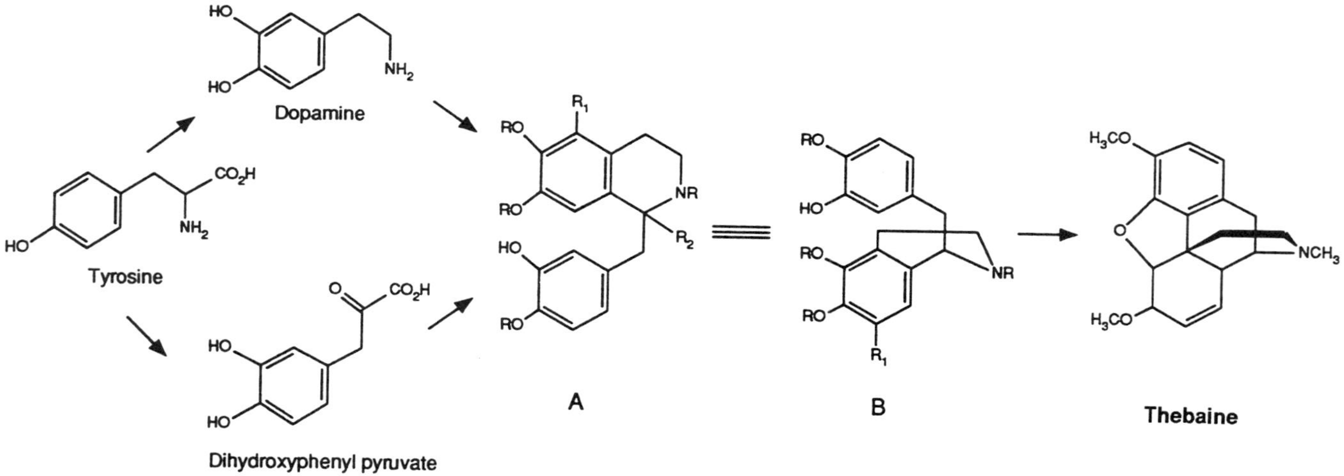

**FIGURE 5.** The biosynthesis of morphine in outline. One molecule of tyrosine is decarboxylated and hydroxylated to form dopamine and another tyrosine molecule is deaminated and hydroxylated to form dihydroxyphenylpyruvate. Condensation of these moieties yields 1-carboxynorlaudanosoline (A: R,R$_1$=H, R$_2$=CO$_2$H). This is decarboxylated to norlaudanosoline (A: R,R$_1$,R$_2$=H), and hydroxylated and methylated to yield reticuline (A: R=CH$_3$,R$_1$=OCH$_3$;R$_2$=H), drawn both (A) conventionally and (B) in a manner stressing its steric resemblance to morphine. Phenolic oxidative coupling of the two rings gives thebaine, followed by minor metabolic changes to morphine.

## 3.2. Neurotoxic Amino Acids in Plants

Numerous unusual, nonproteinaceous amino acids are scattered through the plant kingdom. Examples include GABA, homoserine, or citrulline (Roy, 1981). Most are innocuous in the amounts likely to be ingested. A few are severely neurotoxic. In particular, excitotoxins are found in a number of plants that mimic the actions of glutamate on the central nervous system. Glutamate is often added to foods as a flavor enhancer. It is the cause of the ill-named Chinese restaurant syndrome; ill-named because many foods ranging from canned Peruvian anchovies to Japanese sukiyaki contain levels of glutamate sufficient to precipitate the pounding headaches and lassitude of the syndrome. It is noteworthy that other excitotoxic amino acids, such as tricholomic and ibotenic acids, are also flavor enhancers.

A number of tropical myeloneuropathies are known that are found in association with nutritional, environmental, and climatic factors (Roman et al., 1985). These conditions include peripheral neuropathies, Parkinsonism, dementia, and amyotrophic lateral sclerosis. They all share a dietary factor as a precipitant. Although there is some dispute as to the nature of these factors, the bulk of evidence suggests that they are excitotoxins.

Lathyrism is a disease caused by consumption of the seeds of *Lathyrus* species, such as *L. sativus* (chickling pea), *L. clymenum,* and *L. cicera,* all containing the excitotoxin, β-N-oxalylaminoalanine (Fig. 3). The two major forms of the disease are osteolathyrism, affecting primarily the bones, and neurolathyrism. The latter is a progressive, degenerative motor neuron disease leading to spastic paraplegia (Spencer and Schaumburg, 1983). Pyramidal tract lesions cause damage to upper motor neurons, leading to increased motor tone and exaggerated responses to muscle stretch (Spencer et al., 1986, 1987). There is increasing difficulty with walking, sufferers ultimately being reduced to crawling (Ludolph et al., 1987).

At one time, lathyrism was endemic in Europe and much of Africa and south central and southeast Asia. Although the geographic area in which it occurs is shrinking, the disease still occurs with high prevalence in Bangladesh, India, and Ethiopia (Tekle Heimanot et al., 1990). For India, 100,000 cases were reported in 1975 in men between the ages of 15 and 45 (Liener, 1974). This is probably an underestimate. In affected areas, the incidence can be 2.5% of the population (Ludolph et al., 1987). An unusual outbreak occurred in Europe in the Second World War in German forced-labor camps, when malnourished inmates were given *Lathyrus* flour to eat (Gardner and Sakiewicz, 1963).

*L. sativa* seeds are high in protein (28%), and the plant flourishes in the absence of irrigation or fertilization. It thus becomes an irresistible source of food under famine conditions. Lathyrism develops after weeks or months of seed consumption. The expression of the disease is, therefore, polyfactorial, involving protein and calorie malnutrition, in addition to the consumption of *L. sativa*.

Fed to cynomolgus monkeys, *Macaca fascicularis,* β-N-oxalylaminoalanine produces corticospinal dysfunction in the absence of extrapyramidal lesions, analogous to that seen in humans consuming *L. sativus* (Kurland, 1988; Spencer et al., 1986; Watkins et al., 1966).

To date, attempts to breed a toxin-free variety of *Lathyrus* have not been successful. In areas where rice and wheat supplant *Lathyrus* as a staple in the diet, the incidence of neurolathyrism falls.

*Vicia* (vetch) species contain a neurolathyrogen, β-cyanoalanine (Fig. 3) along with its γ-glutamyl derivative. Both compounds produce hyperactivity and convulsions in weanling rats (Ressler *et al.*, 1969). As *Vicia* seeds sometimes contaminate *Lathyrus* seeds in India, this compound may contribute lathyrism in that country. Although the metabolism of β-cyanoalanine does not appear to have been studied, it is possible that it enters the brain followed by oxidation of the cyano grouping to yield the excitotoxic amino acid, aspartate.

Another neurotoxin-induced degenerative motor disease occurs in the western Pacific (Garruto and Yase, 1986; Kurland, 1988; Rowland, 1987; Spencer *et al.*, 1987; Whiting, 1963; Zhang *et al.*, 1990). The neurotoxin is probably β-N-methylaminoalanine (Fig. 3), a constituent of locally consumed cycad seeds. The well-studied condition it causes has elements of amyotrophic lateral sclerosis and Parkinsonism with dementia. The disease has three geographic loci: It occurs among the Chamorros in the Miriana Islands, including Guam, the Auyu, and Jakai of west New Guinea, now part of Indonesia, and among the Japanese of the Hobara and Kozagawa districts of the Kii peninsula on the main island of Honshu. The rates of amyotrophic lateral sclerosis are the highest in the world in the affected areas of New Guinea, being 150 times higher than the rate for the United States. Forty years ago, the incidence in the Marianas was almost as high (Kurland, 1988). The disease is familial, but not genetic. In the Marianas and Japan, behavioral and cultural changes have led to a decrease in the incidence of disease (Garruto and Yase, 1986). It is noteworthy that no increase in amyotrophic lateral sclerosis or Parkinsonism/ dementia has occurred among the large number of U.S. armed forces who has been stationed on Guam since the war (Brody *et al.*, 1979). Conversely, Guamian-born Chamorros who move to the United States after the age of 18 carry an increased risk of amyotrophic lateral sclerosis, which may appear with a latency of 30 years (Brody *et al.*, 1979).

Pacific amyotrophic lateral sclerosis is similar to the condition originally described by Charcot and is also associated with the presence of neurofibrillary tangles in the brain and spinal cord (Rowland, 1984, 1987). Of Chamorros dying of nonneurological causes, up to 70% show neurofibrillary tangles (Anderson *et al.*, 1975; Chen, 1981; Chen and Yase, 1985). Pacific amyotrophic lateral sclerosis differs from lathyrism in that lesions occur simultaneously in the upper and lower motor neurons. As well as degeneration of the anterior horn cells in the spine, there is degeneration of peripheral motor axons, leading to neurogenic muscle atrophy (Spencer *et al.*, 1987).

The disease is associated with, and in all likelihood caused by, consumption of flour prepared from the cycad palm, *Cycas circinalis,* and related species, such as *C. revoluta.* The latter species, false sago palm, is common in the affected areas of Japan, where it is known as *sotetsu*. These plants should not be confused with the other sago palm, *Metroxylon sagu,* source of the once common but increasingly unfamiliar sago pudding of England (Gilks, 1988).

In Guam, *C. circinalis* has been a traditional food source. During the wartime Japanese occupation of the Marianas, there was an increased consumption of cycad flour, combined with undernutrition of the population. With the changes in life-style brought about by the postwar American military presence on Guam, the use of cycads has fallen dramatically. However, in Japan, cycad seeds are still used in traditional medicine in the Kii peninsula (Spencer *et al.*, 1987).

Recently, a method has been developed allowing analysis of β-N-methylamino-alanine in the low picogram range (Duncan and Kopin, 1989). This has allowed confirmation of the presence of the toxin in a number of *Cycas* species. In seeds from *C. circinalis*, levels of 8.5 μmol/g dry weight were found, and levels of 2.7 and 2.5 μmol/g were found in seeds of *C. revoluta* and *C. media*, respectively. Flour from *Cycas* seeds contained up to 1.2 μmol/g.

Pacific amyotrophic lateral sclerosis has been suggested to be caused by metal intoxication (Duncan *et al.*, 1988; Garruto and Yase, 1986; Garruto *et al.*, 1988), but this theory has been increasingly discounted.

β-N-Methylaminoalanine is unusual among excitatory amino acids in not being acidic. This suggests that the actual toxin may be an acidic metabolite. Cynomolgus monkeys given the acid by gavage develop neurological deficits within 2–12 weeks (Spencer, 1987).

Both β-N-methylaminoalanine and β-N-oxalylaminoalanine are toxic to neuronal cell cultures (Nunn *et al.*, 1987; Spencer *et al.*, 1987), and both produce seizures in neonatal rodents (Olney *et al.*, 1976; Polsky *et al.*, 1972). The effects of β-N-methylaminoalanine take several hours to develop, suggestive of metabolic activation. Furthermore, bicarbonate is required as a cofactor in the expression of β-N-methylaminoalanine toxicity in *in vitro* neuronal cell cultures (Weiss and Choi, 1988). It has been suggested that toxicity is a result of an acidic carbamate grouping forming in solution by reaction of the amine function with bicarbonate (Nunn *et al.*, 1991). The carbamate is stereochemically similar to the neurotoxin, N-methyl-D-aspartate. The formation of carbamates as transient species in solution in the presence of carbon dioxide has been convincingly established by NMR (Morrow *et al.*, 1974; Nunn and O'Brien, 1989). However, it is problematic whether such species are involved in the neurotoxicity of β-N-methylaminoalanine. Amino acids such as alanine are not neurotoxic, although they also form carbamates. Indeed, α-carbamates must be the normal form in which free amino acids and the N-terminal of peptides and proteins exist. Furthermore, it takes several hours for the toxicity of β-N-methylaminoalanine to be manifested in cell cultures, although α-carbamates form rapidly (Morrow *et al.*, 1974).

Intracisternally administered β-N-methylaminoalanine in rats produces a lowering in norepinephrine levels in the hypothalamus without affecting the levels of other monoamines (Lindstrom *et al.*, 1990). Intranigral injections of β-N-oxalylaminoalanine similarly lower norepinephrine levels in the hippocampus.

Neurochemically, both β-N-methylaminoalanine and β-N-oxalylaminoalanine are agonists at glutamate receptors, the latter having the higher potency (Spencer *et al.*, 1987). The action of β-N-oxalylaminoalanine is blocked by the $A_2$ (quisqualate) and $A_3$ (kainate) antagonist, *cis*-2,3-piperidine dicarboxylic acid. The action of β-N-methylaminoalanine is blocked by the $A_1$ (N-methyl-D-aspartate) antagonist, D-2-amino-7-phosphonoheptanoic acid. The D-stereoisomers of the plant amino acids are without toxicity *in vivo* and without potency at the glutamate receptor (Nunn *et al.*, 1987; Spencer *et al.*, 1987).

An algal excitotoxin, domoic acid (Fig. 3), caused an outbreak of poisoning in Canada recently (Snodgrass, 1990; Teitelbaum *et al.*, 1990). Domoic acid was first isolated from a Japanese seaweed, *Chondria armata* (Takemoto, 1978), but was subsequently found to be elaborated by a seaweed, *Nitzschia diatomea*, growing around Prince Edward Island. Mussels grazing on the seaweed were, in turn, consumed by humans.

Domoic acid has high affinity for the kainate subtype of the glutamate receptor. Symptoms of domoic acid intoxication included neurological dysfunction and memory and motor deficits. Neuronal necrosis was apparent on autopsy in the hippocampus and amygdala. Intoxication went through two stages: an initial stage involved neural hyperexcitation, presumably due to the direct neuroexcitatory actions of domoic acid, while the subsequent stage involved loss of function in neural systems suffering excitotoxic degeneration.

Again, however, other factors appear to be involved in the expression of domoic acid toxicity, as no dose-response relationship could be established between the amount consumed and the severity of symptoms (Snodgrass, 1990). The quantity of protein in the diet may affect absorption of domoic acid.

Other neurotoxic amino acids in plants include 2,4-diaminobutyric acid and its γ-oxalyl derivative in *Lathyrus* and *Vicia aurantica,* and 3-nitropropionate in *Indigofera endecaphylla* (Fig. 3) (Roy, 1981).

The latter compound causes lesions of the lateral caudate putamen on i.p. injection in mice (Gould and Gustine, 1982). It is an irreversible inhibitor of succinate dehydrogenase and a competitive inhibitor of fumerase. Nitropropionate therefore blocks energy production by the tricarboxylic acid cycle and disrupts the metabolism of neurotransmitter amino acids. The glucose ester of 3-nitropropionate and the glucoside of 3-nitropropanol (miserotoxin) are present in other legumes of the *Astragulus* and *Coronilla* genera, and are also produced by some fungi, such as *Aspergillus* and *Penicillium*. These nitro compounds are major agricultural problems (Williams and James, 1978).

Kainic acid, an important neurochemical tool, was isolated from the Japanese seaweed, *Digenia simplex* (Takemoto, 1978). Hundreds of tons of this plant per year are used as an ascaricide. Two other excitotoxins have been isolated from Japanese mushrooms: tricholomic acid from *Tricholoma muscarium* and ibotenic acid from *Amanita strobiliformis* and other *Amanita* species (Takemoto, 1978). The former was used by as a food and as a fly killer. These two acids are 20 times more potent than glutamate as flavor enhancers. That so many excitotoxic amino acids have been isolated from Japanese plants must be considered an ethnobotanical rather than a botanical phenomenon.

### 3.3. Neurotoxic Monoterpenes and Terpenoids

Many medical and culinary plants contain terpenes and essential oils that yield a characteristic odor and taste. The fascinating history of the use of such plants can be traced in various monographs (Andrews, 1984; Wheelwright, 1974).

Neurotoxic terpenes tend also to be toxic to other organ systems. Thus, oil of pennyroyal, from *Mentha pulegium,* is often used in attempted abortion. The active terpene, pulegone (Fig. 6), produces hepatic and renal failure, in addition to its effects on the central nervous system. These include hallucinations (Early, 1961). In rats, pulegone causes a neuropathy characterized by lesions in the cerebellum (Olsen and Thorup, 1984).

One of the oldest and most widely distributed psychotomimetic plants is *Cannabis* (Schultes and Hofmann, 1980). This has been cultivated for so long that its botanical origins are unclear. Some think the numerous cultivars comprise one species, *Cannabis sativa,* while others hold that it is a mixture of the three species, *C. sativa, C. indica,* and *C. ruderalis. Cannabis* is a plant of polyvalent uses, serving as the source of hemp, marijuana, and an edible oil. Cultivars have been developed to increase selectively the quality of each of these products.

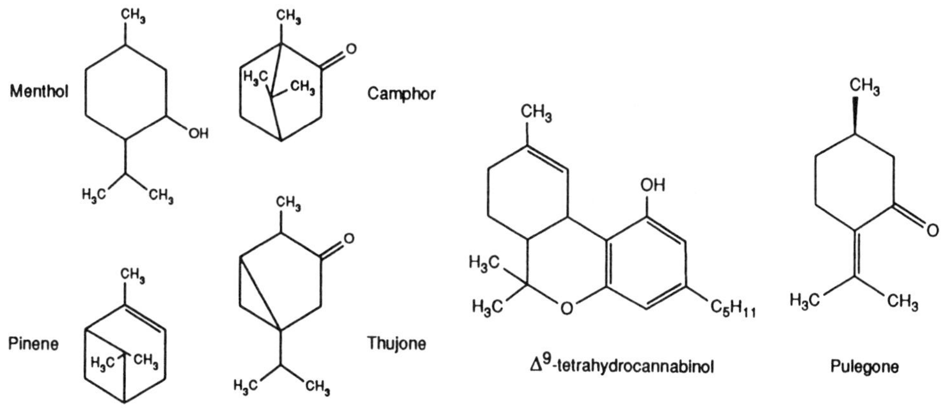

**FIGURE 6.** Some neurotoxic monoterpenes.

In marijuana, the major psychoactive substance is $\Delta^9$-tetrahydrocannabinol (Fig. 6) (Hollister, 1986). This appears to be a combination of a monoterpene with an olivetol fragment. It acts at a specific receptor in the brain, attenuating dopaminergic activity (Howlett et al., 1990; Martin, 1986). The high liposolubility of cannabinol leads to the economical phenomenon of reverse tolerance. As the material accumulates in the central nervous system, less is needed to precipitate a "high." Cannabinoids have antinociceptive and analgetic activities worthy of therapeutic exploitation. The study of synthetic and semisynthetic analogs of the natural cannabinoids has spawned an enormous volume of work (Razdan, 1986).

The wormwood, *Artemisia absinthium*, has been used in Europe and North America as a sedative. Oil of wormwood was an ingredient in the bright green, alcoholic, and hallucinogenic drink, absinthe, banned since the early part of the century. The active principle is the monoterpene, thujone (Fig. 6), which probably acts in the central nervous system at the same receptor as $\Delta^9$-tetrahydrocannabinol (del Castillo et al., 1975). Thujone produces convulsions in rats at 40 mg/kg, and death at 120 mg/kg (Tyler, 1982). In mice, the $LD_{50}$ (s.c.) is 134 mg/kg (Budavari, 1989).

The drinking of absinthe has been fixed on numerous impressionist canvasses, including paintings by Manet, Degas, Toulouse-Lautrec, and van Gogh. In this ritualistic activity, an emerald-green liquid was poured slowly over sugar held in a perforated spoon and diluted into water. The translucent green was replaced by an opaque white as the essential oils held in alcoholic solution precipitated out (Vogt, 1981). Perforated spoons can still be seen in certain European cafés, but these days the purpose is to prevent their theft for free-basing cocaine. The reputation that absinthe had can perhaps be gauged by a quotation from a 1916 letter of Aldous Huxley (1969), ". . . he turned deathly pale and, rushing out of the room, proceeded to be sick . . . And that is what comes of drinking absinthe before dinner." In this case, however, Huxley suspected the drink had been adulterated with methanol.

An extract of *A. absinthium* is extraordinarily bitter, due to the content of absinthin, which has a taste threshold of one part in 70,000. One recalls the nurse in *Romeo and Juliet* who smeared wormwood on her nipples to wean Juliet. The plant has a long medical history. The common name derives from its use in treating intestinal worms, but it was additionally used as a febrifuge and aphrodisiac, the latter action perhaps not unrelated to the popularity of absinthe.

Absinthe drinking was believed to induce a mood of exaltation. It was used by many artists and writers, including Baudelaire, van Gogh, Ernest Dowson, and Verlaine, to enhance their artistic perceptions. The writer, Dawson, refers to "the curious bewilderment of one's mind after much absinthe," and it appears to have been taken as an intellectual or creative stimulant. Prolonged consumption, however, is associated with addiction, auditory and visual hallucinations, and hyperexcitability. The condition was first recognized in the 1850s.

Thujone is found in other genera apart from *Artemisia,* including species of *Salvia, Tanacetum,* and *Thuja* (hence the name) (Albert-Puleo, 1978). It constitutes 40–90% by weight of oil of wormwood (Simonsen, 1949). Thujone is a convulsant, as are the related monoterpenes, camphor, menthol, and pinene (Fig. 6) (Goodman and Gilman, 1958; Sollmann, 1948). Their lethality, however, is low. For camphor, the minimum lethal dose in rats is 2.2 g/kg.

A case has been made that van Gogh suffered from "terpene toxicosis" (Arnold, 1988). He was an habitual imbiber of absinthe, and during one period of abstinence had to be restrained from drinking turpentine. Arnold (1988) points out that turpentine contains monoterpenes such as pinene, and suggests this was an attempt at self-medication of withdrawal symptoms. This raises the further possibility that van Gogh, and perhaps other painters, suffered an occupational addiction caused by the fumes of the turpentine to which they were so frequently exposed.

Part of the attack launched in the columns of medical journals was undoubtedly fueled by the bohemian associations of absinthe drinking. Exaggerated claims about the toxicity of absinthe were made, along the lines of the attacks on "demon" alcohol or the supposed psychosis-precipitating effects of marijuana during Anslinger's 1930–1962 tenure of the U.S. Bureau of Narcotics and Dangerous Drugs. One writer claimed that absinthe was an ignoble poison that brutalized its votaries and made drivelling idiots of them (Beach, 1860). On the other side, it was early argued that the symptoms of absinthism were no different than the symptoms of alcoholism—sleeplessness, tremors, hallucinations, paralysis, and convulsions (Anonymous, 1869).

Dose calculations can illuminate discussion on the cause of absinthism. How much thujone was present in absinthe? Steam distillation of wormwood yields 0.27–0.40% of a bitter, dark-green oil (Guenther, 1952). In a typical recipe for absinthe, 2.5 kg of wormwood were used in preparing 100 liters of absinthe (Arnold, 1989). Typically, 1.5 ounces were consumed (diluted with water) per tipple (Vogt and Montagne, 1982). This is equivalent to 4.4 mg of wormwood oil per drink, or between 2 and 4 mg of thujone. This is far below the level at which acute pharmacological effects are observed. Even chronic administration of 10 mg/kg thujone to rats does not alter spontaneous activity or conditioned behavior (Pinto-Scognamiglio, 1968). The literature on the pharmacology of thujone is, to put it bluntly, second rate, and conclusions as to its effects have been extrapolated far beyond the experimental base. In fact, the supposed chronic neurotoxicity of thujone is by no means well established. Even allowing that a condition not identical to alcoholism existed, agents other than thujone in absinthe could have been responsible. The amount of wormwood used was highly variable. Many other herbs and flavorants were used, including angelica, marjoram, hyssop, mint, fennel, star anise, and calamus. The latter plant, *Acorus calamus,* also has the reputation of being psychedelic, due to its content of asarone (Hoffer and Osmond, 1967). Because the visual esthetics of absinthe drinking were an important part of the ritual, manufacturers did not hesitate to adulterate their product to obtain the correct degree of emerald green, and the appropriate appearance of a white precipitate on dilution with water. Typically, the shade of green was "corrected" with copper sulfate, and the degree of opalescence adjusted by the addition of antimony chloride. Other adulterants included indigo, tumeric, and aniline green. Methanol has been found in absinthe, and some of the neurological effects of absinthe drinking have been ascribed to this (Walton et al., 1986).

Thujone is still to be found in low amounts in drinks such as vermouths, chartreuse, and benedictine, although no addiction comparable to absinthism has been reported. Indeed, the word *vermouth* is but a cognate of the German *Wermuth,* or wormwood. Other drinks, such as raki, arrack, retsina, and ouzo, contain essential oils.

The true nature and cause of absinthism is one of those mysteries that, like that of Edwin Drood, is unlikely ever to be solved. But one can suspect that absinthism was a multifactorial complex of conditions produced partially by adulterants and other ingredients added to the drink, partially by alcohol, and partially by imagination.

The related terpene, camphor (Fig. 6), derives from the tree *Cinnamomum camphora,* indigenous to Japan and Taiwan. Camphor is also a stimulant and convulsant.

The euphoria produced in cats by the odor of catnip, *Nepeta cataria,* is well known. Mood elevation and euphoria also occurs in humans smoking the plant (Jackson and Reed, 1969). The effect, however, is claimed to be proportional to the user's expectations. The activity, at least in cats, is due to nepetalactone (Bates and Sigel, 1963).

## 3.4. Other Plant Neurotoxins

Other volatile substances add flavor and spice to numerous culinary herbs, and some of these are centrally acting. Nutmeg, *Myristica fragrans,* once so important that its geographic source was known simply as the Nutmeg Islands, contains hallucinogenic aromatic ethers such as elemicin (Fig. 7) (Efron et al., 1979; Faguet and Rowland, 1978). The structure is reminiscent of mescaline (Fig. 1). The hallucinogenic action of these ethers may involve their conversion to amphetamine derivatives via oxidation and amination, although this is unproven (Shulgin et al., 1979). Other spices, such as saffron, fennel, dill, anise, and parsley, contain similar psychoactive ethers, including safrole, eugenol, and myristicin (Fig. 7).

*Valeriana officinalis* has been used as a sedative for centuries. Controlled trials have shown its efficacy in humans. Its activity is thought to be due to the sesquiterpenes valeranone, valerenol, and valerenic acid (Hendriks et al., 1981; Leathwood et al., 1982).

*Piper methysticum* is used in the south Pacific to make the drink known as kava, or kava-kava (Ford, 1979). The use of this mild relaxant revolted early missionaries, as its preparation involved the chewing of the root by women and children followed by collection of the expectorate. The active principles are the dihydropyrones, methysticin and kawain (Fig. 7) (Klohs, 1979). Methysticin antagonizes strychnine-induced and electroshock convulsions, and potentiates pentobarbital-induced sleeping time.

Clove cigarettes, prepared from mixtures of tobacco and *Eugenia caryophyllata,* are popular among segments of the American population for the marijuana-type high engendered. The active ingredients are probably eugenol (Fig. 7), acetyleugenol, and related

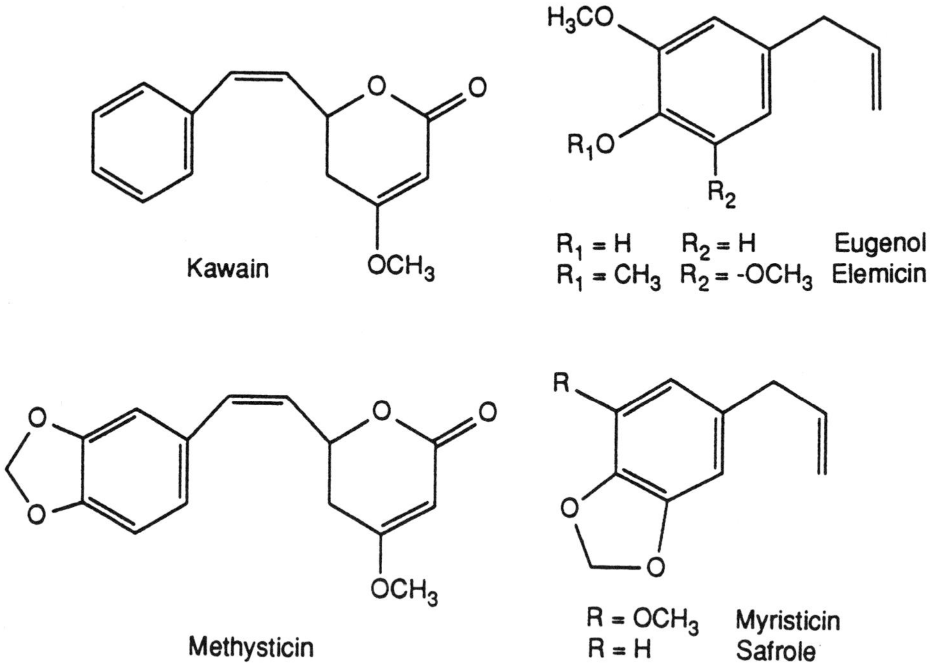

**FIGURE 7.** Some neurotoxic components of essential oils.

compounds. Deaths have resulted from their use. Cloves, however, have a long culinary and medical history, and present little hazard on ingestion.

Chicory, *Chicorium intybus,* has been used as a coffee extender or coffee substitute. It adds its characteristic flavor to New Orleans coffee, where it is viewed as a specialty. In England, after the war, extract of chicory was inflicted as a coffee substitute on a deprived public. A taste of chicory to those so exposed conjures up nothing but a recollection of drabness and perpetual hunger. Such is the importance of a point of view.

Unlike coffee, chicory is sedative. Indeed, it counteracts the stimulation induced by caffeine. The active principle is probably lactucin (Max, 1988b).

One species of the maligned yew, toxic and, like cypress, associated with death and graveyards, has recently come to clinical prominence because of the efficacy of the alkaloid, taxol, as an antineoplastic agent. *Taxus brevifolia* has for years been cleared from American forests as a slow-growing, uneconomic trash tree. Now, however, frantic efforts are being made to increase the supply (Chase, 1991). Taxol exerts its chemotherapeutic effect by inducing microtubule assembly and disrupting cell proliferation. Taxol-induced microtubular assembly in dorsal-root ganglion cells appears to be responsible for the sensory neuropathy that occasionally accompanies its chemotherapeutic use (Lipton *et al.,* 1991).

Neem oil is obtained from the seeds of the Indian tree, *Melia azadirachta* L. (*Azadirachta indica* A. Juss). Although its garlic-like odor limits its culinary use, the oil is widely used in the indigenous, traditional medicines of India, including the Ayurvedic and Unani. It is, however, toxic, producing a syndrome similar to Reye's in children (Sinniah *et al.,* 1989). In experimental animals, it is neurotoxic (Gandhi *et al.,* 1988). The toxic agent may be a monounsaturated fatty acid.

The convulsant, picrotoxinin, in the form of the complex, picrotoxin, is obtained from the east Indian shrub, *Cocculus indicus* (*Anamirta cocculus*). Ethnopharmacologically, it was used as a fish poison. Like the alakaloid, bicuculline, picrotoxinin acts as a GABA antagonist. However, despite its spelling, picrotoxinin contains no nitrogen.

Other important plant neurochemicals include capsaicin, the pungent principle in peppers (*Capsicum* spp.) (Buck and Burks, 1986).

Under certain conditions, thiocyanates derived from plants can cause neuropathies (Roman *et al.*, 1985). Cassava (*Manihot esculenta*) is widely consumed throughout the tropical regions, over 300 million people relying on it as a principal source of calories. In the intensely glutinous form of tapioca, it is even known in England, where it is fed to resisting school children. Cassava has a high content of the cyanohydrin glycoside, linamarin, and has to undergo a labor-intensive washing procedure to make it palatable. Under famine conditions, this washing procedure may be abbreviated, and forms of cassava higher in cyanide may be used. Following consumption, the cyanide is converted to thiocyanate, which produces a variety of health problems, including an ataxic neuropathy. In some cassava-induced outbreaks of ataxic neuropathy in Africa, incidences as high as 34 per 1000 population have occurred. Plasma thiocyanate levels are extremely high in affected individuals. Compared to control levels of 1 $\mu$mol/l, levels of 114 $\mu$mol/l were found in a Nigerian outbreak, and levels ranging from 298 to 336 $\mu$mol/l in an outbreak in Mozambique (Roman *et al.*, 1985).

As with other plant neurotoxicities, consumption of improperly prepared cassava is a necessary but insufficient condition for the disease to develop. Poisoned individuals not only show high plasma levels of thiocyanate, indicating high dietary intake of cyanide, but also low urinary levels of sulfate, indicating low dietary intake of sulfur amino acids. This occurs during periods of food shortage and has been observed in Mozambique, Nigeria, and Tanzania (Cliff *et al.*, 1985). Neighboring populations with the same intake of cyanide combined with normal intake of sulfur amino acids do not develop ataxic neuropathy. Sulfur is needed for detoxification of cyanide via conversion of thiocyanate.

Cassava is not unique in containing cyanogenetic glucosides. These are present in yams, beans, corn, millet, apples, peaches, almonds, and numerous other fruits. Indeed, cyanide is usually described by those who can smell it (80% of the population) as having the odor of almonds (Balbaa *et al.*, 1973). In fact, of course, it is the other way around; almonds smell of cyanide. The almond tree, *Prunus amygdalus*, contains the cyanohydrin, amygdalin. The ataxic neuropathy produced by cassava is, therefore, a cultural problem, brought about by over-reliance on a single cyanogenetic plant for subsistence.

## 4. CONCLUSIONS

Neurotoxicity from plant metabolites is common outside of North America, western Europe, and a few other developed nations. Poisoning often results from a concatenation of circumstance, of which consumption of a neurotoxic plant is only one link in the chain. Climatic factors, such as drought, protein and calorie malnutrition, and economic and cultural factors, all combine in the expression of neurotoxicity. Economic factors are involved in the heavy reliance on one species, such as cassava, for nutrition or the inability to purchase fertilizers for the growing of nontoxic crops. Cultural and political factors were involved in the re-emergence in Europe of lathyrism and ergotism in German forced-labor camps during the Second World War, and in the heavy reliance of *Cycas* flour in the

Mariana Islands during the Japanese occupation in the same war. As with the *Cycas* poisonings, there may be a long latency between exposure to environmental factors and the clinical expression of a disorder (Calne *et al.*, 1986).

In countries having complex industrial economies, occasional epidemics of neurotoxicity occur, as in the recurrence of ergotism in France 40 years ago. However, neurotoxicity in more recent times is usually due to consumption of foods other than plants, as with the outbreak of domoic acid poisoning from contaminated mussels in Canada (although the mussels, in turn, obtained the toxin from a plant). Poisonings due to the deliberate consumption of psychoactive plants or chemical derived from them is common. *Datura* intoxication is well known in emergency rooms and poison control centers in North America.

Fundamental to most cultures is the routine use of stimulants and depressants in pharmacological doses. In western societies, such use is so pervasive that many do not consider such substances to be drugs. But how many among us could get through the diurnal cycle with its ephemeral anxieties and pressures without the assistance of coffee, tea, tobacco, alcohol, or cocoa, or their illegal cousins marijuana, cocaine, or heroin?

Plant neurotoxins have been of inestimable value to pharmacology. The toxicities of one age become the tools of progress of another. Ergot has changed from being a feared and fearsome disease into the source of valuable pharmaceutical agents. Plant excitotoxins are being used to unravel the complexity of amino acid receptors in the brain, cocaine and reserpine were tools in the elucidation of sympathetic function, and caffeine in the parallel study of purinergic receptors. The value to pharmacology of muscarine, nicotine, morphine, atropine, and a Pandora's box of other plant neurotoxins is obvious to any pharmacologist.

The neurotoxicities of plant products may mimic or model other natural processes. This is an increasingly important aspect of research on these compounds. Thus, excitotoxin-induced neuronal degeneration mimics diseases such as Alzheimer's or Parkinson's disease, and may model the process of aging in the central nervous system (Calne *et al.*, 1986).

In the main, knowledge of these valuable compounds has stemmed either from the health problems generated by the plants containing them, or by investigation of plants used ethnobotanically, i.e., for specific cultural uses. What is perhaps not so obvious is that progress in the neurosciences continues to depend on the study of novel natural products. For such progress to continue, the ethnobotanical knowledge of vanishing cultures must be recorded (e.g., see Schultes and Raffauf, 1990) and the accelerating rate of human-induced extinction of plant species slowed.

Man is a poor organic chemist compared to nature, and nature will continue to inspire our synthetic efforts. Within the last 30 years, kainic acid was obtained from an obscure alga, and the potent antineoplastic dolastatins from the insignificant sea hare, *Dolabella auricularia* (Pettit *et al.*, 1982). The clinically important anticancer agents, vincristine and vinblastine, were isolated from the unconsidered Madagascar periwinkle, *Catharanthus roseus*, examined because of its ethnomedical use. Yet the Malagasy Republic on Madagascar encompasses one of the most degraded ecosystems on the planet, one in which numerous unstudied plants have become extinct. From a purely utilitarian point of view, no species can be considered to be without value; a useless species is one for which a use is waiting to be discovered, not one without use. Thus, *Ginkgo biloba,* a plant that fortuitously escaped the extinction of all other species in its family, has proven to be the source of unique pharmacological agents (Max, 1987). We can only wonder at what never-to-be discovered pharmacological agents have been lost forever with the heedless and accelerating extermination of plant species over the last few decades.

## REFERENCES

Agid, Y., Pertuiset, B., and Dubois, B., 1988, Motoneuron disease as manifestation of lupin seed toxicity, *Lancet* 1:1347.
Albert-Puleo, M., 1978, Mythobotany and pharmacology of thujone, *Econ. Bot.* 32:65–74.
Aldridge, A., Aranda, J.V., and Neims, A.H., 1979, Caffeine metabolism in the newborn, *Clin. Pharmacol. Ther.* 25:447–453.
Anderson, E.F., 1980, *Peyote: The Divine Cactus*, University of Arizona, Tucson.
Anderson, F.H., Richardson, E.P., Okazaki, H., and Brody, J.A., 1975, Neurofibrillary degeneration of Guam: Frequency in Chamorros and non-Chamorros with no known neurologic disease, *Brain* 102:65–77.
Andrews, J., 1984, *Peppers: The Domesticated Capsicums*, University of Texas, Austin, TX.
Anonymous, 1869, Absinthe and alcohol. *Lancet* 1:336–336.
Anonymous, 1984, Datura poisoning from hamburger—Canada, *Morbid. Mortal. Week. Rep.* 33:282–283.
Aranda, J.V., Cook, C.E., Gorman, W., Collinge, J.M., Loughnan, P.M., Outerbridge, E.W., Aldridge, A., and Neims, A.H., 1979, Pharmacokinetic profile of caffeine in the premature newborn infant with apnea, *J. Pediat.* 94:663–668.
Arnold, W.N., 1988, Vincent van Gogh and the thujone connection. *JAMA* 260:3042–3044.
Arnold, W.N., 1989, Absinthe, *Sci. Am.* 260:112–117.
Awang, D.V.C., and Kindack, D.G., 1989, Atropine as possible contaminant of comfrey tea, *Lancet* 1:44.
Balbaa, S.I., Zaki, A.Y., Abdel-Wahab, S.M., El-Denshary, E.S.M., and Motazz-Bellah, M., 1973, Preliminary phytochemical and pharmacological investigation of roots of different species of *Chicorium intybus*, *Planta Med.* 24:133–144.
Barger, G., 1931, *Ergot and Ergotism*, Gurney and Jackson, London.
Bates, R.B., and Sigel, C.W., 1963, Terpenoids cis-trans- and trans-cis-nepetalactones, *Experientia* 19:564–565.
Battersby, A.R., Binks, R., Francis, R.J., McCaldin, D.J., and Ramuz, H., 1964, Alkaloid biosynthesis. Part IV. 1-benzylisoquinolines as precursors of thebaine, codeine, and morphine, *J. Chem. Soc.* 3600–3610.
Beach, W., 1860, Absinthism, *Am. J. Pharm.* 40:356–360.
Brenneisen, R., Geisshusler, S., and Schorno, X., 1986, Metabolism of cathinone to (−)-norephedrine and (−)-norpseudoephedrine, *J. Pharm. Pharmacol.* 38:298–300.
Brody, J.A., Edgar, A.H., and Gellapse, M.M., 1979, Amyotrophic lateral sclerosis: No increase among U.S. construction workers in Guam, *JAMA* 240:551–552.
Buck, S.H., and Burks, T.F., 1986, The neuropharmacology of capsaicin: Review of some recent observations, *Pharmacol. Rev.* 38:179–226.
Budavari, S., 1989, *The Merck Index*, 11th ed., Merck & Co., Rahway, NJ.
Calne, D.B., McGeer, E., Eisen, A., and Spencer, P., 1986, Alzheimer's disease, Parkinson's disease, and motoneurone disease: A biotropic interaction between ageing and environment? *Lancet* 2:1067–1070.
Chase, M., 1991, Cancer drug may save many human lives—at cost of rare tree, *Wall Street Journal* April 9:A1–A1.
Chen, K.-M., 1981, Neurofibrillary changes on Guam, *Arch. Neurol.* 38:16–18.
Chen, K.-M., and Yase, Y., 1985, Parkinsonism-dementia, neurofibrillary tangles, and trace elements in the Western Pacific, in: *Senile Dementia of the Alzheimer Type* (J.T. Hutton and A.D. Kenny, eds.), Alan R. Liss, New York, pp. 153–173.
Cliff, J., Lundgrist, P., Mårtensson, J., Rosling, H., and Sörbo, B., 1985, Association of high cyanide and low sulphur intake in cassava-induced spastic parapesis, *Lancet* 2:1211–1212.
Cornish, H.H., and Christman, A.A., 1957, A study of the metabolism of theobromine, theophylline, and caffeine in man, *J. Biol. Chem.* 228:315–323.
Dalvi, R.R., 1986, Acute and chronic toxicity of caffeine: A review, *Vet Hum. Toxicol.* 28:144–150.
Dalvi, R.R., and Bowie, W.C. 1983, Toxicology of solanine: An overview, *Vet. Hum. Toxicol.* 25:13–15.
de Quincey, T., 1948, *The Confessions of an English Opium Eater*, 2nd ed., Folio, London.
Dekant, W., Vamvakas, S., and Anders, M.W., 1989, Bioactivation of nephrotoxic haloalkenes by glutathione conjugation: Formation of toxic and mutagenic intermediates by cysteine conjugate β-lyase, *Drug Metab. Rev.* 20:43–83.
del Castillo, J., Anderson, M., and Rubottom, G.M., 1975, Marijuana, absinthe and the central nervous system, *Nature* 253:365–366.
Dews, P.B., 1984, *Caffeine*, Springer-Verlag, Berlin.
Dobkin de Rios, M., 1984, *Hallucinogens: Cross-Cultural Perspectives*, University of New Mexico, Albuquerque.
Duncan, M.W., and Kopin, I.J., 1989, Quantification of the putative neurotoxin 2-amino-3-(methylamino)propanoic acid (BMAA) in cycadales: Analysis of the seeds of some members of the family cycadaceae, *J. Anal. Toxicol.* 13:169–175.
Duncan, M.W., Kopin, I.J. Garruto, R.M., Lavine, L., and Markey, S.P., 1988, 2-amino-3 (methylamino)-propionic acid in cycad-derived foods is an unlikely cause of amyotrophic lateral sclerosis parkinsonism, *Lancet* 2:631–632.
Early, D.F., 1961, Pennyroyal: A rare case of epilepsy, *Lancet* 2:580–581.
Efron, D.H., Holmstedt, B., and Kline, N.S., 1979, *Ethnopharmacologic Search for Psychoactive Drugs*, Raven Press, New York.
Elmi, A.S., 1983, The chemistry of khat in Somalia, *J. Ethnopharmacol.* 8:163–176.

Emboden, W., 1979, *Narcotic Plants: Hallucinogens, Stimulants, Inebriants, and Hypnotics, their Origins and Uses,* MacMillan, New York.
Faguet, R.A., and Rowland, K.F., 1978, "Spice cabinet" intoxication, *Am. J. Psychiatry* 135:860–861.
Feenaghty, D.A., 1982, Atropine poisoning: Jimsonweed, *J. Emerg. Nurs.* 8:139–141.
Flattery, D., and Schwartz, M., 1989, *Haoma and Harmaline. The Botanical Identity of the Indo-European Sacred Hallucinogen "Soma" and its Legacy in Religion, Language, and Middle Eastern Folklore,* University of California, Berkeley.
Ford, C.S., 1979, Ethnographical aspects of kava, in: *Ethnopharmacologic Search for Psychoactive Drugs,* (D.H. Efron, B. Holmstedt, and N.S. Kline, eds.), Raven Press, New York, pp. 162–181.
Gandhi, M., Lal, R., Sankaranarayanan, A., Banerjee, C.K., and Sharma, P.L., 1988, Acute toxicity study of the oil from *Azadirachta indica* seed (neem oil), *J. Ethnopharm.* 23:39–51.
Gardner, A.F., and Sakiewicz, N., 1963, A review of neurolathyrism including the Russian and Polish literature, *Exp. Med. Surg.* 21:164–191.
Garruto, R.M., and Yase, Y., 1986, Neurodegenerative disorders of the western Pacific: The search for mechanisms of pathogenesis, *TINS* 9:368–374.
Garruto, R.M., Yanagihara, R., and Gajdusek, D.C., 1988, Cycads and amyotrophic lateral sclerosis/parkinsonism dementia, *Lancet* 2:1079.
Geisshüsler, S., and Brenneisen, R., 1987, The content of psychoactive phenylpropyl and phenylpentenyl khatamines in *Catha edulis* Forsk. of different origin, *J. Ethnopharmacol.* 19:269–277.
Gilks, C.F., 1988, Cycads and sago, *Lancet* 1:181–182.
Goodman, L., Gilman, A., Rall, T.W., Nies, A.S., and Taylor, P., 1990, *The Pharmacological Basis of Therapeutics,* 8th ed., Pergamon Press, New York.
Goodman, L., and Gilman, A., 1958, *The Pharmacological Basis of Therapeutics,* 2nd ed., Macmillan, New York.
Gould, D.H., and Gustine, D.L., 1982, Basal ganglia degeneration, myelin alterations, and enzyme inhibition induced in mice by the plant toxin 3-nitropropanoic acid, *Neuropath. Appl. Neurobiol.* 8:377–393.
Grobbee, D.E., Rimm, E.B., Giovannucci, E., Colditz, G., Stampfer, M., and Willett, W., 1990, Coffee, caffeine, and cardiovascular disease in men, *N. Engl. J. Med.* 323:1026–1032.
Guenther, E., 1952, *The Essential Oils, Vol. V,* Van Nostrand, New York.
Hendriks, H., Bos, R., Allersma, D.P., Malingre, T.M., and Koster, A.S., 1981, Pharmacological screening of valerenal and some other components of essential oil of *Valeriana officinalis, Planta Med.* 42:62–68.
Hoffer, A., and Osmond, H., 1967, *The Hallucinogens,* Academic Press, New York.
Hollister, L.E., 1986, Health aspects of cannabis, *Pharmacol. Rev.* 38:1–20.
Hollt, V., 1986, Opioid peptide processing and receptor selectivity, *Ann. Rev. Pharmacol. Toxicol.* 26:59–77.
Holtzman, S.G., 1990, Caffeine as a model drug of abuse, *TIPS* 11:355–356.
Howlett, A.C., Bidaut-Russell, M., Devane, W.A., Melvin, L.S., Johnson, M.R., and Herkenham, M., 1990, The cannabinoid receptor: Biochemical, anatomical and behavioral characterization, *TINS* 13:420–423.
Hughes, J., and Kosterlitz, H.W., 1975, Isolation of an endogenous compound from brain with pharmacological properties similar to morphine, *Brain Res.* 88:295–308.
Huxley, A., 1969, *The letters of Aldous Huxley,* Harper and Row, New York, p. 110.
Huxley, A., 1970, *The Doors of Perception,* Harper and Row, New York.
Huxtable, R.J., 1986, Thiols, disulfides, and thioesters, in: *The Biochemistry of Sulfur* Plenum Press, New York, pp. 199–268.
Huxtable, R.J., 1990a, Activation and pulmonary toxicity of pyrrolizidine alkaloids, *Pharmacol. Ther.* 47:371–389.
Huxtable, R.J., 1990b, The harmful potential of herbal and other plant products, *Drug Safety* 5 (Suppl. 1):126–136.
Jackson, B., and Reed, A., 1969, Catnip and the alteration of consciousness, *JAMA* 207:1349–1350.
Jadhav, S.J., Sharma, R.P., and Salunkhe, D.K., 1981, Naturally occurring toxic alkaloids in foods, *CRC Crit. Rev. Tox.* 9:21–104.
Jones, K., 1990, S'more on Soma, *HerbalGram* 23:46–47.
Kingsbury, J.M., 1964, *Poisonous Plants of the United States and Canada,* Prentice-Hall, Englewood Cliffs, NJ.
Kjaer, A., 1976, Glycosinolates in the Cruciferae, in: *The Biology and Chemistry of the Cruciferae,* (J.G. Vaughan, A.J. MacLeod, and B.M.G. Jones, eds.), Academic Press, London, p. 207.
Kjaer, A., 1978, Glucosinolates and other naturally occurring O-sulfates, in: *Carbohydrate Sulfates* (R.G. Schweiger, ed.), American Chemical Society, Washington, D.C., pp. 19–28.
Klohs, M.W., 1979, Chemistry of kava, in: *Ethnopharmacologic Search for Psychoactive Drugs,* (D.H. Efron, B. Holmstedt, and N.S. Kline, eds.), Raven Press, New York, pp. 126–132.
Koob, M., and Dekant, W., 1991, Bioactivation of xenobiotics by formation of toxic glutathione conjugates, *Chem. Biol. Interact.* 77:107–136.
Kurland, L.T., 1988, Amyotrophic lateral sclerosis and Parkinson's disease complex on Guam linked to an environmental neurotoxin, *Trends Neurosci.* 11:51–54.
Leathwood, P.D., Chauffard, F., Heck, E., and Munoz-Box, R., 1982, Aqueous extract of valerian root (*Valeriana officinalis* L.) improves sleep quality in man, *Pharmacol. Biochem. Behav.* 17:65–71.
Liener, I.E., 1974, The nutritional significance of naturally occurring toxins in plant foodstuffs, in: *Toxic Constituents of Animal Foodstuffs,* Academic Press, New York, pp. 72–94.
Liener, I.E., 1983, Naturally occurring toxicants in foods and their significance in the human diet, *Arch. Toxicol.* Suppl. 6:153–166.

Lindstrom, H., Luthman, J., Mouton, P., Spencer, P., and Olson, L., 1990, Plant-derived neurotoxic amino acids (β-N-methylamino-L-alanine): Effects on central neurons, *J. Neurochem.* 55:941–949.

Lipton, R.B., Apfel, S.C., Dutcher, J.P., Rosenberg, R., Kaplan, J., Berger, A., Einzig, A.I., Wiernik, P., and Schaumburg, H.H., 1991, Taxol produces a predominantly sensory neuropathy, *Neurology* 39:368–373.

Ludolph, A.C., Hugon, J., Dwivedi, M.P., Schaumburg, H.H., and Spencer, P.S., 1987, Studies on the aetiology and pathogenesis of motor neuron diseases, *Brain* 110:149–165.

Majno, G., 1977, *The Healing Hand: Man and Wound in the Ancient World*, Harvard University Press, Cambridge, MA, p. 111.

Manno, B.R., and Manno, J.E., 1977, Toxicology of ipecac: A review, *Clin. Toxicol.* 10:221–242.

Martin, B.R., 1986, Cellular effects of cannabinoids, *Pharmacol. Rev.* 38:45–74.

Matossian, M.K., 1989, *Poisons of the Past: Molds, Epidemics and History*, Yale University Press, New Haven, CT.

Max, B., 1986, This and that: Please the patient and pass the coffee, *TIPS* 7:12–14.

Max, B., 1987, This and that: Survival and certainty, *TIPS* 8:290–292.

Max, B., 1988a, This and that: Thanatomimetics, bradychronotoxins, osmocides and ototoxins, *TIPS* 9:353–356.

Max, B., 1988b, This and that: An odorless crime and the mystery of a poet's heart, *TIPS* 9:276–278.

McCaleb, R., 1990, The search for soma, *HerbalGram* 22:14–15.

McIntyre, A.R., 1972, History of curare, in: *Neuromuscular Blocking and Stimulating Agents, Vol. I. International Encyclopedia of Pharmacology and Therapeutics* (J. Cheymol, ed.), Pergamon Press, Oxford, pp. 187–203.

Merlin, M.D., 1984, *On the Trail of the Ancient Opium Poppy*, Fairleigh Dickinson University, London.

Morrow, J.S., Keim, P., and Gurn, F.R.N., 1974, $CO_2$ adducts of certain amino acids, peptides, and sperm whale myoglobin studied by carbon 13 and proton nuclear magnetic resonance, *J. Biol. Chem.* 249:7484–7494.

Myerhoff, B.G., 1974, *Peyote Hunt: The Sacred Journey of the Huichol Indians*, Cornell University Press, Ithaca, NY.

Nakamoto, T., Hartman, A.D., and Joseph, F., Jr., 1989, Interaction between caffeine intake and nutritional status on growing brains in newborn rats, *Ann. Nutr. Metab.* 33:92–99.

Nunn, P.B., and O'Brien, P., 1989, The interaction of β-N-methylamino-L-alanine with bicarbonate: An $^1$H-NMR study, *FEBS Lett.* 251:31–35.

Nunn, P.B., Seelig, M., Zagoren, J.C., and Spencer, P.S., 1987, Stereospecific acute neuronotoxicity of "uncommon" plant amino acids linked to human motor-system diseases, *Brain Res.* 410:375–379.

Nunn, P.B., Davis, A.J., and O'Brien, P., 1991, Carbamate formation and the neurotoxicity of L-α amino acids, *Science* 251:1619.

Olney, J.W., Misra, C.H., and Rhee, V., 1976, Brain and retinal damage from *Lathyrus* excitotoxin, β-N-oxalyl-L-α,β-diaminopropionic acid, *Nature* 264:659–661.

Olsen, P., and Thorup, I., 1984, Neurotoxicity in rats dosed with peppermint oil and pulegone, *Arch. Toxicol.* 57:408–409.

Pettit, G.R., Kamano, Y., Brown, P., Gust, D., Inoue, M., and Herald, C.L., 1982, Structure of the cyclic peptide dolastatin 3 from *Dolabella auricularia*, *J. Am. Chem. Soc.* 104:905–907.

Pinto-Scognamiglio, W., 1968, Effects of thujone on spontaneous activity and conditioned behavior in rats, *Boll. Chim. Farm.* 107:780–791.

Polsky, F.I., Nunn, P.B., and Bell, E.A., 1972, Distribution and toxicity of α-amino-β-methylaminopropionic acid, *Fed. Proc.* 5:1473–1475.

Razdan, R.K., 1986, Structure-activity relationships in cannabinoids, *Pharmacol. Rev.* 38:75–149.

Ressler, C., Nigam, S.N., and Giza, Y.-H., 1969, Toxic principle in vetch: Isolation and identification of γ-L-glutamyl-L-β-cyanoalanine from common vetch seeds. Distribution in some legumes, *J. Am. Chem. Soc.* 91:2758–2765.

Roman, G.C., Spencer, P.S., and Schoenberg, B.S., 1985, Tropical myeloneuropathies: The hidden endemias, *Neurology* 35:1158–1170.

Rowland, L.P., 1984, Motor neuron diseases and amyotrophic lateral sclerosis, *TINS* 7:110–112.

Rowland, L.P., 1987, Motor neuron diseases and amyotrophic lateral sclerosis: Research progress, *TINS* 10:393–398.

Roy, D.N., 1981, Toxic amino acids and proteins from *Lathyrus* plants and other leguminous species: A literature review, *Nutr. Abstr. Rev.* A 51:691–707.

Schultes, R.E., and Hofmann, A., 1979, *Plants of the Gods: Origins of Hallucinogenic Use*, McGraw-Hill, New York.

Schultes, R.E., and Hofmann, A., 1980, *The Botany and Chemistry of Hallucinogens*, 2nd ed., Charles C. Thomas, Springfield, IL.

Schultes, R.E., and Raffauf, R.F., 1990, *The Healing Forest: Medicinal and Toxic Plants of the Northwest Amazonia*, Dioscorides Press, Portland, OR.

Sharma, R.P., and Salunkhe, D.K., 1989, Solanum glycoalkaloids, in: *Toxicants of Plant Origin, Vol. I Alkaloids* (P.R. Cheeke, ed.), CRC Press, Boca Raton, FL, pp. 179–236.

Shulgin, A.T., Sargent, T., and Naranjo, C., 1979, The chemistry and psychopharmacology of nutmeg and of several related phenylisopropylamines, in: *Ethnopharmacologic Search for Psychoactive Drugs* (D.H. Efron, B. Holmstedt, and N.S. Kline, eds.), Raven Press, New York, pp. 201.

Siegel, R.K., 1976, Herbal intoxication: Psychoactive effects from herbal cigarettes, tea and capsules, *JAMA* 236:473–476.

Simonsen, J.L., 1949, *The Terpenes, Vol. 2*, University Press, Cambridge.

Sinniah, R., Sinniah, D., Chia, L., and Baskaran, G., 1989, Animal model of margosa oil ingestion with Reye-like syndrome. Pathogenesis of microvesicular fatty liver, *J. Pathol.* 159:255–264.

Snodgrass, S.R., 1990, Neurologic sequelae after ingestion of mussels contaminated with domoic acid, *N. Engl. J. Med.* 323:1631.

Sollmann, T.A., 1948, *Manual of Pharmacology and its Applications to Therapeutic Toxicology*, 7th ed., W.B. Saunders, Philadelphia.

Spencer, P.S., 1987, Guam ALS/Parkinsonism-dementia: A long-latency neurotoxic disorder caused by "slow toxin(s)" in food? *Can. J. Neurol. Sci.* 14:347–357.

Spencer, P.S., and Schaumburg, H.H., 1983, Lathyrism: A neurotoxic disease, *Neurobehav. Toxicol.* 5:625–629.

Spencer, P.S., Ludolph, A., Dwidedi, M.P., Roy, D.N., Hugon, J., and Schumburg, H.H., 1986, Lathryism: Evidence for role of the neuroexcitatory amino acid BOAA, *Lancet* 2:1066–1067.

Spencer, P.S., Hugon, J., Ludolph, A., Nunn, P.B., Ross, S.M., Roy, D.N., and Schaumburg, H.H., 1987, Discovery and partial characterization of primate motor-system toxins, *CIBA Foundation Symposium* 126:221–238.

Spencer, P.S., Nunn, P.B., Hugon, J., Ludoph, A.C., Ross, S.M., Roy, D.N., and Robertson, R.C., 1987, Guam amyotrophic lateral sclerosis-Parkinsonism-dementia linked to a plant excitant neurotoxin, *Science* 237:517–522.

Spencer, P.S., Ohta, M., and Palmer, V.S., 1987, Cycad use and motor neurone disease in Kii peninsula of Japan, *Lancet* 2:1462–1463.

Spencer, P.S., Ross, S.M., Nunn, P.B., Roy, D.N., and Seelig, M., 1987, Detection and characterization of plant-derived amino acid motorsystem toxins in mouse CNS cultures, in: *Model Systems in Neurotoxicology: Alternative Approaches to Animal Testing* (A. Sahar and A.M. Goldberg, eds.), Alan R. Liss, New York, pp. 349–361.

Spiller, G.A., 1984, *The Methylxanthine Beverages and Food: Chemistry, Consumption and Health Effects*, Alan R. Liss, New York.

Stavric, B., 1988a, Methylxanthines: Toxicity to humans. 2. Caffeine, *Food Chem. Toxicol.* 26:645–662.

Stavric, B., 1988b, Methylxanthines: Toxicity to humans. 3. Theobromine, paraxanthine and the combined effects of methylxanthines, *Food Chem. Toxicol.* 26:725–733.

Sturtevant, E.L., 1919, *Sturtevant's Notes on Edible Plants*, New York Agricultural Experimental Station, Geneva, NY.

Swain, T., 1975, *Plants in the Development of Modern Medicine*, Harvard University Press, Cambridge, MA.

Takemoto, T., 1978, Isolation and structural identification of naturally occurring excitatory amino acids, in: *Kainic Acid as a Tool in Neurobiology* (E.G. McGeer, J.W. Olney, and P.L. McGeer, eds.), Raven Press, New York, pp. 1–15.

Teitelbaum, J.S., Zatorre, R.J., Carpenter, S., Gendron, D., Evans, A.C., Gjedde, A., and Cashman, N.R., 1990, Neurologic sequelae of domoic acid intoxication due to the ingestion of contaminated mussels. *N. Engl. J. Med.* 322:1781–1787.

Tekle Heimanot, R., Kidane, Y., Wuhib, E., Kalissa, A., Alemu, T., Zein, Z.A., and Spencer, P.S., 1990, Lathyrism in rural northwestern Ethiopia: A highly prevalent neurotoxic disorder, *Int. J. Epidemiol.* 19:664–672.

Trollope, A., 1983, *The Letters of Anthony Trollope, Vol. 2, 1871–1882*, Stanford University Press, Stanford, CA, p. 982.

Tyler, V.E., 1963, Poisonous mushrooms, *Prog. Chem. Toxicol.* 1:339–384.

Tyler, V.E., 1982, *The Honest Herbal: A Sensible Guide to Herbs and Related Remedies*, George F. Stickley Co., Philadelphia.

Urich, R.W., Bowerman, D.L., Levisky, J.A., and Pflug, J.L., 1982, *Datura stramonium*: A fatal poisoning, *J. Forensic Sci.* 948–954.

Vogt, D.D., 1981, Absinthium: A nineteenth-century drug of abuse, *J. Ethnopharmacol.* 4:337–342.

Vogt, D.D., and Montagne, M., 1982, Absinthe: Behind the emerald mask, *Int. J. Addict.* 17:1015–1029.

Walton, J., Beeson, P.B., and Scott, R.B., 1986, *The Oxford Companion to Medicine, Vol. I A–M*, Oxford University Press, Oxford.

Wasson, R.G., 1968, *Soma: Divine Mushroom of Immortality*, Harcourt, Brace & World, The Hague.

Wasson, R.G., 1979, Fly agaric and man, in: *Ethnopharmacologic Search for Psychoactive Drugs* (D.H. Efron, B. Holmstedt, and N.S. Kline, eds.), Raven Press, New York, pp. 405–414.

Wasson, R.G., 1980, *The Wondrous Mushroom: Mycolatry in Mesoamerica*, McGraw-Hill, New York.

Watkins, J.C., Curtis, D.R., and Biscoe, T.J., 1966, Central effects of $\beta$-N-oxalyl-$\alpha,\beta$-diaminopropionic acid and other *Lathyrus* factors, *Nature* 211:637.

Weiss, J.L., and Choi, D.W., 1988, Beta-N-methylamino-L-alanine neurotoxicity: Requirement for bicarbonate as a cofactor, *Science* 241:973–975.

Wheelwright, E.G., 1974, *Medicinal Plants and their History*, Dover Publications, New York.

Whiting, M.G., 1963, Toxicity of cycads, *Econ. Bot.* 17:271–302.

Williams, M.C., and James, L.F., 1978, Livestock poisoning from nitro-bearing *Astragalus*, in: *Effects of Poisonous Plants on Livestock* (R.F. Keeler, K.R. VanKampen, and L.F. James, eds.), Academic Press, New York, pp. 379–389.

Zhang, Z., Anderson, D.W., and Mantel, N., 1990, Geographic patterns of Parkinsonian-dementia complex on Guam, *Arch. Neurol.* 47:1069–1074.

Chapter 5

# "Malnutrition" and the Vulnerable Brain

## What a Difference a Molecule Makes

*Roger W. Russell*

## 1. FROM MOLECULES TO BEHAVIOR

"... we are what we eat. More correctly, we are the atoms we eat" (Spallholz, 1989). "What we are" includes measurable properties from molecules to the behavior of the "integrated organism" as it adjusts to its physical and psychosocial environments (Russell, 1990). The latter are the final outcome of a sequence of events, among which initial binding of a molecule to its receptor is the first. Food can only produce effects at any of these levels as a result of physiochemical interactions between the molecules of which it is composed and receptor sites on biologically active molecules present in the body (Doull, 1980). The former may range greatly in the structures of their atoms. However, they may also closely resemble each other, having only one difference in chemical structure (isomers) or in the arrangements of their atoms (stereoisomers). A quarter century ago, "... it was shown that brain neurochemistry could be readily altered by the composition of food consumed" (Krasnegor *et al.*, 1990). The ingestion of many substances is essential to maintaining the health and general well-being of the organism. Others may be detrimental, even life threatening (Albert, 1987). As its title indicates, this chapter is concerned primarily with the latter.

It is essential at the very beginning of our discussion to differentiate clearly between the meanings of *malnutrition* and *undernutrition*. Within the present context *malnutrition* (as defective nutrition) differs from *undernutrition*. The latter refers to an insufficient

---

Roger W. Russell • Center for the Neurobiology of Learning and Memory and Department of Psychobiology, University of California, Irvine, California 92717.
*The Vulnerable Brain and Environmental Risks, Volume 1: Malnutrition and Hazard Assessment*, edited by Robert L. Isaacson and Karl F. Jensen. Plenum Press, New York, 1992.

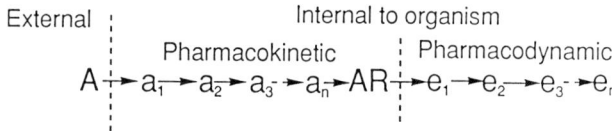

**FIGURE 1.** Schematic representation of the sequence of events occurring between the ingestion of a substance into the body and its neurobehavioral effects. Substance A is transported to its site of action, $a_1$ to $a_n$, where it binds to its specific receptor, R, initiating an extensive series of events, $e_1$ to $e_n$, ending eventually with its effects on behavior. Biotransformation may occur during $a_1$ to $a_n$; thus, binding to R may involve A's metabolic product(s) rather than A in its original form.

intake of substances necessary to maintain normal growth, maintenance, and repair of the body and its constituent parts, i.e., to a caloric deficit. As the term is used here, *malnutrition* always involves dietary imbalance (Scrimshaw and Gordon, 1968). It includes both the ingestion of substances that are inadequate or excessive for, or toxic to, normal nutritional requirements and also aberrant conditions within the organism that interfere with the normal metabolism of substances included in the normal diet.

Effects of malnutrition thus defined may be evidenced at any of many points in the chain of events connecting the ingestion of a substance to its neurobehavioral endpoint(s). This progression is shown schematically in Figure 1. Events $a_1$ to $a_n$ represent processes by which a chemical, A, reaches its site of action. The transport of A to its receptor may involve progress through several different membranes and chemical milieu. During this period, A is a target for biotransformation, which, as we shall see, may produce a molecule that is much different in terms of its neurobehavioral effects than the parent substance. The binding of A to its receptor may be reversible or irreversible. If irreversible, receptors must be synthesized de novo before their normal population numbers are re-established. Effects $e_1$ to $e_n$ following formation of the AR complex are independent of those preceding it, but may be influenced by interactions with other processes within the body that are underway simultaneously. *Malnutrition* in its present meaning may involve events occurring at any one or several points in this overall schema. The size of the literature relevant to this broad range of topics is very considerable. Obviously it has not been possible to include it all in this brief review. Therefore, the paragraphs that follow look at representative examples only.

Anyone studying effects of malnutrition cannot but be impressed by the magnitude of changes in behavior that may be associated with even very small differences in molecular structures. If you have ever, in confusion, put castor oil rather than olive oil on your salad, you know the differences in effects of behavior! Yet, the only difference between the two molecules is a hydroxyl group in the same basic molecule. Small differences in molecular structure may also affect the "vulnerable brain," with consequent effects on behavior. Molecules may enter the body through several different routes. For present purposes, however, our discussion will concentrate on substances ingested. These include not only food and drink, but also chemicals taken for therapeutic purposes or for "kicks." It will be important to keep in mind that there are individual differences in reactions to such compounds: "There are inherent risks in eating that we must take in order to live" (Kilgore and Li, 1980). Adverse effects may not appear immediately. Some may become apparent only after chronic or repeated exposures, i.e., as "neurobehavioral time bombs"

## 2. DIFFERENCES IN MOLECULAR "CONFIGURATION"

Two or more compounds may possess the same molecular or structural formulas but be different in configuration, i.e., in the spatial relationships of their atoms, as illustrated by the position of the OH group in Figure 2 (Testa and Mayer, 1988). Differential effects of the "stereoisomers" on the CNS and, hence, on behavior may, however, be very significant. The introduction of levodopa (L-dihydroxyphenylalanine) for the treatment of Parkinson's disease provides an excellent example of compensation for a CNS deficiency by the selective ingestion of a particular stereoisomer. Behaviorally Parkinson's syndrome is characterized by chronic progressive motor disfunction, evidenced particularly as tremor, rigidity, and akinesia. The discovery that striatal dopamine concentrations are one tenth or less than normal in the brains of patients with parkinsonism linked the neurotransmitter dopamine to these behavioral anomalies (Hornykiewicz, 1966). Dopamine was known to be the predominant transmitter of the mammalian extrapyramidal system. An obvious means for correcting the deficiency would be to raise central dopaminergic levels. However, it was also known that dopamine could not cross the blood–brain barrier. An alternative was to administer its precursor, dopa, which did have this capability. Early trials in patients with Parkinson's disease using high oral doses of DL-dopa reported equivocal results. These were followed by trials with L-dopa, the active isomer, which was found to be less toxic and clearly effective to the extent that it gained approval for general therapeutic use. Much experimental research involving the use of animal models has focused on differentiating neurobehavioral effects of other stereoisomers, such as D- and L-amphetamine (Segal, 1975). These examples illustrate how the ingestion of molecules with the same molecular constitution and that differ only in their spatial configurations can lead to very diverse behavioral effects.

## 3. A MISSING MOLECULE: GENETIC ERRORS OF METABOLISM

". . . some individuals, or, indeed, some groups of humankind may find it difficult to deal with certain types of food because of inherited errors of metabolism" (Patrice *et*

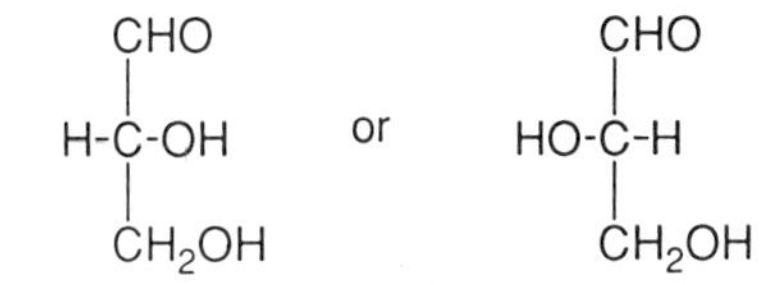

**FIGURE 2.** Differences in molecular "configuration" may have significantly disparate neurobehavioral effects. Different spatial relationships are shown in the OH group of the two stereoisomers of this relatively simple molecule.

$$\begin{array}{ccc} \text{CHO} & & \text{CHO} \\ | & & | \\ \text{H-C-OH} & \text{or} & \text{HO-C-H} \\ | & & | \\ \text{CH}_2\text{OH} & & \text{CH}_2\text{OH} \\ \textit{dextro-isomer} & & \textit{levo-isomer} \end{array}$$

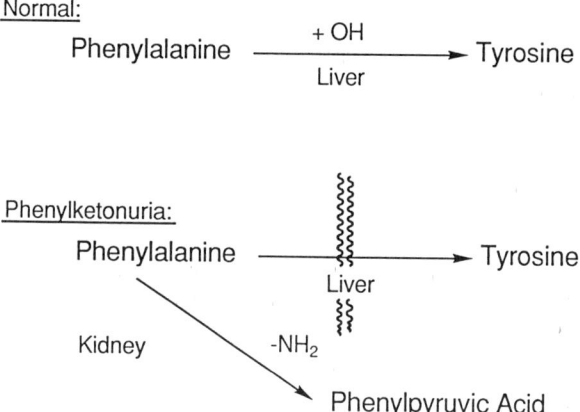

**FIGURE 3.** Phenylketonuria, a genetic error of metabolism, results from an absence of the enzyme phenylalanine hydroxylase, which is required for the breakdown of phenylalanine during its normal conversion to tyrosine. This disrupts the synthesis of the catecholaminergic neurotransmitters, which are essential for normal behavior. Effects are evidenced neurobehaviorally as mental retardation.

*al.*, 1982). One of the difficulties may appear as very significant neurobehavioral malfunctions. A genetic fault that results in failure to produce an enzyme essential to normal CNS functioning serves as an example. In the preceding section attention was focused on the ingestion of a substance as a means of reversing a neurochemical deficiency in the CNS and its adverse neurobehavioral consequences. The present example illustrates how restrictions on food ingested may be used to offset another kind of neurochemical error.

For many years it has been known that inherited metabolic faults observable in humans are understandable if it is assumed that in each case the body fails to carry out one particular step in a normal series of biochemical events. Perhaps best known of these faults is the disorder phenylketonuria (PKU). As illustrated in Figure 3, in this case the error occurs in the breakdown of the amino acid, phenylalanine, during its normal conversion to tyrosine en route to the synthesis of the catecholaminergic neurotransmitters (dopamine, noradrenaline, and adrenaline). The condition results from the missing enzyme, phenylalanine hydroxylase, and is identified by excretion in urine of excessive amounts of phenylalanine and its conversion products. One or more of these are toxic, especially in infants, in whom high blood concentrations produce brain damage, resulting in such neurobehavioral abnormalities as mental retardation. Very early diagnosis can lead to dietary controls designed to lower the blood concentration of phenylalanine and, thus, to eliminate the adverse neurobehavioral effects of PKU.

There are other examples of inborn errors of metabolism, e.g., alkaptonuria, in which a metabolic block, even in the same major pathway as PKU, leads to the accumulation of toxic precursors. In some cases the disorder is not usually manifest until the third decade of life or later, and may not involve overt neurobehavioral effects until then. Clinically, alkaptonuria generally appears during middle life in the form of degenerative joint changes. PKU illustrates the fact that even the foods that are innocuous to the majority of eaters can be health endangering to a significant minority.

## 4. A SINGLE CHANGE IN MOLECULAR STRUCTURE

Much remains to be learned about the "cascade" of events that must follow the binding of a molecule to its receptor site. Such being the case, it is impressive when neurobehavioral effects that follow ingestion of a particular substance are predictable. Furthermore, it is remarkable that a single change in the structure of a molecule may produce effects that are radically different from those of its parent. Such phenomena are clearly illustrated by an extensive series of experiments in which the substitution of a false precursor in the diet led to the synthesis of a false transmitter, with amazing neurobehavioral effects (Jenden et al, 1987; Knusel et al., 1990; Newton and Jensen, 1986).

The approach in these experiments was to create a hypocholinergic condition in an animal model (rat) by replacing the normal precursors, choline (Ch), in the diet with a much less efficient analog, N-aminodeanol (NADe). Figure 4 shows that the only difference between the two molecular structures was the substitution of an amine ($NH_2$) group for a single methyl ($CH_3$) group in the parent molecule. Results of a number of neurochemical experiments demonstrated that NADe is taken up by the Ch transport system in competition with Ch, acetylated by the synthesizing enzyme, stored in vesicles, and released on stimulation of the nerve. The normal neurotransmitter, acetylcholine (ACh), is replaced by acetyl aminodeanol (Ac NADe), which is inactivated by the normal hydrolyzing enzyme, acetylcholinesterase (AChE). AcNADe interacts with muscarinic and nicotinic receptors, but with potencies of only 4% and 17%, respectively, of ACh (Newton et al., 1985). Neurobehavioral functions showed strikingly different effects as time on the NADe diet increased (Russell et al., 1990). Basic physiological ("vegetative") processes (e.g., core body temperature) adapted very rapidly. Sensory-reflexive (e.g., acoustic-startle reflex mediated within the spinal core and brainstem) and sensory-perceptual processes (e.g., exploratory behavior) were significantly affected early in the dietary treatment, with cognitive functions (e.g., learning and memory) being most sensitive and showing the least adaptability. The time frame for recovery from these effects ranged from hours for the basic homeostatic processes to failure of the more complex behaviors to return to control levels through the duration of the experiments. Replacing the NADe with the normal control diet after the hypocholinergic state had been well established (e.g., 210 days) resulted in recovery of all biochemical and physiological functions to or toward control levels within 30–60 days. However, the behavioral variables showed no such recovery. Findings of these kinds suggest that the effects may be related to

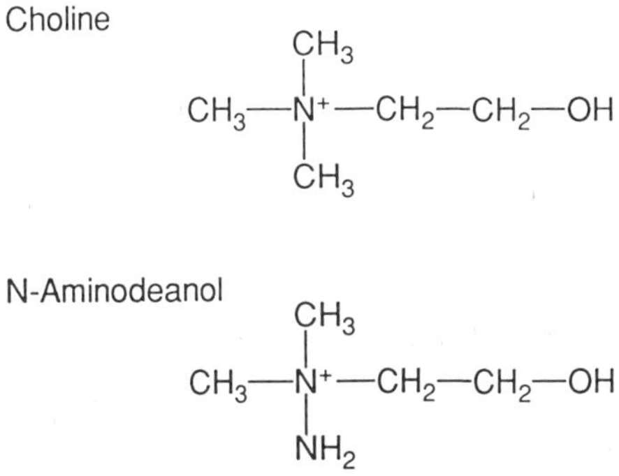

**FIGURE 4.** Choline is a component in the synthesis of the essential neurotransmitter acetylcholine. In experimental animal models, substitution of only a single group, i.e., $NH_2$ or $CH_3$, produces a different molecule, which when replacing choline in the diet changes normal behavior to that analogous to progressive degenerative dementia.

Choline

$$CH_3-\underset{\underset{CH_3}{|}}{\overset{\overset{CH_3}{|}}{N^+}}-CH_2-CH_2-OH$$

N-Aminodeanol

$$CH_3-\underset{\underset{NH_2}{|}}{\overset{\overset{CH_3}{|}}{N^+}}-CH_2-CH_2-OH$$

morphological changes in the CNS or may be associated with adaptive processes in other neurochemical events in the CNS, hypotheses still to be tested. Viewed overall, the effect of the change of a single group in the Ch molecule had induced the major signs of progressive degenerative dementia (Russell et al., 1990).

## 5. FUNCTIONAL RECEPTORS

Earlier we noted that molecules of exogenous substance entering the body by any route must themselves or through their biotransformation products reach specific binding sites in biologically active molecules if they are to have neurobehavioral effects. Indeed, it is a basic presumption in receptor theory that biological effects occur when molecules of the substance or of its product(s) are bound to their receptors. Chemicals ingested may affect the number of receptors available for such binding. Thus, the time course of the effects when receptor binding is reversible corresponds to the association and dissociation of the binding. The situation is different when the binding is irreversible, i.e., covalent (the ligand and the receptor share electrons). Non-functional receptors must then be replaced by de novo synthesis (Ehlert et al., 1984).

When molecules of natural substances ingested bind irreversibly, differential effects on various neurobehavioral functions may be observed that have important implications for the organism affected. It became clear early in the use of radioligands that there was only a finite number of binding sites of high affinity for any particular ligand. That there are such limits can be seen when, with increasing concentrations of a ligand, an asymptote is reached when all binding sites have been occupied (evidenced empirically in "saturation curves"). Molecules that bind irreversibly have been used experimentally to observe relations between the state of a receptor population (receptor density) and effects on a variety of biological functions. The significance of such relationships when malnutritions are involved is suggested by the following example.

Because of personal knowledge of its details, the example chosen comes from our own laboratory (Russell, et al., 1986). This particular series of experiments was designed to test the hypothesis that different neurotransmitter and physiological "endpoints" require different densities ("threshold") of receptor occupancy to function normally. If correct, the probability of a threshold being reached should be related to the density of the receptor population. In the experiments an irreversible cholinergic agonist was administered i.v. in the rat subjects. The number of functional muscarinic receptors (mAChR) was reduced to less than 10% of normal. Recovery to normal population density occurred exponentially over a period of 8 days, as shown by $[^3H](-)$QNB binding (Figure 5). Quinuclidinyl benzilate, QNB, is a reversible anticholinergic that binds selectively to muscarinic receptors and is used as a standard means for labelling such sites. During the recovery period, thresholds (mAChR densities) for normal functioning of the sample of variables measured returned in a hierarchical order. Physiological ("vegetative") variables (including tremor, chromodacryorrhea, salivation, core body temperature), affected in less than 5 min after injection, returned to their pretreatment baselines within minutes. Sensory-perceptual processes, e.g., nociceptive thresholds, showed peak changes of +230% and returned to normal within hours. Motoric responses recovered in 3–4 days. Learned responses and those requiring temporal discrimination took 8–11 days to recover and were the only variables to parallel the return of the receptors to their normal population levels. In other words, those cognitive functions had little if any "receptor reserve."

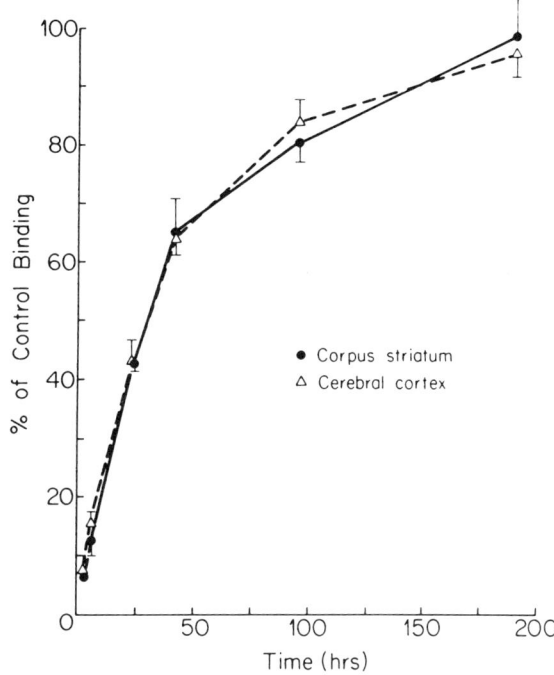

**FIGURE 5.** Different neurobehavioral functions require different densities of receptor populations in order to function normally. This figure shows the time characteristics of the recovery of muscarinic cholinergic receptors following treatment with an irreversible agonist (BM123). During the recovery period neurobehavioral functions returned to normal in a hierarchial order, with physiological processes recovering first (fewer receptors required) and cognitive processes last (little if any receptor reserve).

## 6. BIOTRANSFORMATION

"Investigation of biotransformation processes has been a rapidly expanding aspect of xenobiotic metabolism. This has been brought about by the increasing realization of the important influence of biotransformation on pharmacological activity and toxicity . . ." (Hawkins, 1988). When discussing Figure 1, attention was called to the possibilities that a compound entering the body may undergo change before the resulting product(s) reaches its sites of action. The chemical transformation of exogenous compounds by various enzymes present in the organism is referred to as *biotransformation*. The enzymes carry out their functions by a variety of chemical actions and interactions (Dauterman and Hodgson, 1980). Chemical transformations may also occur in the environment whenever appropriate physicochemical conditions are present, and the product(s) are then ingested in foods for human consumption. An example of each of these should make clearer their roles in malnutrition and the neurobehavioral implications of their actions.

"Parathion has the dubious distinction of being the pesticide most frequently involved in fatal poisonings" (Murphy, 1980). It is one of the organophosphorus insecticides, synthesized in the mid-1940s in the search for more stable compounds for use in agriculture. These compounds function by reducing the activity of the enzyme acetylcholinesterase (AChE), which is responsible for inactivating the neurotransmitter ACh after its release from presynaptic neurons. Reducing AChE activity elevates ACh levels in the brain. Parathion finds its way into the food chain as a contaminant. It has high mammalian toxicity by all routes of entry into the body. However, parathion per se is not the real villain. It is one of the organophosphorus compounds containing bonds between phosphorous and sulfur (P=S), groups that are relatively nontoxic until the P=S is oxidized to P=O. This is accomplished within the body by microsomes, converting parathion to paraoxon, which is many thousandfold more toxic. Other organophosphorus compounds follow similar pathways, the biotransformation products being responsible for the main physiological and neurobehavioral effects observed (Cohen, 1948). Because of the wide uses of organophosphate for the control of insect pests and because of the frequent opportunities for human exposures, an extensive clinical and research literature has developed. Reports of human occupational or adventitious exposure describe general symptoms, including loss in sensory-perceptual discrimination performance, difficulty in concentration and expressing thoughts, confusion, disorientation, and signs of anxiety and depression. Early experiments using animal models concluded that exposure to anti-ChEs produced differential effects on behavior, some, e.g., cognitive functions, being more sensitive than others. However, because of their action on the cholinergic neurotransmitter system, their neurobehavioral effects are widespread, as noted in a critical review of information entitled *Handbook of Drug and Chemical Stimulation of the Brain* (Myers, 1974): "Most impressive is the singular fact that ACh is the only substance that can influence every physiological or behavioral response thus far examined."

An example of chemical transformation in the external environment entering the food chain to the detriment of human consumers is the tragedy that occurred at Minamata Bay in Japan in the 1950s and 1960s. The story is so well known that only its major features need be recalled for our present purposes. Here, as in several other cases, environmental contamination occurred involving organic forms of mercury, principally methyl mercury. Mercury, entering the water in industrial effluents, was biotransformed (methylated) by the action aquatic organisms, initiating transfers and bioconcentration of the products up the food chain to fish used for human consumption. The most consistent and pronounced effects of ingesting methyl mercury are on the CNS. At Minamata, and at other sites where similar pollution has occurred, extensive behavioral symptoms have been observed: severe disturbance of speech and gait, loss of normal hearing, narrowing of the visual field and other sensory disturbances, and occasionally, hallucinations (Government of Japan, 1972).

This too brief discussion of the importance of biotransformation in molecular events affecting neurobehavioral functions should conclude by calling attention to the fact that ". . . extrapolation of activity in vitro pharmacological screens to animals in vivo and finally to man can be improved by consideration of the impact of biotransformation on the compound in different systems" (Hawkins, 1988).

## 7. NATURAL TOXICANTS

Foods of plant origin may contain potent natural toxicants (Kingsbury, 1980). There is considerable diversity in the variety of these toxic principles, whether viewed in terms of their chemical structures or of their physiological effects. The latter are, in turn, evidenced by neurobehavioral syndromes in human and infrahuman animals. The syndromes may involve the liver and kidney, and the the central and autonomic nervous systems. Damage to the liver may affect phospholipid metabolism, with consequent effects on the availability of choline, on ACh synthesis, and hence, on behaviors serviced by the muscarinic cholinergic system. Using autoradiography it has been possible to identify brain areas with rates of local glucose utilization altered by peripheral administration of nicotine (London et al., 1988). Stimulation occurred primarily in areas known to have nicotine binding sites ("true receptors"), an effect observed at dose levels that are discriminated by the rat subjects and produce changes in behavioral and physiological variables. Another example of a rather circuitous route by which a natural toxicant may influence neurobehavioral functions is interference with normal glycolysis and the synthesis of the second precursor in the synthesis of ACh, i.e., acetyl-coenzyme A. Following ingestion, mammals metabolize plant compounds in a wide variety of different ways that result in bioconcentration of natural toxicants, some of which may have significant neurobehavioral effects (Scheline, 1991).

One of the most striking "detective" efforts in the search for natural toxicants has been reported in detail by Spencer (1990). "This is a story about a remarkable and terrible affliction that sometimes presents at onset as motor neuron disease (amyotrophic lateral sclerosis) and, in other instances, as parkinsonism, presenile dementia, or various combinations of all three" (Spencer, 1990). The discovery that the disorders appeared in three areas of the Western Pacific Ocean suggested the possibility of a common etiology. In all three areas the neurobehavioral disorders were discovered to be associated with exposure to the untreated seed kernel of *Cycas* plants. Uses of cycads in the high-risk areas of the Pacific include medicinal purposes, food, beverage, confection, and as childrens' playthings. Characteristic of human exposure to cycad toxins is the fact that the onset of clinical symptoms may follow by years or even decades. Intensive probing of the kind that has led to the identification of the cycad as containing natural neurotoxins with such devastating effects, combined with intensive laboratory studies, may lead to the discovery of whether ". . . neurotoxins are driving us crazy in developed countries, just as they are tragically the apparent cause of dementia in certain communities of the western Pacific" (Spencer, 1990).

Abraham Lincoln's mother ". . . may have been the most famous person ever to die in the 'milk sick' . . ." (Duffy, 1990). Milk sickness, first named a separate disease in 1810, is characterized neurobehaviorally by anorexia and general motor debilitation. In rural areas during the early years of the last century, it was observed that where cattle grazed in rich woodlands, they often developed "trembles." In some of these areas high death rates occurred in human populations after drinking their milk. By elimination the responsible toxicant was associated with milk from cattle feeding on the plant white snakeroot (*Eupatorium rugosum*). Biochemical analyses later showed that the plant contains a variety of chemicals, among which is tremetal, an unsaturated alcohol with constituents not toxic in themselves. Tremetal is biotransformed to tremetone, a chemical similar in structure to rotenone, also a powerful botanical insecticide. The neurobehavioral effects are due to the fact that tremetone blocks the normal reconversion of lactic acid to glycogen in the liver, thus interfering with the body's source of energy. This example illustrates two basic principles emphasized in the title of this chapter: "What a Difference a Molecule Makes." The first principle is that of biotransformation, by which a molecule of little if any toxic capability is altered to a similar molecule that is highly toxic. Secondly, it illustrates how a molecule that, although causing symptoms that are nonlethal in its

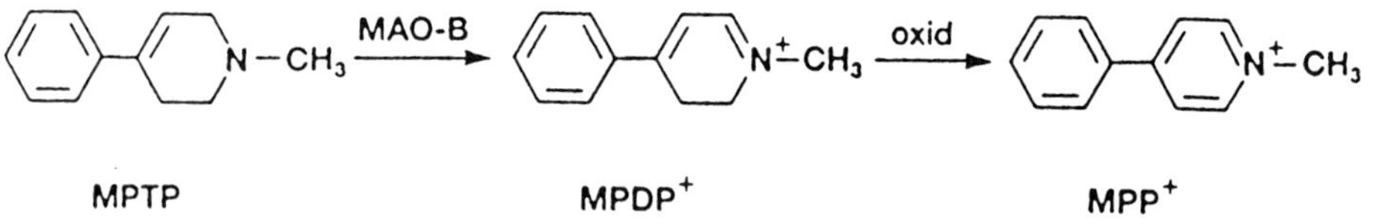

MPTP → (MAO-B) → MPDP⁺ → (oxid) → MPP⁺

**FIGURE 6.** A human error in preparing a synthetic heroin produced a contaminant, MPTP, which was converted to the metabolite MPP⁺. The latter is highly toxic to the same neurons that show damage in Parkinson's disease.

original host, may induce severe toxicity in another organism: "the secondary poisoning can be more severe than that in the lactating animal because of the concentration of the poisoning [in the milk] and the lesser ability of the nonlactating consumer to eliminate it" (Kinsbury, 1980).

## 8. A HUMAN ERROR IN SYNTHESIS

It was not the first time, nor is it likely to be the last, that a human error in synthesis resulted in tragic neurobehavioral effects. The error produced a contaminant in what was intended to be a synthetic heroin. The contaminant, MPTP, is converted to a metabolite, MPP⁺, which is highly toxic to the same neurons that show damage in Parkinson's disease (Hornykiewicz and Kish, 1986). The sequence of neurochemical events involved are diagrammed in Figure 6. MPTP is converted to the intermediate product, MDPD, by the enzyme, monoamine oxidase. MPDP can be further oxidized to MPP⁺, which is taken up by mitochondria, where it blocks respiration. MPP⁺ is the preferred candidate for the ultimate toxin. Evidence supporting this hypothesis comes from clinical observations in humans and from experimental studies with nonhuman primates (Langston *et al.*, 1984). Both clinically and experimentally, MPP⁺ produces destruction of neurons in the nigral compacta and induces the clinical syndrome of dopamine deficiency characteristic of parkinsonism. Research with mice has shown greater neuropathy in older animals, implicating age as a contributing factor. Other studies suggest that genetic components may add to the complex series of events leading from the molecule to behavior. As evidence continues to accumulate, it becomes quite clear that "sloppiness" in synthesis had led not only to varying degrees of parkinsonian symptoms in humans exposed to MPTP, but also to an animal model for understanding the disease that has such devastating effects on the substantial numbers of persons afflicted.

## 9. NEUROBEHAVIORAL EFFECTS OF FOOD PROCESSING

### 9.1. Energy and Molecular Changes

There is an enormous flow of energy in the biosphere. Solar energy is used in photosynthetic organisms by converting it into the chemical energy of glucose and other organic products. These products are then used as precursors of structural biomolecules and as energy-rich fuels needed by the organisms for activities that require the expenditure of energy. Energy is also used in food processing, and it is with such usages that we are presently concerned (Bender, 1978).

Energy passing through food substances can induce significant molecular changes (Devins, 1988). The validity of this obvious statement is apparent when, during the course of preparing a meal, the changes produced when heat is applied are clearly visible. Foods are subjected to a vast number of processes that have such effects. Some involve radiation, which directly or indirectly produces ions (e.g., gamma radiation), and others that do not (e.g., microwave, infrared). Because the uses of these sources of energy frequently result in chemical changes, "It is therefore not surprising that hazardous molecules can be produced during cooking . . ." (Caldwell and Sangster, 1985). It is also not surprising that some of these molecules are associated with neurobehavioral effects.

Food processing (Mudgett, 1988) involves the application of a wide spectrum of energy sources. This includes both *nonionizing* and *ionizing* radiation, the former referring to electromagnetic waves below ultraviolet (UV) and the latter to UV and higher frequency waves e.g., X-rays and γ-rays. Both may have profound and often irreversible effects on inorganic and organic substances.

A major difficulty in seeking to relate molecular changes induced during food processing to neurobehavioral effects lies in the large number of such changes from which to select prime candidates. To complicate the task further is the fact that quantities of the altered materials available for assay are often below the limits of present techniques to capture and to measure (Miller, 1987).

Although a considerable part of our food undergoes one or more of the several (nonionizing) heat-processing techniques in common use, relatively little information about neurobehavioral effects is available. Thus, as recently as 5 years ago, it could be stated that ". . . no definitive conclusions are available regarding the health significance of heat-processing practices in human disease" (Larson *et al.*, 1987). As research builds a body of information, conclusions generally accepted at one time may become suspect, as, for example, has the widely accepted view that removal of caffeine from coffee reduces such risks to health as heart disease. Preliminary evidence now suggests that decaffeination, by exposing coffee to superheated water, may produce molecular changes more threatening than coffee without such treatment. Caffeine can produce neurobehavioral effects, e.g., improvements in behaviors that have been affected adversely by fatigue or sleep deprivation (Tarka and Shively, 1987). To what extent these effects are related to caffeine per se or to molecules created by methods of preparing coffee and how they are influenced by the decaffeination process are still open questions. The possibility that nonionizing radiation during food processing may induce molecular changes of a toxic nature becomes a matter of importance for research when the emerging evidence cannot categorically assert that there is no risk, but also that there is no basis for predicting a significant risk (Gamberale, 1990; Lovely, 1988; Wilkening and Sutton, 1990).

The use of ionizing radiation in food processing was first tested in Sweden in 1916 as a means of preservation for strawberries (Murray, 1990). Its use generally has been a subject of debate and research. The debate has been clouded by the fact that "irradiation" suffers from a very unfavorable image. The distinction has not always been made between "radioactive food" and "food exposed to irradiation." In fact, the process of irradiation does not make food radioactive. However, it may alter biologically important molecules, with consequent effects on neurobehavioral functions. Very little is known about the risks of such effects. Both irradiated and non-irradiated foods are chemically complex. "Since there may be hundreds of discrete chemical species present . . . their complete chemical characterization and quantification is not feasible" (Elias, 1985). Observations of changes that have been induced in food by ionizing irradiation have led some investigators to conclude that the effects are quantitatively very small to minute (Murray, 1990). Others strongly disagree. That much more attention must be given to expanding present knowledge is reflected in debates by those responsible for regulating the uses of ionizing radiation during food processing, e.g., the United States and the European Economic Community. This need is further supported by recent reports on effects of whole-body exposures, both acute (e.g., Bogo, 1988) and chronic (e.g., Fry and Fry, 1990; Salon, 1987). The need takes on a new kind of urgency as concerns about "global changes" in radiation continue to grow. Charged particles entering the solar system and secondary radiation they produce in the Earth's atmosphere (galactic cosmos radiation) have the potential of inducing changes in foodstuffs (Friedberg *et al.*, 1989).

"Several trends in food processing seem likely to predominate into the twenty-first century . . ." (Fennema, 1990). If they do, concern must be directed to much fuller understanding of the neurobehavioral effects induced by chemicals developed in foods during processing, handling, and storage.

## 9.2. Food Additives and Contamination

Contamination may be introduced during food preparation, resulting in undesirable neurobehavioral effects. The contamination may occur intentionally or unintentionally (Nriagu and Simmons, 1990). The former are natural or synthetic compounds added to the original food during commercial or home processing for specific purposes. Unintentional additives are substances not present in the food as produced and not introduced for particular purposes in the finished product. In either case, the substance may be biologically hazardous in its own right, may undergo biotransformation to a toxic form within the organization, or may interact with other materials to form a threatening complex. Further complications arise when the age variable is considered, young organisms tending to be more susceptible (Dobbing, 1981; Weiner *et al.,* 1983). Contaminants ". . . run the gamut from sand to pesticides to radioactive fallout, with a corresponding range in toxicity from harmless to acutely toxic compounds" (Kilgore and Li, 1980). Potentially hazardous microbial and fungal contaminants may also be present (Kilgore and Li, 1980). This very brief overview of potential sources of contamination in foods indicates how complex are the tasks of providing continuous surveillance and of developing the kinds of sensitive and reliable techniques required to do so.

*Food additives* may be hazardous, as well a beneficial to health. The intentional use of additives goes far back in human history, at least as far as the salting of meats for preservation. During the years since then a wide variety of other substances have been added to foods for coloring and flavoring, as well as preservation. Because some of these proved to be highly toxic, e.g., dyes, questions were raised during the 20th century about the safety of chemical preservatives that then included such compounds as formaldehyde and salicylic acid. Eventually public laws were passed requiring strict testing of all substances proposed as food additives before their approval for marketing.

Despite such testing, problems may arise from two major sources that deserve special mention here. One is due to the range of individual differences in sensitivities to chemical substances. Earlier in the present discussion, the point was made that there are individuals who are supersensitive to ingestion of foods that have no observable effects on the majority of the population. The effects on such individuals may appear as physical and/or neurobehavioral symptoms. The second source of problems is one that may affect individuals at any level of sensitivity. Some centuries ago Paracelsus, one of the "great physicians" in medical history, commented, "All things are poisons, for there is nothing without poisonous qualities. It is only the dose which makes a thing a poison" (Sigerist, 1958). A premise on which the concept of "neurobehavioral toxicity" depends is that some low magnitude exists for all chemical substances that will not produce an effect no matter how long the exposure. Coupled with this is the corollary that *all* substances will produce a neurobehavioral effect at some higher dose level. Exposure–effect relations for any food additive are further complicated by such variables as the duration of the exposure and the stage of an organism's development when the exposure occurs. Ingestion of vitamin A will serve as an example. Vitamin A occurs naturally in foods in its basic form or as the carotenes that serve as precursors for its synthesis. Extensive research has demonstrated the involvement of vitamin A in visual processes and in growth. Both of these roles have their neurobehavioral effects, the first by directly influencing the visual sensory modality and the second indirectly by affecting the development of motoric capabilities. Vitamin A may produce abnormalities when its content in the diet is either overly restricted or when it is used excessively. For example, deficiency is evidenced neurobehaviorally by the failure of vision in dim light ("night blindness"). Effects of "overdosing" with vitamin A have been most clearly apparent during early stages of development. Doses relatively low compared to acceptable daily uptakes for adults have been toxic when infants have been given the vitamin supplement.

*Contaminants,* unintentional additives, may enter the food chain during production, during processing, and/or during packaging and storage. Possible contaminants include a very broad range of molecular forms, both organic and inorganic. Production practices are designed to prevent the inclusion of hazardous molecules or to ensure that they are kept below toxic levels. "Problems arising from pathogenic organisms and their toxic metabolites in food are many and varied" (Kilgore and Li, 1980). For example, the highly lethal toxins produced by *Clostridium botulinum,* perhaps the most feared of the food-borne intoxications, have been shown to produce inhibition of transmitter release from cholinergic nerve endings (Gunderson, 1980). The neurobehavioral effects are those associated with presynaptic events in that transmitter system (Russell, 1988), including effects on the efficiency of cognitive processes.

The recent establishment of new standards for levels of lead (Pb) in drinking water by the U.S. Environmental Protection Agency makes Pb a timely example of contamination by metals found widely as nonintentional food additives. The toxic effects of Pb at high doses have been known for centuries. Today's questions are directed more specifically toward the definition of thresholds for adverse health effects (Singhal and Thomas, 1980). As with other additives and contaminants, effects of the ingestion of organic Pb show wide individual differences. Toxicities have been shown to occur from both acute and chronic exposures. The human child is the most vulnerable subgroup in the population, with workers exposed to Pb in second place (Needleman, 1990). Adverse neurobehavioral effects have received particular attention, measures of such effects showing changes throughout the range of behaviors from peripheral sensorimotor to central cognitive.

## 10. DEFENSE AGAINST FOOD TOXICANTS

Within limits there occurs a balance between toxicants in food and the capacity of natural defense mechanisms in the body to maintain homeostasis. Many of these mechanisms involve the actions of enzymes and/or microorganisms. The actions of such "scavengers" result in the transformation of toxicants into compounds that are less threatening or nonthreatening. They may be excreted from the body by several different routes, e.g., urine, feces, expired air, perspiration. Biotransformation may have benevolent, as well as malevolent, roles to play! The ease with which compounds are excreted depends to a great extent on their solubility in water. Toxic compounds that are more lipid soluble tend to accumulate in mammalian tissues, thus disrupting cellular processes and leading to adverse neurobehavioral consequences. A number of the "scavengers" referred to above are capable of metabolizing these compounds in such ways as to make them more water soluble, thus more readily excreted, and hence, less threatening to neurobehavioral functions.

Neurobehavioral defense against food toxicants includes modifications in normal biochemical processes to compensate for changes induced by the toxicants. A specific example to which some reference has already been made will serve to illustrate such compensatory capabilities. Recognizing the basic roles played by receptors in the sequence of events extending from ingestion of a chemical to its neurobehavioral effects suggests that changes in functional receptors could be involved as a homeostatic mechanism. Evidence supporting this general hypothesis came from research reports by three independent laboratories at about the same time (Russell and Overstreet, 1987). By far the most common and consistent finding in these and subsequent studies of the neurobehavioral effects of pesticide residues has been a reduction in the number of muscarinic receptors, i.e., significant decreases in receptor densities. The evidence indicates that the extent of reduction is related to the dose level to which the subject is exposed, with recovery to normal receptor population levels occurring after the exposure is terminated. In more general terms, there appears to be a finely tuned process involving downregulation of postsynaptic muscarinic receptors when the cholinergic system is affected by the actions of direct or indirect agonists. Further studies have shown that this process is also capable of responding to cholinergic antagonists, the entry into the body of such compounds producing an upregulation of receptors (Russell *et al.*, 1986). Both upregulation and downregulation are accompanied by behavioral tolerance.

There is a third important means of defense against food toxicants. The fact ". . . that behavioral changes during acute intoxication are often modified too quickly to allow a recourse to the more obvious explanations, such as those based on the chemicals disposition . . ." (Bignami, 1979) or on its pharmacodynamics suggests that biochemical mechanisms may be supplemented by a "behaviorally augmented "component (Corfield-Sumner and Stolerman, 1978; Le Blanc *et al.*, 1973). In other words, behavioral compensation may occur before biochemical adjustments can be made. Such compensation involves selecting alternative behaviors from an already acquired pool or learning new behaviors that maintain homeostatic mechanisms within their "normal" ranges.

Such covariations between neurochemical and behavioral functions illustrate mechanisms by which neurobehavioral defenses may be mounted against food toxicants. However, they still leave unanswered many questions about events that transduce neurochemical to behavioral changes in the defense mechanisms.

## 11. IN CONCLUSION

Some quarter century ago the importance of understanding neurobehavioral effects of malnutrition began to filter significantly into thinking about human interactions with the biophysical environment. At about that time a courageous physician, employed by a large industrial firm, published a challenge entitled, "Functional Testing for Behavioral Toxicity: A Missing Dimension in Experimental Toxicology" (Ruffin, 1963). Soon thereafter a committee of the U.S. National Research Council (NRC) published in their report, "Problems of regulating chemicals in the environment are particularly beset with information characterized by a high degree of uncertainty. For some aspects of these problems there exists no information at all" (U.S. National Research Council, 1975). Information about neurobehavioral effects per se had received but little attention, the major criteria for toxic effects being carcinogenesis and mutagenesis (Buckholtz and Panem, 1986). The view that behavior should be another important endpoint in the study of malnutrition is supported by at least two major considerations: (1) Adjustments to the biophysical environment ultimately involve the behavior of the total, integrated organism, and (2) many research results have demonstrated that parameters of behavior provide sensitive and noninvasive measure of toxicity. A major objective of the present chapter has been to indicate how the "uncertainties" worrisome to the NRC may be narrowed by basic and clinical research designed to understand the neurochemical mechanisms by which exposures to toxicants affect neurobehavioral functions. Rational development of procedures for averting malnutrition and for treating its consequences depends upon much more knowledge about these mechanisms than we now possess, and there are reasons for believing that there is some urgency in the need to know.

The International Council of Scientific Union's (ICSU) International Geosphere-Biosphere Program, A Study of Global Change, has described the era in which we live as a period of potentially stressful changes in our global environment in ways that we are only now beginning to understand. The International Social Service Council has developed a program to parallel and supplement the ICSU effort: Framework for Research on the Human Dimensions of Global Environmental Change. The World Health Organization (1975) has expressed the view that health is more than merely the prevention of disease: it includes the behavioral capabilities needed to carry on one's chosen activities at work and at play. Will global changes interfere with such "rights"? A very recent report from a panel established by the U.S. National Academy of Sciences has reinforced still further the view that there should not be an excuse for delaying action to discover the nature of the "stressful changes" in the global environment. For example, there appears to be a "reasonable chance" that, by the middle of next century, global temperatures will rise 2–9°F. Radiation produced by such a change could, by mechanisms discussed above, cause significant molecular changes in the human food chain that would have important neurobehavioral effects.

The preceding discussion has viewed "malnutrition" as involving dietary imbalances that include both (1) the ingestion of foods that are inadequate or toxic to normal nutritional requirements and (2) aberrant conditions within the organism that interfere with the metabolism of substances included in the normal diet. The general model within which malnutrition has been viewed is one in which the behavioral property of living organisms is inextricably bound to other basic properties, i.e., biochemical, elecrophysiological, and morphological. Neurobehavioral effects following ingestion of a toxic or potentially toxic substance are the final endpoints in a "cascade" that includes kinetic (biotransformation) and dynamic changes. The latter begin with interactions between molecules of the substance and receptor sites on bioactive molecules in the body. In a sense, such interactions are the "pacemakers" in a long series of biodynamic events. This view is the source of the subtitle of the chapter: "What a Difference a Molecule Makes." The main body of the chapter has been devoted to examples of ways in which even small differences in the molecular structures of food may result in very significant differences in their neurochemical and neurobehavioral effects. In terms of our model, the small differences in structure at the molecular level may be greatly amplified as the dynamic effects of molecules run their various courses. These courses affect the capabilities of living organisms to adjust their behaviors to meet the demand of their constantly changing physical and psychosocial environments. The inclusion of behavioral endpoints as criteria in research on malnutrition and in regulations generated by the research has begun to receive the attention that a quarter century of evidence and predictions of global change suggest is needed, and indeed, is overdue.

Acknowledgments.    I with to express my appreciation to Ms. Marla Lay for her valiant efforts to make this chapter presentable from the manuscripts I provided.

## REFERENCES

Albert, A., 1987, *Xenobiosis: Foods, Drugs, and Poisons in the Human Body*, Chapman and Hall, New York.
Bender, A. E., 1978, *Food Processing and Nutrition*, Academic Press, New York, p. 243.
Bignami, G., 1979, Methodological problems in the analysis of behavioral tolerance in toxicology, *Neurobehav. Toxicol.* 1(Suppl. 1):179–186.
Bogo, V., 1988, Early behavioral toxicity produced by acute ionizing radiation, *Fund. Appl. Toxicol.* 11(4):578–579.
Buckholtz, N.S., and Panem, S., 1986, Regulation and evolving science: Neurobehavioral toxicology, *Neurobehav. Toxicol. Teratol.* 8:89–96.
Caldwell, J., and Sangster, S.A., 1985, Are unprocessed food any safer?, in: *Food Toxicology—Real or Imagined Problems?* (G.G. Gibson and R. Walker, eds.), Taylor and Francis, London, pp. 379–387.
Cohen, S.D., 1984, Mechanisms of toxicological interactions involving organophosphate insecticides, *Fund. Appl. Toxicol.* 4:315–324.
Corfield-Sumner, P.K., and Stolerman, I.P., 1978, Behavioral tolerance, in: *Contemporary Research in Behavioral Pharmacology* (D.E. Blackman and D.J. Sanger, eds.), Plenum Press, New York, pp. 391–448.
Dauterman, W.C., and Hodgson, E., 1980, Chemical transformations and interactions, in: *Introduction to Environmental Toxicology* (F.E. Guthrie and J.J. Perry, eds.), Elsevier, New York, pp. 358–374.
Devins, D.W., 1988, *Energy: Its Physical Impact on the Environment*, Wiley, New York.
Dobbing, J., 1981, Nutritional growth restriction and the nervous system, in: *The Molecular Basis of Neuropathology* (R.H.S. Thomson and A.N. Davison, eds.), Edward Arnold, London, pp. 221–233.
Doull, J., 1980, Factors influencing toxicology, in: *Toxicology: The Basic Science of Poisons* (J. Doull, C.D. Klaasen, and M.O. Amour, eds.), New York, Macmillan, pp. 70–83.
Duffy, D.C., 1990, Land of milk and poison, *Natural History* 7:4–8.
Ehlert, F.J., Jenden, D.J., and Ringdahl, G., 1984, An alkylating derivative of oxotremorine interacts irreversibly with the muscarinic receptors, *Life Sci.* 34:985–991.
Elias, P.S., 1985, Food irradiation and radiolytic products, in: *Food Toxicology—Real or Imagined Problems?* (G.G. Gibson and R. Walker, eds.), Taylor and Francis, London, pp. 362–378.
Fennema, U., 1990, Influence of food-environment interactions on health in the twenty-first century, *Env. Health Persp.* 86:229–232.
Fry, R.J., and Fry, S.A., 1990, Health effects of ionizing radiation, *Med. Clin. North Amer.* 74(2):475–488.
Friedberg, W., Faulkner, D.N., Snyder, L., Darden, E.B., Jr., and O'Brien, K., 1989, Galactic cosmos radiation exposure and associated health risks for air carrier crewmembers, *Air. Space Environ. Med.*, 60:1104–1108.
Gamberale, F., 1990, Physiological and psychological effects of exposure to extremely low-frequency electric and magnetic fields on humans, *Scand. J. Work. Environ. Health* 16(Suppl. 1):51–54.
Government of Japan, 1972, Pollution Related to Diseases and Relief Measures in Japan, Environment Agency, Tokyo.
Gunderson, C.B., 1980, The effects of botulinum toxin on the synthesis, storage and release of acetycholine, *Prog. Neurobiol.* 14:99–119.

Hawkins, D.R. (ed.), 1988, *Biotransformations: A Survey of the Biotransformations of Drugs and Chemicals in Animals*, Vol. 1, The Royal Society of Chemistry, London, p. 511.

Hornykiewicz, O., 1966, Dopamine (3-hydroxy-tyramine) and brain function, *Pharmacol. Rev.* 18:925–964.

Hornykiewicz, O., and Kish, S.J., 1986, *Biochemical Pathophysiology of Parkinson's Disease* (M.D. Yahr and K.J. Bergmann, eds.), Raven Press, New York, pp. 19–34.

Jenden, D.J., Russell, R.W., Booth, R.A., Lauretz, S.D., Knusel, B.J., George, R., and Waite, J.J., 1987, A model hypocholinergic syndrome produced by a false choline analog, N-aminodeanol, *J. Neural Transm.* 24:325–329.

Kilgore, W.W., and Li, M-Y, 1980, Food additives and contaminants, in: *The Basic Science of Poisons* (J. Doull, C.D. Klaassen, and M.O. Amdur, eds.), Macmillan, New York, pp. 593–607.

Kingsbury, J.M., 1980, Phytotoxicology, in: *Toxicology: The Basic Science of Poisons* (J. Doull, C.D. Klaassen, and M.O. Amdur, eds.), Macmillan, New York, pp. 578–590.

Knusel, B., Jenden, D.J., Lauretz, S.D., Booth, R.A., Rice, K.M., Roch, M., and Waite, J.J., 1990, Global in vivo replacement of choline by N-aminodeanol: Testing a hypothesis about progressive degenerative dementia. I. The dynamics of choline replacement, *Pharmacol. Biochem. Behav.* 37:799–809.

Krasnegor, N.A., Miller, G.D., and Simopoulos, A.P., (eds.), 1990, *Diet and Behavior: Multidisciplinary Approaches*, Springer-Verlag, London, pp. 234.

Langston, J.W., Langston, E.B., and Irwin, I., 1984, MPTP-induced parkinsonism in human and non-human primates—clinical and experimental aspects, *Acta Neurol. Scand.* 100:49–54.

Larson, J.C., and Poulsen, E., 1987, Mutagens and carcinogens in heat-processed foods, in: *Toxicological Aspects of Food* (K. Miller, ed.), Elsevier Applied Science, London, pp. 205–252.

LeBlanc, A.E., Gibbins, R.J., and Kalant, H., 1973, Behavioral augmentation of tolerance to ethanol in the rat, *Psychopharmacology* 39:117–122.

London, E.D., Connolly, R.J., Szikszay, M., Wamsley, J.K., and Dam, M., 1988, Effects of nicotine on local cerebral glucose utilization in the rat, *J. Neurosci.* 8:3920–3928.

Lovely, R.H., 1988, Recent studies in the behavioral toxicology of ELF electric and magnetic fields, *Prog. Clin. Biol. Res.*, 257:327–347.

Miller, K. (ed.), 1987, *Toxicological Aspects of Food*, Elsevier Applied Science, London, p. 458.

Needleman, H.L., 1990, Lessons from the history of childhood plumbism for pediatric neurotoxicology, in: *Advances in Neurobehavioral Toxicology: Applications in Environmental and Occupational Health* (B.L. Johnson, ed.), Lewis Publishers, Chelsea, MI, pp. 331–338.

Mudgett, R., 1988, Electromagnetic energy and food processing, *J. Microwave Power Electromag. Ener.* 23:225–230.

Murphy, S.D., 1980, Pesticides, in: *The Basic Science of Poisons*, 2nd ed. (J. Poull, C.D. Klaassen, and M.O. Amdur, eds.), Macmillan, New York, pp. 357–408.

Murray, D.R., 1990, *Biology of Food Irradiation*, John Wiley, New York, pp. 255.

Myers, R.D., 1974, *Handbook of Drug and Chemical Stimulation of the Brain*, Van Nostrand, New York, pp. 651–660.

Newton, M.W., and Jenden, D.J., 1986, False transmitters as presynaptic probes for cholinergic mechanisms and function, *Trends Pharmacol. Sci.* 7:316–320.

Newton, M.W., Crosland, R.D., and Jenden, D.J., 1985, In vivo metabolism of a cholinergic false precursor after dietary administration to rats, *J. Pharmacol. Exp. Ther.* 235:157–161.

Nriagu, J.O., and Simmons, M.S., 1990, *Food Contamination from Environmental Sources*, Wiley, New York.

Patrice, E.F., Jelliffe, E., and Jelliffe, D.B., (eds.), 1982, *Adverse Effects of Foods*, Plenum Press, New York.

Salon, L.R., 1987, Health aspects of low-level ionizing radiation, *Ann. N.Y. Acad. Sci.*, 502:32–42.

Ruffin, J.B., 1963, Functional testing for behavioral toxicity: A missing dimension in experimental environmental toxicology, *J. Ocup. Med.* 5:117–121.

Russell, R.W., 1988, Behavioral correlates of presynaptic events in the cholinergic neurotransmitter system, *Prog. Drug Res.* 32:43–130.

Russell, R.W., 1990, Neurobehavioral time bombs: Their nature and their mechanisms, in: *Behavioral Measures of Neurotoxicity* (R.W. Russell, P. Ebert Plattau, and A.M. Pope, eds.), U.S. National Academy Press, Washington, D.C., pp. 206–225.

Russell, R.W., and Overstreet, D.H., 1987, Mechanisms underlying sensitivity to organophosphorus anticholinesterase compounds, *Prog. Neurobiol.* 28:97–129.

Russell, R.W., Smith, C.A., Booth, R.A., Jenden, P.J., and Waite, J.J., 1986, Behavioral and physiological effects associated with changes in muscarinic receptors following administration of an irreversible cholinergic agonist (BM123), *Psychopharmacology* 90:308–315.

Russell, R.W., Jenden, D.J., Booth, R.A., Lauretz, S.D., Rice, K.M., and Roch, M., 1990, Global in vivo replacement of choline by N-amenodeanol: Testing a hypothesis about progressive degenerative dementia. II. Physiological and behavioral effects, *Pharmacol. Biochem. Behav.* 37:811–820.

Scrimshaw, S., and Gordon, J.E., (eds.), 1968, *Malnutrition, Learning and Behavior*, MIT Press, Cambridge, MA, p. 568.

Segal, D.S., 1975, Behavioral characterization of d- and l-amphetamine: Neurochemical implications, *Science*, 190:475–477.

Scheline, R.R., 1991, *CRC Handbook of Mammalian Metabolism of Plant Compounds*, CRC Press, Boca Raton, FL, p. 512.

Sigerist, H.E., 1958, *The Great Doctors*, Doubleday, New York.

Singhal, R.L., and Thomas, J.A., eds., 1980, *Lead Toxicity*, Urban and Schwarzenberg, Baltimore, p. 514.

Spallholz, J.E., 1989, *Nutrition: Chemistry and Biology*, Prentice Hall, Englewood Cliffs, NJ, p. 288.

Spencer, P.S., 1990, Are neurotoxins driving us crazy? Planetary observations on the causes of neurodegenerative diseases in old age, in: *Behavioral Measures of Neurotoxicity* (R.W. Russell, P.E. Flattau, and A.M. Pope, eds.), National Academy Press, Washington, D.C., pp. 11–36.

Tarka, S.M., Jr., and Shively, C.A., 1987, Methylxanthines, in: *Toxicological Aspects of Food* (K. Miller, ed.), Elsevier Applied Science, London, pp. 373–423.

Testa, B., and Mayer, J.M., 1988, Stereo-selective drug metabolism and its significance in drug research, *Prog. Drug Res.* 32:249–303.

U.S. National Research Council, 1975, *Decision Making for Regulation of Chemicals in the Environment*, National Academy of Science Press, Washington, DC.

Weiner, S.G., Robinson, L., and Levine, S., 1983, Influence of perinatal malnutrition on adult physiological and behavioral reactivity in rats, *Physiol. Behav.* 39:41–50.

Wilkening, G.M., and Sutton, C.H., 1990, Health effects of nonionizing radiation, *Med. Clin. North Am.* 74(2):489–507.

World Health Organization, 1975, *Early Detection of Health Impairment in Occupational Exposure to Health Hazards*, World Health Organization Report Series, Geneva, No. 571.

*Part II*

**Methods**

Chapter 6

# Animal Models of Cognitive Development in Neurotoxicology

*Mark E. Stanton*

## 1. INTRODUCTION

It is estimated that 5–10% of U.S. citizens suffer from some form of developmental learning disability, at great human and financial cost to our society. The magnitude of this problem has generated widespread concern among government agencies and private organizations over the need for research to examine the etiology, prediction, and treatment of mental retardation and/or developmental learning disorders (Kavanaugh and Truss, 1988; *Learning Disabilities: A Report to the U.S. Congress*, 1987). The etiology of these disorders is largely unknown, although a variety of factors have been implicated, including genetic, environmental, and sociocultural factors. One environmental factor for which there is very clear evidence for a role in the etiology of mental retardation is exposure to chemicals during the prenatal and early postnatal period (Kimmel *et al.*, 1990). As indicated in Table 1, there are a variety of chemical compounds (and other agents) that are neurotoxic to developing humans. Moreover, a common, if not cardinal, feature of the human clinical syndrome that follows developmental exposure to these compounds is impaired cognitive development. For example, in the case of environmental lead, it has been claimed that, of all the various neurotoxic effects of this compound, cognitive dysfunction in infants and children occurs at the lowest levels of exposure (Davis *et al.*, 1990). Indeed, in the case of lead, cognitive development has impacted on the regulatory

---

Disclaimer: This chapter has been reviewed by the Health Effects Research Laboratory, U.S. Environmental Protection Agency, and approved for publication. Mention of trade names or commercial products does not constitute endorsement or recommendation for use.

---

*Mark E. Stanton* • Neurotoxicology Division, Health Effects Research Laboratory, U.S. Environmental Protection Agency, Research Triangle Park, North Carolina 27711.
*The Vulnerable Brain and Environmental Risks, Volume 1: Malnutrition and Hazard Assessment,* edited by Robert L. Isaacson and Karl F. Jensen. Plenum Press, New York, 1992.

**TABLE 1.** Generally Recognized
Human Developmental Neurotoxicants

---
Ethanol
Methylmercury
Lead
Heroin
Methadone
Cocaine
Diphenylhydantoin
PCBs
X-irradiation

---

From Rees *et al.* (1990), with permission.

process. Recently promulagated and proposed standards for the level of lead legally permitted in the environment by the U.S. Environmental Protection Agency have been, in large part, based on findings from several studies that used a clinical test of intelligence, the Bayley's Mental Development Index (MDI), performed in 6-month-old infants (Bellinger *et al.*, 1987; Davis *et al.*, 1990; U.S. EPA, 1991). Although it would be unwise to overgeneralize to all developmental neurotoxicants, the experience with lead has encouraged a view that developmental exposure may have qualitatively different and/or more severe neurotoxic effects than adult exposure. An extension of this view is that developmental assessment may provide the most sensitive means of detecting such effects (Davis, 1990; Spear, 1990).

Recognition that neurotoxicant exposure can impair cognitive development in humans has naturally motivated research attempting to demonstrate similar effects in laboratory animals. Such studies permit experimental confirmation of relationships that are typically correlative in human studies, they permit basic research into the toxicological and neurobiological mechanisms of these effects, and they provide for safety evaluation of chemicals that permit human risk assessment in the absence of actual human exposure (Kimmel *et al.*, 1990).

Animal studies do, however, raise problems of cross-species extrapolation in developmental neurotoxicology (Kimmel *et al.*, 1990). Central to this issue is the concept of animal models. What properties should they have? What are their goals? How should they be developed and used? It has recently been suggested (Stanton and Spear, 1990) that the implementation and use of animal models in developmental neurotoxicology may benefit from consideration of logical criteria proposed for animal models of other neurological phenomena and/or disorders. Examples of such phenomena include the development of psychotherapeutic drugs and/or the attempt to understand memory loss associated with aging (Bartus and Dean, 1987; Solomon and Pendlebury, 1988). The purpose of this chapter is to use data from my laboratory to illustrate the use of these criteria in constructing an animal model of cognitive development in neurotoxicology.

## 2. CRITERIA OF ANIMAL MODEL

I will focus on four logical criteria (Table 2). These criteria are adapted from those proposed for the study of aging-related memory disorders (Bartus and Dean, 1987; Sol-

**TABLE 2.**  Criteria for Animal Model of Cognitive Development in Neurotoxicology

1. Conceptual or operational similarities should exist between behavioral measure of cognition in developing animals and humans.
2. Developmental profile of cognitive capacity should resemble that found in humans.
3. Developmental profile of neurobiological changes resembles that found in humans, particularly those that underlie the cognitive capacity in question.
4. Treatments that alter neural or behavioral maturation in humans should cause similar alterations in the animal model.

omon and Pendlebury, 1988). The primary modification has been to change the period in the life span from aging to early development. Several assumptions underly this set of criteria. First, it is assumed that cognition is ultimately a behavioral phenomenon and that the animal model must employ behavioral measures. Second is the assumption that cognition has a neural basis and that cognitive development can be related to neural maturation. Another assumption is that when neurotoxicants alter behavioral development, they do so through their effects on the nervous system. Finally, there is the assumption that there are central aspects of neurocognitive development and its disruption by neurotoxicants that are common to humans and laboratory animals. This last assumption may appear too tautological or circular to even mention (i.e., an assumption of animal models is that one can have animal models). However, it is important to emphasize the notion of commonality across species, because it points to constraints or limitations of this approach to animal models. There are doubtless aspects of brain and behavior, particularly in the area of cognition, that are unique to a given species. It would be difficult, for example, to develop a rodent model of language development or performance of school children on the California Achievement Test (CAT, a test that reveals effects of fetal alcohol exposure). The human neuropsychology of CAT performance is probably not understood, and the CAT requires behavioral capacities that simply do not exist in laboratory animals. Conversely, the abilities of migrating birds to navigate on the basis of electromagnetic fields (Walcott et al., 1979) is a complex behavioral adaptation that is probably not shared by humans. The present framework, then, assumes that there are basic processes of cognition, for example, memory, that are homologous across mammalian species, in the sense of sharing common neural mechanisms and evolutionary origins. If developmental exposure to a neurotoxicant disrupts these basic processes in an animal, it is assumed that this disruption would appear in humans in the same way, and perhaps in uniquely human ways as well. These and other methodological issues associated with the complex problem of modeling phenomena in human (neuro)psychology with animals are more fully discussed elsewhere (Coyle, 1987; Davey, 1983; Olton et al., 1985).

It should also be pointed out that the criteria outlined in Table 2 are best thought of as properties of a particular behavioral paradigm. There may be several paradigms that fulfill these criteria for the purposes of modeling different cognitive phenomena. One could also use these criteria to compare different paradigms for their effectiveness as animal models. Finally, these criteria can be used as a blueprint to guide parallel studies in animals and humans, for the purposes of establishing a particular paradigm as an animal model (Solomon and Pendlebury, 1988). Indeed, it is recent research on memory in *human* infants, research conducted quite independently by other investigators (but motivated by the same zeitgeist as my own), that has made this chapter possible.

## 3. SPATIAL DELAYED ALTERNATION AS A RODENT MODEL SYSTEM

In the present chapter, I will discuss spatial delayed alternation in the rodent in relation to the logical criteria outlined in Table 2. In delayed alternation, rats choose one of two spatial locations in a T-maze on the basis of recent memory for one of those locations (see below). This task belongs to a family of memory tasks that have a long tradition of use in (what is now called) behavioral neuroscience, both in rodents (Kolb, 1984; Olton, 1983; Thomas, 1984) and primates (Fuster, 1989; Goldman-Rakic and Selemon, 1986; Oscar-Berman *et al.*, 1982). I will describe recent developmental research in my laboratory involving this task as it may relate to recent investigations of the developmental psychobiology of memory in human and nonhuman primates. My thesis is that the commonalities among rodents, monkeys, and humans that emerge from this body of research make spatial delayed alternation a good rodent model of cognitive development in neurotoxicology.

## 4. CONCEPTUAL/OPERATIONAL APPROACH TO BEHAVIORAL CAPACITY

The first logical criterion states that conceptual/operational similarities should exist between the behavioral measure of cognition in developing animals and humans. In view of the neurobiological aspects of the present approach, it makes sense to begin with conceptualizations of memory taken from human neuropsychology (Squire, 1987). A long tradition of research on human amnesia, and attempts to study its neural basis in animals, indicates that memory is probably not a single entity but is rather best divided into two or more systems (Mishkin *et al.*, 1984; O'Keefe and Nadel, 1978; Olton, 1983; Schacter, 1984; Squire *et al.*, 1988; Sutherland and Rudy, 1989). There appear to be some aspects of memory that are preserved in human amnesia, whereas others are severely impaired. Indeed, a dual-process view of memory has been advanced by a number of investigators, representing a variety of research traditions. Table 3 lists some of the memory dichotomies that have been proposed. Some of these dichotomies are incompatible, whereas others are difficult to distinguish, particularly at an operational level. The task of theroetically pursuing these various dichotomies, although important in the long run, is not the immediate priority of a practical animal model. However, the consensus represented in Table 3 suggests that attempting to capture, in a general way, the dual-process nature of memory *would* be a desirable goal of an animal model. Clinical research with humans and experimental studies in monkeys also suggests that the limbic system and certain thalamocortical systems (e.g., medial dorsal thalamus and prefrontal cortex; anteroventral thalamus and cingulate cortex) are critically involved in memory. Precisely what elements of these systems are involved and for which aspects of memory are issues that will continue to evolve with further research progress. However, it certainly makes sense at present for an animal model to broadly capture the role of these brain systems in memory.

How have dual-process approaches to the neuropsychology of memory been operationalized? Figure 1 illustrates two paradigms that have been used for this purpose. Both paradigms involve two tasks, that is, they employ a task dissociation (Olton, 1985). One is the delayed-nonmatch-to-sample vs. object discrimination (DNMTS vs. OD) paradigm (Figure 1, left) that has been advanced as a monkey model of human amnesia (Mishkin,

TABLE 3. Two Kinds of Memory

| | |
|---|---|
| Fact memory | Skill memory |
| Declarative | Procedural |
| Memory | Habit |
| Explicit | Implicit |
| Knowing that | Knowing how |
| Cognitive mediation | Semantic |
| Conscious recollection | Skills |
| Elaboration | Integration |
| Memory with record | Memory without record |
| Autobiographical memory | Perceptual memory |
| Representational memory | Dispositional memory |
| Vertical association | Horizontal association |
| Locale | Taxon |
| Episodic | Semantic |
| Working | Reference |

From Squire (1987), with permission.

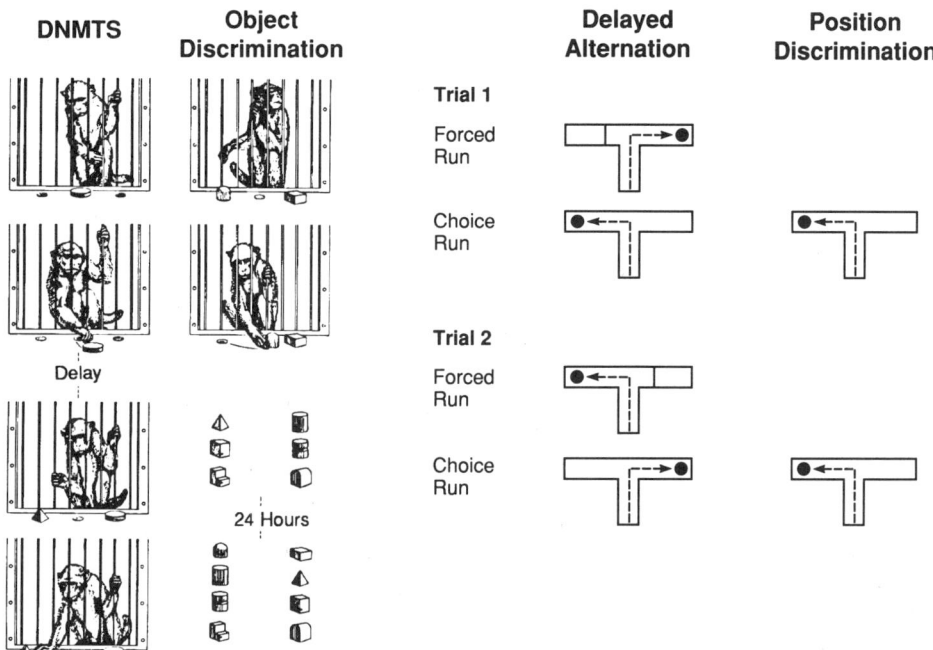

FIGURE 1. Two task distinctions used to study the neuropsychology of memory in human and nonhuman primates (left) and in rodents (right). In primates, delayed-nonmatch-to-sample (DNMTS) is contrasted with object discrimination. In rodents, delayed alternation is contrasted with position discrimination. In both delayed alternation and DNMTS, a sample stimulus is presented, a delay is interposed, and then a choice is offered between the stimulus and an alternative. Reward occurs when the alternative (not the sample) is chosen. For primates, stimuli consist of visual objects, whereas for rodents they consist of spatial locations in the T-maze. Each of these tasks is contrasted with a simpler discrimination task: object discrimination for primates and position discrimination for rodents (see text for further explanation). Illustration of primate tasks from Mishkin and Appenzellar (1987); rodent tasks adapted from Olton (1983), with permission.

1978; Mishkin *et al.*, 1984; Squire *et al.*, 1988). Monkeys with lesions of the medial temporal lobe are impaired on DNMTS but not OD, and indeed, recently human amnesics have been studied with these same tasks and show a similar pattern of results (Chen *et al.*, 1988). The other is the delayed alternation vs. position discrimination (DA vs. PD) paradigm that has been used to study the neural mechanisms of memory in adult rodents (Olton, 1983; Thomas, 1984) and has been adapted for use with developing rats in my laboratory (Freeman and Stanton, 1991; Green and Stanton, 1989; Stanton *et al.*, 1991). Adult rats with damage to the limbic system (Olton, 1983) or prefrontal cortex (Kolb, 1984) are impaired on DA but not PD.

In DNMTS, a monkey is presented with a trial consisting of two phases: a sample phase and, following a delay, a matching phase. During the sample phase, a single object is placed over a center food well and the monkey is rewarded for displacing the object (Figure 1, top left). Following the delay, two objects are presented, one of which is the former sample object and the other is a novel object. During this phase of the trial, the monkey is rewarded if it chooses the novel (nonmatching) object. In object discrimination (OD), trials consist of a single choice phase. The animal is presented with two objects, one of which is always associated with reward. A large set of unique pairs of objects is presented each day until the discrimination is learned.

Delayed alternation (Figure 1, right) resembles DNMTS in that trials also consist of two phases or runs: a forced run, in which the animal is allowed to enter only one arm of the T-maze and, following a delay, a choice run, in which both arms of the T-maze are available. If the rat chooses the arm alternate to that entered on the forced run, it receives a reward. This procedure is repeated across many subsequent trials, with the direction of the forced run varying according to an irregular, counterbalanced sequence. Thus, the only stimulus that can guide choice on a particular trial is the memory of the arm entered on the immediately preceding forced run. DA is contrasted with PD. The PD task is like OD in the monkey paradigm in that trials consist only of a single choice phase. In PD, rats are rewarded for entering only one arm of the T-maze (left or right, counterbalanced across rats). These two task dissociations (DNMTS vs. OD and DA vs. PD) are similar in some respects and different in others. In both cases, choice behavior guided by information in memory over a delay is contrasted with simple choice behavior guided by a consistent relationship between a stimulus (and/or response) and subsequent reward. DNMTS and DA are also similar in that the correct response is to choose the stimulus other than the one presented during the earlier phase of the trial. The monkey and rodent paradigms differ, however, in that, for monkeys, stimuli consist of visual objects and are trial unique (the same stimuli do not reappear in typically hundreds of trials), whereas for rodents stimuli consist of spatial locations and are not trial unique. In fact, the same set of two stimuli (left and right arms of the T-maze) appear on every trial. These differences may be important for some purposes. However, we will see that the rodent and monkey paradigms share developmental and neurobiological properties that suggest the common procedural features of these two paradigms may be more important.

In addition to its relevance to the concept of dual memory systems, task dissociations of the kind described here offer the advantage of addressing the memory vs. performance distinction (Olton, 1985); that is, the simple discrimination tasks (OD or PD) make the same sensory, motivational, and motor demands on the subject as do the memory tasks (DNMTS or DA). Thus, when biological variables such as development, brain damage, or neurotoxicant exposure impair performance on the memory tasks but not the simple discrimination tasks, one can more confidently conclude that these variables affected cognitive processes involved in the memory tasks. This is an important feature of animal models of memory (Olton, 1985).

In summary, we have seen that recent research in behavioral neuroscience has demonstrated that there are forms of memory that are impaired and others that are preserved in human amnesia. The DNMTS vs. OD paradigm seems to capture this property of the neuropsychology of memory. In addition, the spatial DA vs. PD paradigm in rodents shares conceptual, operational, and neurobiological similarities with this primate task distinction. Thus, rodent DA appears to satisfy the first criterion of an animal model (Table 2).

## 5. DEVELOPMENTAL PROFILE OF BEHAVIOR

We now turn to the second criterion of animal models (Table 2), similarity of developmental profile. Is the dual-process approach to memory relevant to behavioral ontogeny?

Bachevalier and Mishkin (1984) performed a study of DNMTS and OD in developing rhesus monkeys. The results for DNMTS appear in Figure 2. Clearly, there is an increase in the rate of acquisition of this task during early ontogeny. For example, 3-month-old monkeys required three times the number of training blocks as 1-year-olds to achieve a criterion of 90% correct responding. In contrast, 3-month-olds learned the OD task very rapidly and at approximately the same rate as adults (data not shown).

More recently, Overman (1990), who was trained in the DNMTS procedure in Mishkin's laboratory, used a procedure that was as similar as possible to that used with infant monkeys to examine memory development in human infants. Specifically, infant monkeys in the Bachevalier and Mishkin study were moderately food deprived and were rewarded with banana pellets, whereas the infant humans in Overman's (1990) study were not deprived and were rewarded with Cheerios and verbal praise ("good boy" for correct responses). Otherwise, the monkey and human studies involved nearly identical procedures (Overman, 1990). Data from human infants appear in Figure 3. There was a pattern of results that was strikingly similar to that seen with monkeys: 12- to 15-month-old human infants required over three times as much training as 22- to 32-month olds to reach training criterion. Overman (1990) also found that 12- to 15-month-old human

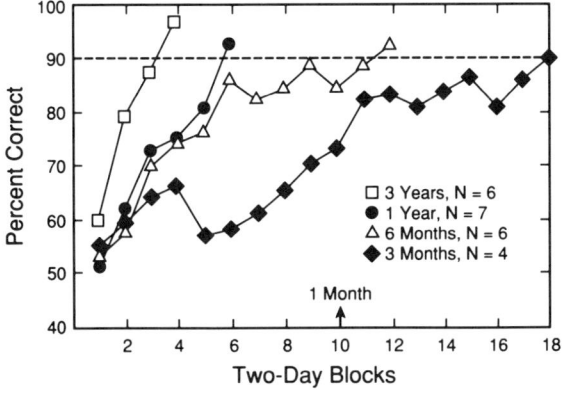

**FIGURE 2.** Results of a study of the ontogeny of delayed-nonmatch-to-sample in monkeys. Monkeys were trained beginning at ages 3 months, 6 months, 1 year, or 3 years (adult). There was a clear age-related increase in the rate of acquisition of this task. From Bachevalier and Mishkin (1984), with permission.

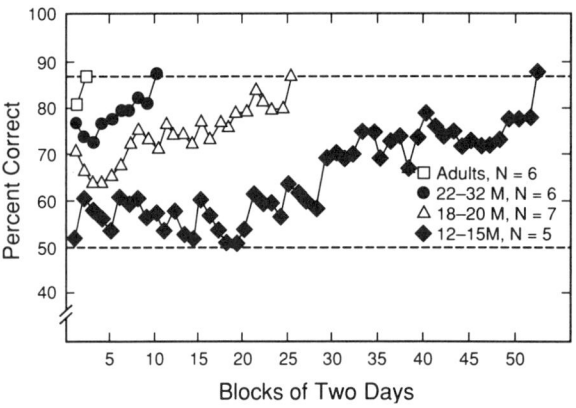

**FIGURE 3.** Results of a study of the ontogeny of delayed-nonmatch-to-sample in human infants. Infants were trained beginning at ages 12–15 months, 18–20 months, or 22–32 months and were compared with adults. There was a clear age-related increase in the rate of acquisition of this task. From Overman (1990), with permission.

infants acquired the OD very rapidly and at a rate similar to that of older infants (data not shown). Together, these two studies show that there is differential ontogeny of DNMTS and OD in human and nonhuman primates. This has been interpreted as evidence that there are early-developing (nonlimbic) and late-developing (limbic) memory systems (Bachevalier and Mishkin, 1984).

Does a similar phenomenon exist in developing rodents? If DA vs. PD can serve as a rodent model of primate memory, then perhaps differential ontogeny on these two tasks can be demonstrated in developing rodents. This question was addressed by Green and Stanton (1989). The basic finding is illustrated in Figure 4. Rat pups aged 15, 21, or 27 days were trained on either DA or PD tasks (Expmnt), as outlined in Figure 1. Their performance was contrasted with control groups that were treated identically, except that reward was given regardless of choice (Control). Rat pups were able to learn the PD task (Position Habit, Figure 4, right panels) at all three ages. This is indicated by the high (>90%) levels of responding in the Expmnt groups and the large difference between their performance and that of their noncontingently rewarded controls. The DA task, on the other hand (Figure 4, left panels), revealed a pattern of late postnatal ontogeny. At 15 days, experimental animals failed to differ from chance or their controls. At 21 or 27 days, in contrast, animals trained on DA achieved high (>90%) performance levels at the end of training, levels that exceeded both chance (50%) and control performance. It thus appears that in the rat, as in human and nonhuman primates, there are early- and late-developing memory systems; and this can be revealed with the spatial DA model.

## 6. NEURAL SUBSTRATES OF BEHAVIORAL DEVELOPMENT

We now turn to the third criterion of animal models: common neural substrates of behavioral development. If the neural systems that are involved in human memory continue to mature during infancy, it is reasonable to suppose that this maturation might contribute to cognitive development. Maturation of these systems in animals has been studied for many years, and many investigators have argued that both the limbic system (Altman et al., 1973; Amsel and Stanton, 1980; Bachevalier and Mishkin, 1984; Douglas, 1975; Rudy et al., 1987; Nadel and Zola-Morgan, 1984) and prefrontal cortex (Goldman-

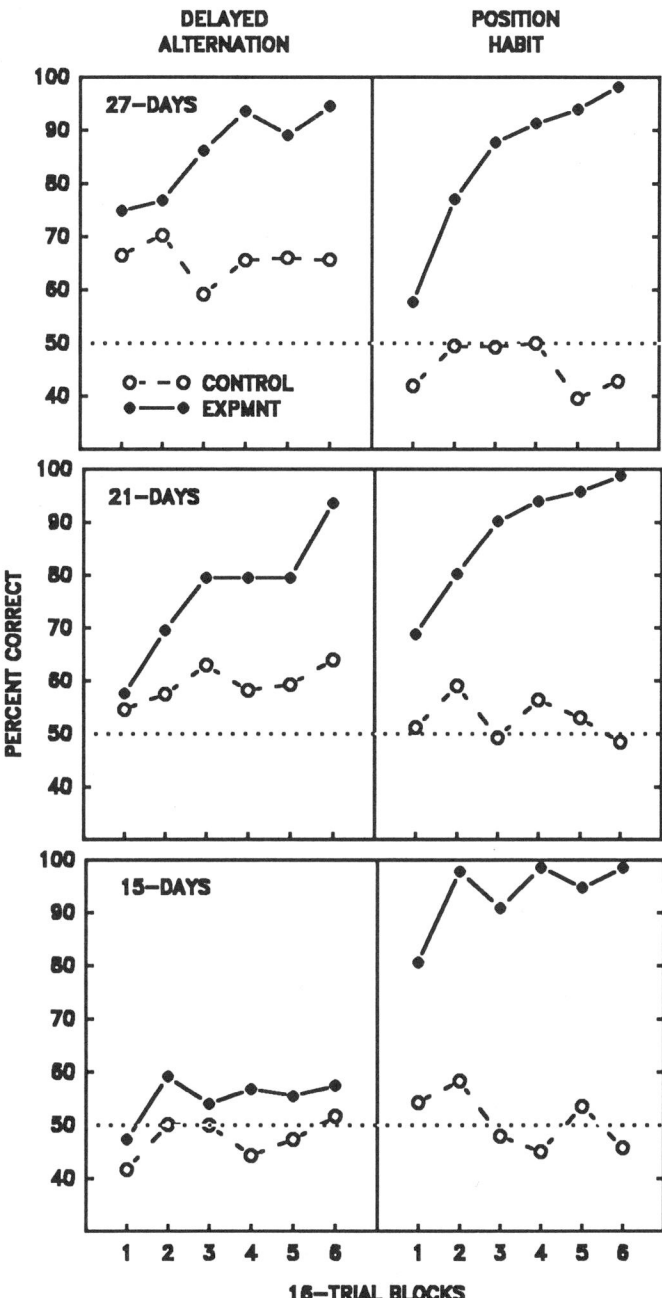

**FIGURE 4.** Results of a study of the ontogeny of delayed alternation (left panels) and position discrimination (right panels) in rats aged 15 (lower panels), 21 (middle panels), or 27 days (upper panels) at the start of training. Groups of rat pups trained on these tasks (Expmnt) were compared with control groups (Control) that were treated identically, except that reward occurred regardless of choice. Learning is indicated by differences between the Expmnt and Control groups that emerge across trial blocks. The dotted line at 50% indicates chance performance. After Green and Stanton (1989), with permission.

Rakic *et al.*, 1983; Nonneman *et al.*, 1984; Van Eden and Uylings, 1985) play a role in the ontogeny of memory, at least in animals.

In the case of the limbic system, these arguments have been based largely on either (1) parallels in the time course of hippocampal maturation (Altman and Bayer, 1975; Rakic and Nowakowski, 1981) and the ontogeny of behaviors, which, on the basis of adult lesion studies, are thought to involve the hippocampus; or (2) the effects of early limbic damage on behavior in adulthood (Brunner *et al.*, 1974). Only recently have the effects of limbic damage on *infant* learning and memory begun to be examined (Bachevalier, 1990; Freeman and Stanton, 1991; Lobaugh *et al.*, 1985; Nicolle *et al.*, 1989; Saperstein *et al.*, 1989). Evidence on the role of limbic maturation and behavior in humans is very recent and relatively limited. For example, it has been reported that hippocampal volume continues to increase through approximately the 15th postnatal month in humans (Kretschmann *et al.*, 1986). This finding, combined with the behavioral data of Overman (1990) described above, suggest a possible correlation between hippocampal maturation and the ontogeny of memory.

This question has been further pursued in a lesion study involving infant monkeys (Bachevalier, 1990). This study showed that combined lesions of the amygdala and hippocampus performed at 1–2 weeks of age produced impairments on a test of DNMTS performed at 10 months of age. These findings combined with the Kretschman *et al.* (1986) study and the close parallels between monkeys and humans in the postnatal development of DNMTS (Figures 2 and 3) strongly suggest that limbic system development contributes to the ontogeny of memory in humans. However, interactions of limbic areas with other (cortical) regions probably best account for the developmental time course of DNMTS (Bachevalier, 1990; Diamond, 1990b).

In the case of prefrontal cortex, the extensive work of Pat Goldman-Rakic and her colleagues (Goldman-Rakic *et al.*, 1983) employing behavioral, electrophysiological, neuropharmacological, and neuroanatomical techniques, has very clearly established a role of the prefrontal cortex in cognitive development in nonhuman primates. Again, however, only recently has evidence for this role in human infants begun to emerge (Diamond, 1990c) (Figure 5). This evidence is primarily behavioral and is based on developmental changes in the performance of Piaget's A-not-B task. This task is very similar to the delayed response paradigm that reveals deficits in prefrontally damaged monkeys. Briefly, subjects watch while an A well is baited and, after a delay, are rewarded for reaching to that well. After a correct response is made, the B well is baited and, after a delay, subjects commit A-not-B error by incorrectly reaching for the A well. Both infant monkeys and humans show age-related improvement in the memory components of this task; dorsolateral prefrontal lesions in adult monkeys produce errors typical of those that appear in very young infants, and early prefrontal lesions impair performance of A-not-B and delayed response tasks in infant monkeys (Diamond, 1990c).

There is reasonable evidence, then, that maturation of the limbic system and prefrontal cortex are involved in the ontogeny of human memory. Can spatial DA capture these effects in the developing rat? Recently, Freeman and Stanton (1991, 1992) performed a pair of studies examining this question. In one study, rat pups received fimbria-fornix transections at 10 days of age and were then tested for DA or PD at 23 days of age. The results appear in Figure 6. This early limbic lesion had no effect on acquisition of the PD task (upper) but completely disrupted DA learning (lower, see Freeman and Stanton, 1991). A similar effect occurs when medial prefrontal cortex lesions are performed at 10 days of age (Freeman and Stanton, 1992). These studies suggest that spatial DA vs. PD is

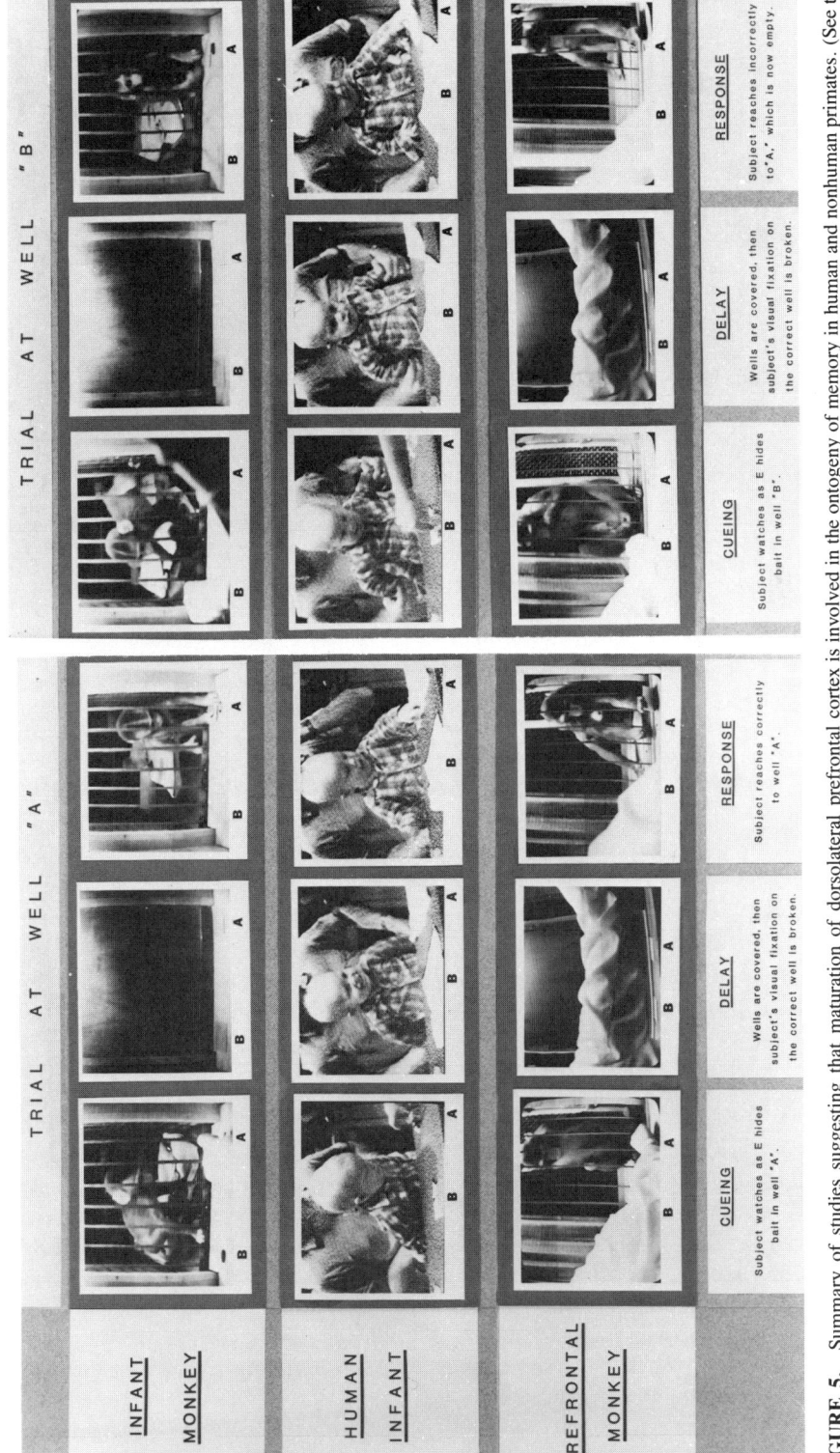

**FIGURE 5.** Summary of studies suggesting that maturation of dorsolateral prefrontal cortex is involved in the ontogeny of memory in human and nonhuman primates. (See text for further explanation.) From Diamond (1990c), with permission.

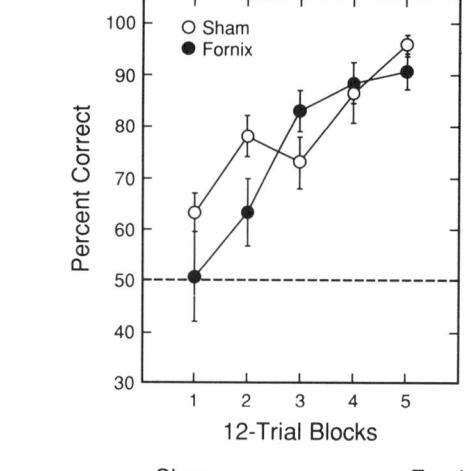
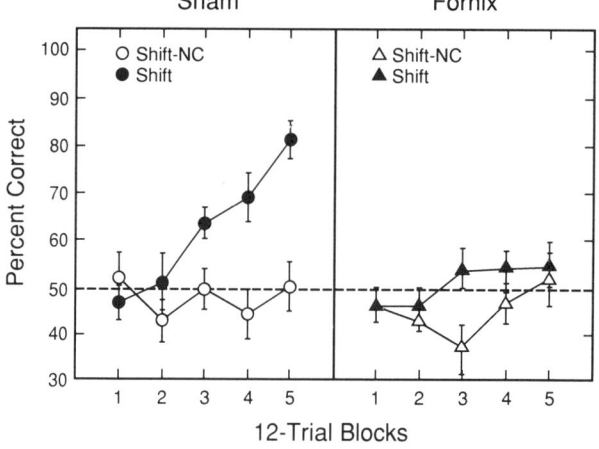

**FIGURE 6.** Results of study on the effects of neonatal fimbria-fornix transection on acquisition of position discrimination (upper panel) or delayed alternation (lower panels) in 23-day-old rat pups. Data points depict mean ± SEM. This transection selectively impaired delayed alternation. (See text for further explanation.) From Freeman and Stanton (1991), with permission.

a rodent model of cognitive development that depends on the integrity of neural systems that are important for the ontogeny of memory in humans (Criterion 3).

## 7. NEUROTOXICANT EFFECTS ON DEVELOPING BRAIN AND BEHAVIOR

Finally, we turn to the fourth criterion of animal models: common effects of neurotoxicants on cognitive development in humans and animals. For illustrative purposes, and to return to the example of lead raised at the beginning of this chapter, we will consider heavy metals. This discussion will be more general than in the previous sections because there is currently, to my knowledge, no information on rodents, monkeys, and humans tested on the same memory paradigm following developmental exposure to the same neurotoxicant. We know that early exposure to lead impairs performance on a clinical measure of cognition (Bayley's MDI) (Davis *et al.*, 1990) in human infants; and performance of spatial delayed alternation in mature monkeys (Levin and Bowman, 1986; Rice and Gilbert, 1990). In this section, I present recent studies from my laboratory involving developmental exposure to the organotin compounds, trimethyltin (TMT) and triethyltin (TET), on the ontogeny of spatial delayed alternation. These compounds were used because they have been subject to much multidisciplinary study (Miller, 1984; Miller and O'Callaghan, 1984; O'Callaghan and Miller, 1988, 1989; Reuhl and Cranmer, 1984; Ruppert, 1986; Ruppert et al., 1983, 1984, 1985) and because they may be representative of heavy metals as a general class of development neurotoxicant. These studies illustrate general methodological principles or themes from developmental neurotoxicology, including the large body of literature on lead (Davis et al., 1990).

## 7.1. Early Detection of Neurobehavioral Impairment

It is perhaps ironic that early assessment has a longer history in human studies of developmental neurotoxicology than in animal studies. In the case of environmental lead, or the fetal alcohol syndrome (FAS), for example, impaired mental function was noted in children and infants first, and only now are we getting the news that these effects persist into adulthood (USA Today, 1991; Needleman, 1991). This is understandable when one realizes that FAS was first clinically described about 19 years ago (Jones and Smith, 1973), and the first human cases are only now entering adulthood. In the meantime, animal research in developmental neurotoxicology has to a large extent remained oblivious to recent advances in developmental psychobiology (Kail and Spear, 1984; Krasnegor et al., 1986; Spear and Campbell, 1978) and continues to be guided by the misconception that complex forms of learning and memory can only be studied in juveniles and adults (see Riley et al., 1985; Spear, 1990; Stanton and Spear, 1990, for further discussion).

If the limbic system is involved in late-developing forms of memory in animals and humans, as reviewed in previous sections of this chapter, then exposure to neurotoxicants that produce early damage to the limbic system should also produce memory impairments at the point in ontogeny when they first appear. Administration of TMT in the rodent a few days after birth produces damage to the hippocampus that is apparent at least by 13 days of age (Chang, 1987; Miller and O'Callaghan, 1984), and this effect persists into adulthood (Miller and O'Callaghan, 1984). Assessment of spatial working memory in juvenile rats with the radial-arm maze has shown that neonatal TMT exposure impairs performance on this task (Miller and O'Callaghan, 1984). Recently, we have shown that this impairment can be demonstrated in the preweanling rat and that the impairment is selective for this form of memory and is not a general performance deficit (Stanton et al., 1991).

Rat pups were injected on PND10 with 6 mg/kg TMT (i.p.) or saline vehicle and then tested for acquisition of DA or PD (Position Habit) on PND18 (Figure 7). Regardless of TMT administration, pups trained on the PD task (SAL-EXP, TMT-EXP) performed significantly better than chance (50%) or their noncontingently rewarded controls (SAL-NC, TMT-NC) by the end of training (Figure 7, right panels). In the case of delayed alternation, on the other hand, TMT produced a marked failure of learning. Saline-injected controls (Figure 7, lower left) showed characteristic acquisition of DA (SAL-EXP) relative to noncontingently rewarded controls (SAL-NC) and performed at greater than 80% correct by the end of training. Their TMT counterparts (TMT-EXP), however, failed to improve across blocks and never differed from their control group (TMT-NC) or from chance (Figure 7, upper left). Histological examination of the brains of these animals

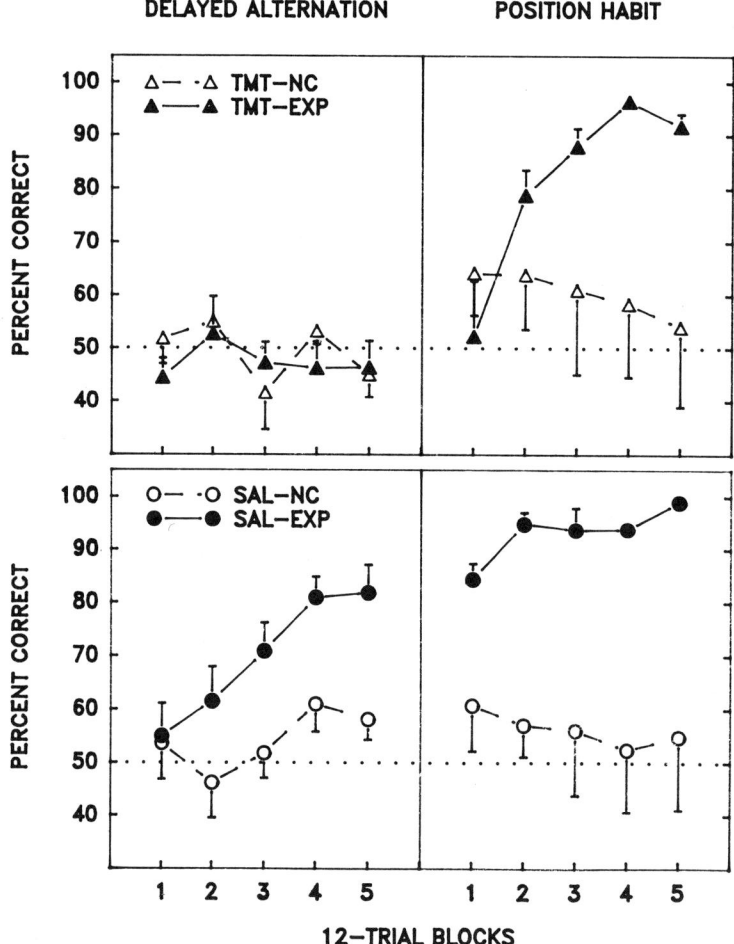

**FIGURE 7.** Acquisition of delayed alternation (left panels) or position discrimination (position habit, right panels) in infant rats following neonatal exposure to the neurotoxic organometal compound trimethyltin (TMT, upper panels) or saline (SAL, lower panels). TMT administration selectively impaired delayed alternation. EXP = contingently rewarded; NC = noncontingently rewarded. Data points depict mean ± SEM. (See text for further explanation.) From Stanton et al. (1991), with permission.

confirmed previous reports (Chang, 1987; Miller and O'Callaghan, 1984) of pyramidal cell loss in the CA3 region of hippocampus (Figure 8). Although such cell loss is not the only consequence of TMT exposure (Balaban et al., 1988; Miller and O'Callaghan, 1984), the similarity of these results to those obtained after neonatal damage to the septohippocampal pathway by Freeman and Stanton (1991; see above) suggest that hippocampal damage may be sufficient to account for the early cognitive deficit.

These findings indicate that developmental exposure to a neurotoxic heavy metal produces clear impairments in our rodent model of cognitive development. They also show that it is possible to study this impairment at relatively early stages of postnatal development and in a way that permits contact with knowledge of brain–behavior relations obtained from developmental psychobiology.

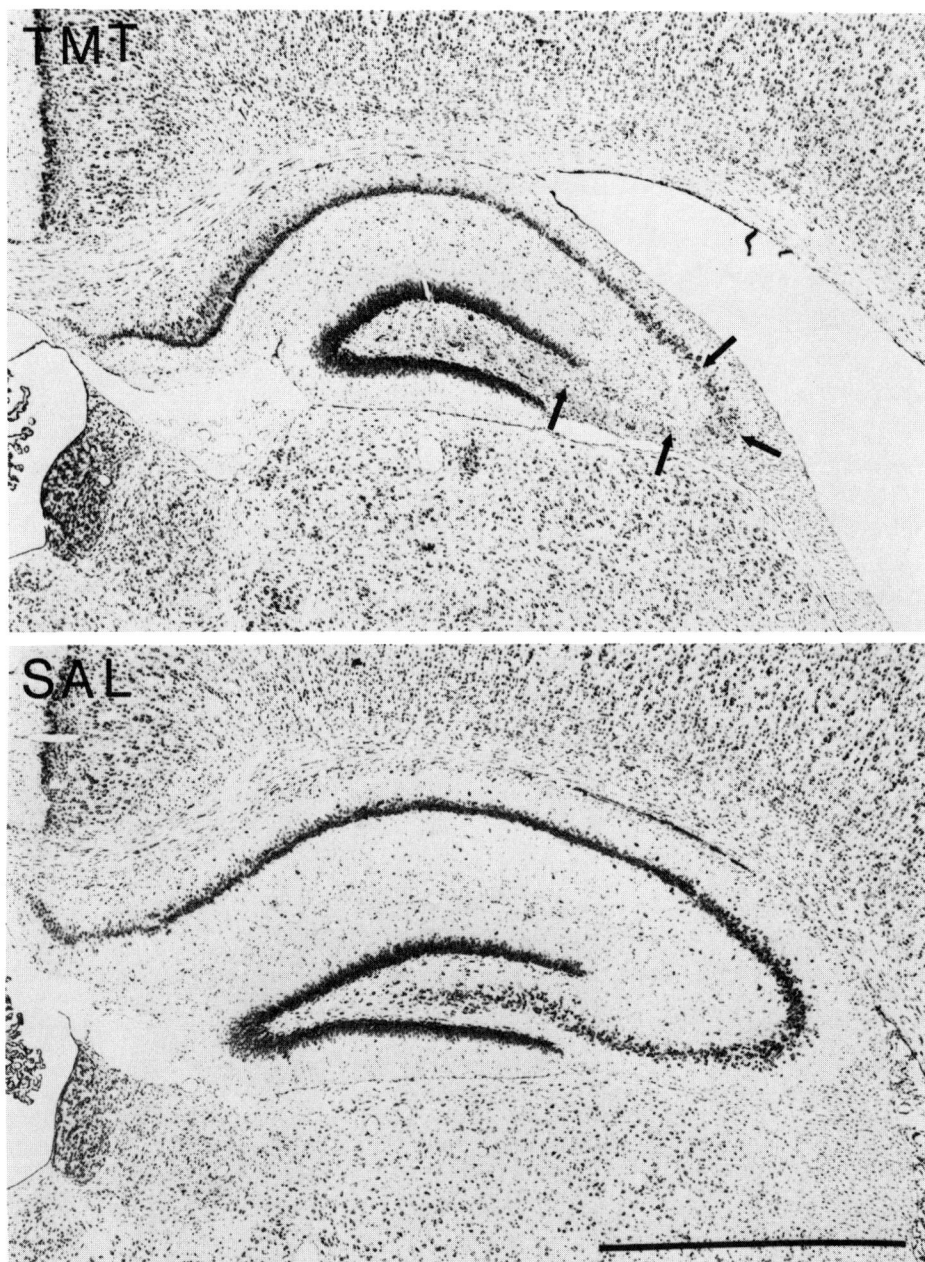

**FIGURE 8.** Cresyl-violet stained, coronal sections through the dorsal hippocampus of representative vehicle-treated (SAL, lower panel) and TMT-treated (TMT, upper panel) rat pups. A reduction in the size of the hippocampus and loss of pyramidal cells in areas CA3-CA4 (arrows) are evident following neonatal exposure to TMT. Scale = 1 mm.

## 7.2. Special Effects of Developmental Exposure

One of the reasons that research with lead has brought so much attention to developmental neurotoxicology is that many of its most noticeable neurotoxic properties occur only with developmental exposure. There is an acute lead toxicity syndrome following adult exposure, but in general, cognitive deficits are more clearly seen following developmental exposure (Davis, 1990). Can a similar phenomenon be shown in our rodent model system? A recent study involving developmental exposure to TET (Stanton et al., 1990) suggests that it can. TET is neurotoxic to both adult and developing organisms. However, there is evidence that the neurotoxicity following developmental exposure is qualitatively different from that seen with adult exposure. Specifically, adult exposure to this compound produces a reversible demyelination (Suzuki, 1971; Watanabe, 1980), whereas there is evidence that developmental exposure produces limbic damage as well, damage similar to that seen with TMT (O'Callaghan and Miller, 1988). In our study (Stanton et al., 1990), rat pups were injected (i.p.) with 5 mg/kg TET or saline vehicle on PND5 and then tested on DA or PD on PND23. TET produced a selective impairment of DA similar to that observed with TMT (Figure 7). Of greater interest were the effects of age of exposure. Figure 9 shows the performance of 28-day-old rats on DA (Shift) or its control condition involving noncontingent reward (Shift-NC) following exposure to saline or TET on PND5 (SAL-5, TET-5; lower panels) or 1 week later on PND12 (SAL-12, TET-12, upper panels). DA learning was impaired only when TET was administered on PND5 (Figure 9, lower right panel). These findings indicate that spatial DA is a rodent model of cognitive

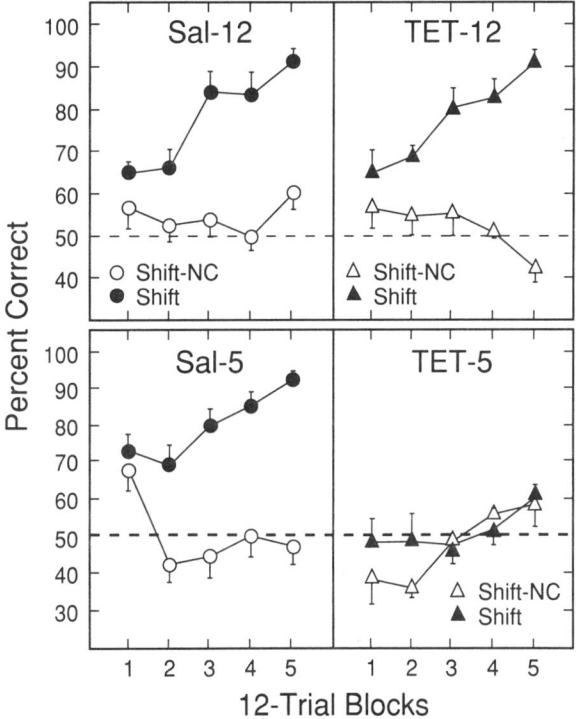

**FIGURE 9.** Acquisition of delayed alternation in weanling rats that received injections of the neurotoxic organometal compound, triethyltin (TET, right panels) or saline (SAL, left panels) at 5 days of age (lower panels) or 12 days of age (upper panels). TET impaired delayed alternation only when it was administered at 5 days of age. SHIFT = contingently rewarded; SHIFT-NC = noncontingently rewarded. Data points depict mean ± SEM. (See text for further explanation.) From Stanton et al. (1990), with permission.

development that can reveal neurotoxic effects of developmental exposure to a heavy metal that depend on the stage of development when exposure occurs.

### 7.3. Special Sensitivity of Early Assessment

Another concept that has emerged in developmental neurotoxicology is the notion that cognitive impairments may be seen at lower levels of exposure when behavioral assessments are performed early rather than at later points in ontogeny (Davis, 1990; Spear, 1990). A provisional look at this issue can be achieved by comparing the results of our study of TET (Stanton et al., 1990) with an earlier one carried out by Miller (1984). Miller (1984) injected rat pups with 0, 3, or 6 mg/kg TET on PND5 and then tested them in the radial-arm maze from 37 to 53 days of age. Stanton et al. (1990) exposed pups to 0, 3, 4, or 5 mg/kg TET on PND5 and tested them for DA at 23 days of age. Thus, similar doses of the compound were given on the same day of development, but one study (Miller, 1984) employed an arguably more complex spatial memory task with older animals, whereas the other (Stanton et al., 1990) examined the effects of TET at an age when spatial DA learning is first emerging. Comparison of the results of these two studies (Figure 10) suggest that early assessment may detect neurotoxic effects at lower exposure levels; that is, Stanton et al. (1990) found an impairment of DA learning at doses of TET as low as 3 mg/kg, whereas Miller (1984) found impaired radial-arm-maze performance at the 6 mg/kg but not the 3 mg/kg dose. This comparison must be made with extreme caution, since it involves a comparison of studies performed with different tasks by different investigators at different times. Thus, it will be important for my laboratory to reexamine this question with the same DA-learning paradigm in older subjects. Neverthe-

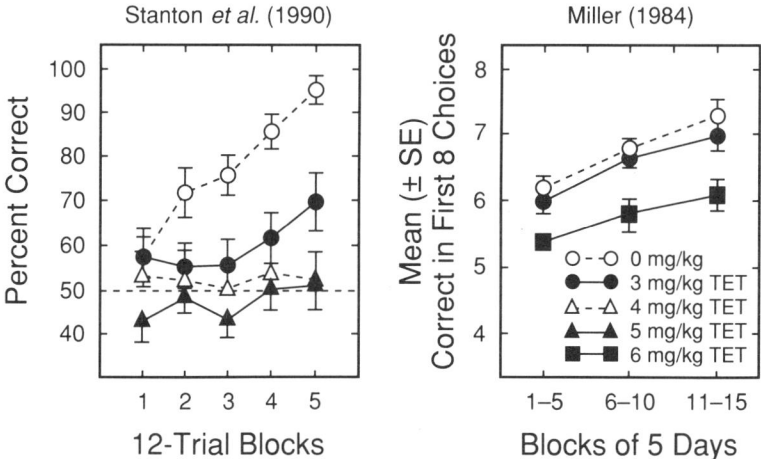

**FIGURE 10.** Effects of neonatal exposure to various doses of triethyltin (TET) on performance of two spatial memory tasks, assessed at different stages of development. T-maze delayed alternation was assessed at 23 days of age and was impaired at the 3 mg/kg dose of TET. Data points depict mean ± SEM. Radial-arm-maze performance was assessed at 37–53 days of age and was impaired only at a dose of 6 mg/kg. Early assessment appears to reveal effects at lower doses of TET, despite the fact that the task used in the older animals is arguably more complex. From Stanton et al. (1990), with permission.

less, there is a suggestion that our rodent model of cognitive development may reveal a special sensitivity of early assessment (Spear, 1990).

## 8. SUMMARY AND CONCLUSIONS

The thesis of this chapter has been that spatial delayed alternation vs. position discrimination learning can serve as a valuable rodent model of cognitive development in neurotoxicology. This model captures dual-process conceptualizations of memory in human neuropsychology and involves procedures that are operationally very similar to those that have been used to address these conceptualizations in human and nonhuman primates. This model also captures the developmental profile and, at least in a general way, common neural mechanisms of cognitive development in human and nonhuman primates. Finally, this model reveals the effects of heavy metals on cognitive development that would have been predicted from knowledge of the neuroanatomical effects of developmental exposure to these compounds. In addition, some of this work reveals properties of developmental neurotoxicity that resemble those claimed for environmental lead (Davis, 1990). In sum, this model system fulfills in a general way the criteria for animal models proposed earlier (and by investigators of other neurobehavioral disorders, such as Bartus and Dean, 1987; Solomon and Pendlebury, 1988). Further use of this model may better permit investigation of the basic mechanisms of developmental neurotoxicity as it relates to impaired cognitive development. Use of this model for regulatory purposes (safety evaluation, risk assessment) may also provide greater confidence concerning the applicability of rodent data to human risk than is possible on the basis of other rodent test methods.

ACKNOWLEDGMENTS.   The author wishes to thank the volume editors and J. Michael Davis for comments on an earlier draft of this chapter.

## REFERENCES

Altman, J., and Bayer, S., 1975, Postnatal development of the hippocampal dentate gyrus under normal and experimental conditions, in: *The Hippocampus,* Part 1 (R. Isaacson and K.H. Pribram, eds.), Plenum Press, New York, pp. 95–122.

Altman, J., Brunner, R.L., and Bayer, S., 1973, The hippocampus and behavioral maturation, *Behav. Biol.* 8:557–596.

Amsel, A., and Stanton, M., 1980, Ontogeny and phylogeny of paradoxical reward effects, in: *Advances in the Study of Behavior* (J.S. Rosenblatt, R.A. Hinde, C. Beer, and M. Busnel, eds.), Academic Press, New York, pp. 227–274.

Bachevalier, J., 1990, Ontogenetic development of habit and memory formation in primates, in: *The Development and Neural Basis of Higher Cognitive Functions* (A. Diamond, ed.), New York Academy of Sciences Press, New York, pp. 457–484.

Bachevalier, J., and Mishkin, M., 1984, An early and late developing system for learning and retention in infant monkeys, *Behav. Neurosci.* 98:770–778.

Balaban, C.D., O'Callaghan, J.P., and Billingsley, M.L., 1988, Trimethyltin-induced neuronal damage in the rat brain: Comparative studies using silver degeneration stains, immunocytochemistry and immunoassay for neuronotypic and gliotypic proteins, *Neuroscience,* 26:337–361.

Bartus, R.T., and Dean, G.L., 1987, Animal models of age-related memory disturbances, in: *Animal Models of Dementia* (J.T. Coyle, ed.), Alan R. Liss, New York, pp. 69–79.

Bellinger, D., Leviton, A., Waternaux, C., Needleman, H.L., and Rabinowitz, M., 1987, Longitudinal analysis of prenatal and postnatal lead exposure and early cognitive development, *N. Engl. J. Med.* 316:1037–1043.

Brunner, R.L., Haggbollom, S.J., and Gazzara, R.A., 1974, Effects of hippocampal x-irradiation-produced granule-cell agenesis on instrumental runway performance in rats, *Physiol. Behav.* 13:485–494.

Chang, L.W., 1987, Neuropathological changes associated with accidental or experimental exposure to organometallic compounds: CNS effects, in: *Neurotoxicants and Neurobiological Function: Effects of Organoheavy Metals* (H.A. Tilson and S.B. Sparber, eds.), New York, Wiley, pp. 82–116.

Coyle, J.T., 1987, *Animal Models of Dementia*, Alan R. Liss, New York.
Davey, G.C.L., 1983, *Animal Models of Human Behavior: Conceptual, Evolutionary, and Neurobiological Perspectives*, John Wiley, New York.
Davis, J.M., 1990, The sensitivity of children to lead. Paper presented at an EPA/ILSI conference on "Similarities and Differences between Children and Adults: Implications for Risk Assessment," Hunt Valley, MD, November 5–7, 1990. A manuscript of this presentation is in preparation.
Davis, J.M., Otto, D.A., Weil, D.E., and Grant, L.D., 1990, The comparative developmental neurotoxicity of lead in humans and animals, *Neurotoxicol. Teratol.* 12:215–230.
Diamond, A., 1990a, *The Development and Neural Basis of Higher Cognitive Functions*, New York Academy of Sciences Press, New York.
Diamond, A., 1990b, Infant's and young children's performance on delayed non-match-to-sample (direct and indirect) and visual paired comparison, in: *The Development and Neural Basis of Higher Cognitive Functions*, (A. Diamond, ed.), New York Academy of Sciences Press, New York.
Diamond, A., 1990c, The developmental and neural bases of memory functions as indexed by the AB and delayed response tasks in human infants and infant monkeys, in: *The Development and Neural Bases of Higher Cognitive Functions* (A. Diamond, ed.), New York Academy of Sciences Press, New York, pp. 267–319.
Douglas, R., 1975, The development of hippocampal function: Implications for theory and therapy, in: *The Hippocampus*, Part 1, (R. Isaacson and K.H. Pribram, eds.), Plenum Press, New York.
Dyck, R.H., Sutherland, R.J., and Buday, M.R., 1985, The ontogeny of mapping and non-mapping spatial strategies following neonatal hippocampal damage in rats, *Soc. Neurosci. Abstr.* 11:832.
Freeman, J.H., Jr., and Stanton, M.E., 1991, Fimbria-fornix transections disrupt the ontogeny of delayed alternation but not position discrimination in the rat, *Behav. Neurosci.* 105:386–395.
Freeman, J.H., Jr., and Stanton, M.E., 1992, Medial prefrontal cortex lesions and spatial delayed alternation in the developing rat: Recovery or sparing? *Behav. Neurosci.*, (in press).
Fuster, J.A., 1989, *The Prefrontal Cortex: Anatomy Physiology, and Neuropsychology of the Frontal Lobe*, Raven Press, New York.
Goldman-Rakic, P., and Selemon, L.D., 1986, Topography of corticostriatal projections in nonhuman primates and implications for functional parcellation of the neostriatum, in: *Cerebral Cortex, Vol. 5* (E.G. Jones and A. Peters, eds.), Plenum, New York, pp. 447–466.
Goldman-Rakic, P.S., Isseroff, A., Schwartz, M.L., and Bugbee, N.M., 1983, The neurobiology of cognitive development, in: *Handbook of Child Psychology: Infancy and Developmental Psychobiology* (P. Mussen, ed.), Wiley, New York, pp. 282–344.
Green, R.J., and Stanton, M.E., 1989, Differential ontogeny of working and reference memory in the rat, *Behav. Neurosci.* 103:98–105.
Jones, K.L., and Smith, D.W., 1973, Recognition of the fetal alcohol syndrome in early infancy, *Lancet* 2:999–1001.
Kail, R., and Spear, N.E., 1984, *Comparative Perspectives on the Development of Memory*, Lawrence Erlbaum, Hillsdale, NJ, 1984.
Kavanaugh, J.F., and Truss, T.J., 1988, *Learning Disabilities: Proceedings of the National Conference*, York Press, Parkton, MD.
Kimmel, C.A., Rees, D.C., and Francis, E.Z., 1990, Qualitative and quantitative comparability of human and animal developmental neurotoxicity. *Neurotoxicol. Teratol. (Special Issue)* 12:173–292.
Kolb, B., 1984, Functions of the frontal cortex of the rat: A comparative review, Brain Res. Rev. 8:65–98.
Krasnegor, N.A., Blass, E.M., Hofer, M.A., and Smotherman, W.P., 1986, *Perinatal Development: A Psychobiological Perspective*, Academic Press, New York.
Kretschmann, H.J., Kammradt, G., Krauthausen, I., Sauer, B., and Wingert, F., 1986, Growth of the hippocampal formation in man, *Bibliob. Anat.* 28:27–52.
*Learning Disabilities: A Report to the U.S. Congress*, 1987, Prepared by the Interagency Committee on Learning Disabilities. National Institutes of Health, Washington DC.
Levin, E.D., and Bowman, R.E., 1986, Long-term lead effects on the Hamilton Search Task and delayed alternation in monkeys, *Neurobehav. Toxicol. Teratol.* 8:219–224.
Lobaugh, N.J., Bootin, M., and Amsel, A., 1985, Sparing of patterned alternation but not partial reinforcement effect after infant and adult hippocampal lesions in the rat, *Behav. Neurosci.* 99:46–59.
Miller, D.B., 1984, Pre- and postweaning indices of neurotoxicity in rats: Effects of triethyltin (TET), *Toxicol. Appl. Pharmacol.* 72:557–565.
Miller, D.B., and O'Callaghan, J.P., 1984, Biochemical, functional and morphological indicators of neurotoxicity: Effects of acute administration of trimethyltin to the developing rat, *J. Pharmacol. Exp. Ther.* 231:744–751.
Mishkin, M., 1978, Memory in monkeys severely impaired by combined but not separate removal of amygdala and hippocampus, *Nature* 273:297–298.
Mishkin, M., and Appenzeller, T., 1987, Anatomy of memory, *Sci. Am.* 256:80–89.
Mishkin, M., Malamut, B., and Bachevalier, J., 1984, Memory and habits: Two neural systems, in: *Neurobiology of Learning and Memory* (G. Lynch, J.L. McGaugh, and N.M. Weinberger, eds.), Guilford Press, New York, pp. 66–77.
Nadel, L., and Zola-Morgan, S., 1984, Infantile amnesia: A neurobiological perspective, in: *Infant Memory* (M. Moscovitch, ed.), Plenum, New York, pp. 145–172.

Needleman, H.L., 1991, Long term effects of early asymptomatic lead exposure, *Toxicologist* 11:3.
Nicolle, M.M., Barry, C.C., Veronesi, B., and Stanton, M.E., 1989, Fornix transections disrupt the ontogeny of latent inhibition in the rat. *Psychobiology* 17:349–357.
Nonneman, A.J., Corwin, J.V., Sahley, C.L., and Vicedomini, J.P., 1984, Functional development of the prefrontal system, in: *Early Brain Damage*, Vol. 2 (S. Finger and R. Almli, eds.), Academic Press, New York, pp. 139–153.
O'Callaghan, J.P., and Miller, D.B., 1988, Acute exposure of the neonatal rat to triethyltin results in persistent changes in neurotypic and gliotypic proteins, *J. Pharmacol. Exp. Ther.* 244:368–378.
O'Callaghan, J.P., and Miller, D.B., 1989, Assessment of chemically-induced alterations in brain development using assays of neuron- and glia-localized proteins, *Neurotoxicology* 10:393–406.
O'Keefe, J., and Nadel, L., 1978, *The Hippocampus as a Cognitive Map*, Oxford University Press, London.
Olton, D.S., 1983, Memory functions and the hippocampus, in: *Neurobiology of the Hippocampus* (W. Seifert, ed.), Academic Press, London.
Olton, D.S., 1985, Strategies for the development of animal models of human memory impairments, in: *Memory Dysfunctions: An Integration of Animal and Human Research from Preclinical and Clinical Perspectives* (D.S. Olton, E. Gamzu, and S. Corkin, eds.), *Ann. N.Y. Acad. Sci.* 444:113–121.
Olton, D.S., Gamzu, E., and Corkin, S., 1985, Memory dysfunctions: An integraion of animal and human research from preclinical and clinical perspectives. *Ann. N.Y. Acad. Sci.* 444:1–553.
Oscar-Berman, M., Zola-Morgan, S.M., Oberg, R.G.E., and Bonner, R.T., 1982, Comparative neuropsychology and Korsakoff's syndrome. III-Delayed response, delayed alternation and DRL performance, *Neuropsychologia* 20:187–202.
Overman, W.H., 1990, Performance on traditional match-to-sample, non-match-to-sample, and object discrimination tasks by 12 to 32 month old children: A developmental progression, in: *The Development and Neural Basis of Higher Cognitive Functions* (A. Diamond, ed.), New York Academy of Sciences Press, New York.
Rakic, P., and Nowakowski, R.W., 1981, The time of origin of neurons in the hippocampal region of the rhesus monkey, *J. Compar. Neurol.* 196:99–128.
Rees, D.C., Francis, E.Z., and Kimmel, C.A., 1990, Scientific and regulatory issues relevant to assessing risk for developmental neurotoxicity: An overview, *Neurotoxicol. Teratol.* 12:175–182.
Reuhl, K.R., and Cranmer, J.M., 1984, Developmental neuropathology of organotin compounds, *Neurotoxicology* 5:187–204.
Rice, D.C, and Gilbert, S.G., 1990, Effect of lead exposure during different periods of development on spatial delayed alternation in monkeys, *Toxicologist* 10:301.
Riley, E.P., Hannigan, J.H., and Balaz-Hannigan, M.A., 1985, Behavioral teratology as the study of early brain damage: Considerations for the assessment of neonates, *Neurobehav. Toxicol. Teratol.* 7:635–638.
Rodier, P.M., 1984, Time of exposure and time of testing in developmental neurotoxicology, *Neurotoxicology* 7:69–76.
Rudy, J.W., Stadler-Morris, S., and Albert, P., 1987, Ontogeny of spatial navigation behaviors in the rat: Dissociation of "proximal"- and "distal"-cue based behaviors, *Behav. Neurosci.* 101:62–73.
Ruppert, P.H., 1986, Postnatal exposure, in: *Neurobehavioral Toxicology* (Z. Annau, ed.), Johns Hopkins University Press, Baltimore, pp. 170–189.
Ruppert, P.H., Dean, K.F., and Reiter, L.W., 1983, Comparative developmental toxicity of triethyltin using split-litter and whole-litter dosing, *J. Toxicol. Environ. Health* 12:73–87.
Ruppert, P.H., Dean, K.F., and Reiter, L.W., 1984, Neurobehavioral toxicity of triethyltin in rats as a function of age at postnatal exposure, *Neurotoxicology* 5:9–22.
Ruppert, P.H., Dean, K.F., and Reiter, L.W., 1985, Development of locomotor activity of rat pups exposed to heavy metals, *Toxicol. Appl. Pharmacol.* 78:69–77.
Saperstein, L.A., Kucharski, D., Stanton, M.E., and Hall, W.G., 1989, Developmental change in reversal learning of an olfactory discrimination. *Psychobiology* 17:293–299.
Schacter, D.L., 1984, Toward the multidisciplinary study of memory: Ontogeny, phylogeny, and pathology of memory systems, in: *Neuropsychology of Memory* (L.R. Squire, and N. Butters, eds.), Guilford Press, New York, pp. 13–24.
Solomon, P.R., and Pendlebury, W.W., 1988, A model systems approach to age-related memory disorders, *Neurotoxicology* 9:443–462.
Spear, L.P., 1990, Neurobehavioral assessment during the early postnatal period, *Neurobehav. Toxicol. Teratol.* 12:489–496.
Spear, N.E., and Campbell, B.A., 1979, *Ontogeny of Learning and Memory*. Lawrence Erlbaum, Hillsdale, NJ.
Squire, L., 1987, *Memory and Brain*, Oxford University Press, New York.
Squire, L.R., and Butters, N., 1984, *Neuropsychology of Memory*, Guilford Press, New York.
Squire, L.R., Zola-Morgan, S., and Chen, K.S., 1988, Human amnesia and animal models of amnesia: Performance of amnesic patients on tests designed for the monkey, *Behav. Neurosci.* 102, 210–221.
Stanton, M.E., and Spear, L.P., 1990, Workshop on the Qualitative and Quantitative Comparability of Human and Animal Developmental Neurotoxicity, Work Group I Report: Comparability of Measures of Developmental Neurotoxicity in Humans and Laboratory Animals, *Neurotoxicol. Teratol.* 12:261–267.
Stanton, M.E., Barry, C., and Keck, C., 1990, Neonatal exposure to triethyltin (TET) disrupts the ontogeny of working memory in the rat, *Toxicologist* 10:109.
Stanton, M.E., Jensen, K.F., and Pickens, C.V., 1991, Neonatal exposure to trimethyltin impairs spatial delayed alternation in preweanling rats. *Neurotoxicol. Teratol.* 18:525–530.
Sutherland, R.J., and Rudy, J.W., 1989, Configural association theory: The role of the hippocampal formation in learning, memory, and amnesia, *Psychobiology* 17:129–144.

Suzuki, K., 1971, Some new observations in triethyltin intoxication of rats, *Exp. Neurol.* 31:207–213.
Thomas, G.J., 1984, Memory: Time binding in organisms, in: *Neuropsychology of Memory* (L.R. Squire and N. Butters, eds.), Guilford Press, New York, pp. 374–384.
U.S. EPA, 1991, Maximum contaminant level goals and national primary drinking water regulations for lead and copper; final rule, *Fed. Reg.* 40 CFR, Parts 141 and 142.
Van Eden, C.G., and Uylings, H.B.M., 1985, Postnatal volumetric development of the prefrontal cortex in the rat, *J. Compar. Neurol.* 241:268–274.
Walcott, C., Gould, J., and Kirschvink, J., 1979, Pigeons have magnets, *Science* 205:1027–1029.
Watanabe, I., 1980, Organotins (triethyltin), in: *Experimental and Clinical Neurotoxicology* (P.S. Spencer and H.H. Schaumburg, eds.), Williams and Wilkins, Baltimore, pp. 545–557.

Chapter 7

# The Evaluation of Behavioral Changes Produced by Consumption of Environmentally Contaminated Fish

*Helen B. Daly*

## 1. INTRODUCTION

Is dilution the solution to pollution? All over the world toxic chemicals have been released into the rivers and lakes with the assumption that these chemicals would become so dilute that they would cause no harm. Unfortunately, this disposal technique does not work for persistent (long-lasting) toxic chemicals such as PCBs, DDT, dioxin, organic lead, and mercury, etc. because they bioaccumulate and biomagnify. The chemicals are picked up by the phytoplankton and zooplankton, and small fish feed on the plankton. Larger fish eat many of the small fish, and the larger and older the fish, the more concentrated the chemicals become. If wildlife, such as the bald eagle, and humans, who are on the top of the food chain, consume many of the large fish, they can accumulate large quantities of the chemicals.

Bioaccumulation of persistent toxic chemicals is having an impact even in large bodies of water such as the Great Lakes in the northeastern United States (e.g., Lake

---

*Helen B. Daly* • Department of Psychology and Center for Neurobehavioral Effects of Environmental Toxins, State University of New York College at Oswego, Oswego, New York 13126.
*The Vulnerable Brain and Environmental Risks, Volume 1: Malnutrition and Hazard Assessment,* edited by Robert L. Isaacson and Karl F. Jensen. Plenum Press, New York, 1992.

Michigan and Lake Ontario). The concentrations of toxins in the fish are so high that wildlife feeding on these fish have reproductive problems. For example, there are far fewer bald eagle nests along the Great Lakes than inland and the eagles are not reproducing. There are many more birth deformities seen in double-crested cormorant embryos along the shores of the Great Lakes than in inland areas (see Colborn *et al.,* 1990, for a review). A report produced by the National Wildlife Federation recommends severe restrictions on consumption of Lake Michigan fish (Glenn and Foran, 1989–90), and the New York State Department of Health warns sports fishermen to curtail their consumption of Lake Ontario fish (especially the large salmon and trout). Commercial fishing on Lake Ontario is prohibited. State programs, however, continue to stock Pacific salmon and lake trout in these lakes to support the large sports-fishing industry, and sports fishermen report eating these fish (Dawson and Brown, 1989).

Restrictions on consumption of fish contaminated with persistent toxic chemicals are based primarily on potential physical health effects (e.g., cancer). Does their consumption also cause *behavioral changes? Yes!* The present chapter reviews research that supports this conclusion.

## 2. RESEARCH APPROACHES

At the Center for Neurobehavioral Effects of Environmental Toxins (SUNY Oswego) we are using a four-pronged approach to determine the behavioral changes caused by consumption of the chemicals found in Lake Ontario fish:

|  |  | Adults | Offspring |
|---|---|---|---|
| (correlational) | Humans |  |  |
| (experimental) | Rats |  |  |

We are testing adults and offspring of humans and laboratory rats who have eaten Lake Ontario fish, and are comparing their behavior with appropriate control groups. For ethical reasons, the research with humans is restricted to the correlational approach: Only the relationship between fish consumption and behavior are determined, making it difficult to establish that consumption of the fish *causes* behavioral changes. Humans cannot be randomly assigned to the experimental group and forced to eat Great Lakes fish, or to the control group and prevented from eating these fish. People decide if they are going to eat the fish, and the reasons that made them decide to do this could also be the cause of the behavioral differences. For example, poor people may eat the fish from the Great Lakes because it is free, and poor people may also not be able to provide as rich a developmental environment for their children, e.g., to purchase as many educational toys. The lack of such an environment may be the cause of the behavioral deficits found in the human offspring, rather than the toxic chemicals present in the mother. To attempt to solve this problem, many possible confounding variables are measured (e.g., income, education level, age, home environment, substance abuse, etc.), and statistical techniques are used to factor out their possible influence. The problem is that one can never be sure that all the appropriate confounding variables have been measured. Therefore, it is extremely difficult, and probably impossible, to prove a cause-and-effect relationship using the correlational approach.

To establish a cause-and-effect relationship, however, the experimental method can be used with animals. We have been using laboratory rats, because a large number of well-established behavioral testing procedures have been developed for this species by experimental psychologists. Rats are randomly assigned to one of three groups. The experimental group is fed Lake Ontario salmon fillets (a 30% ground fish and 70% ground rat-chow mash mixture) for 20 days (called LAKE). One of the control groups is fed a diet consisting of 30% Pacific Ocean salmon (called OCEAN), and the other (not included in all studies) is fed a no-salmon rat-chow mash diet (called MASH). They are then taken off the fish diet and tested in various behavioral tasks. To our surprise, a consistent pattern of behavioral changes has emerged. When "life was pleasant" there were no behavioral differences, but when "life was made unpleasant" the rats fed Lake Ontario salmon reacted more to the negative (aversive) events than control rats fed Pacific Ocean salmon or no salmon. Similar results have been found with the *offspring* of rats fed Lake Ontario salmon. Since we have never found behavioral differences between the two control groups, and the differences are always between the experimental group and the two control groups, we conclude that a fish diet per se does not influence behavior. The major difference between Pacific salmon raised in Lake Ontario vs. those raised in the Pacific Ocean is the amount of persistence toxic chemicals (see Section 5). Some combination of these chemicals is, therefore, the likely cause of the behavioral differences.

Although our research has focused on testing behavioral changes in rats, we have recently begun testing adult humans and their offspring. The initial test phase will be completed by 1994. If the same pattern of results is found in humans as in rats, then we will have a firmer basis for concluding that the correlational evidence with humans is based on a cause-and-effect relationship.

## 3. RESEARCH RESULTS

### 3.1. Human Offspring

There has been only one major study completed (the "Jacobson" study) to determine the behavioral differences between children of mothers who ate Great Lakes fish vs. those who did not. The Jacobsons tested the behaviors of offspring whose mothers had eaten two to three Lake Michigan fish meals per month for at least a 6-year period. In 1980–81 they interviewed mothers in four western Michigan hospitals on the day following delivery. They obtained fish-consumption histories, demographic information, and the PCB level in umbilical cord blood. At birth, the higher the mother's consumption of Lake Michigan fish, the lower the birth weight, the smaller the head circumference, the shorter the gestational age, and the lower the neuromuscular maturity (Fein *et al.*, 1984). On the third day after birth, the babies were given the Brazelton Neonatal Behavioral Assessment Scale (NBAS). In addition to finding that exposed babies had "greater motoric immaturity, poorer lability states, a greater amount of startle, and more abnormally weak (hypoactive) reflexes, . . . the most highly exposed infants were more likely than controls to be classified as 'worrisome' on three NBAS clusters" (Jacobson et al., 1984, p. 523): automatic maturity, reflexes, and range of state. The results were significant, even when the physical differences at birth and other possible confounding variables were factored out.

At 7 months of age the babies were given the Fagan Test of Visual Recognition (also called the Fagan Test of Infant Intelligence). Two identical photos of human faces were presented to the baby, and then a new face was switched with one of the original faces. Normal babies prefer to look at the novel face. The higher the cord serum PCB level, however, the lower the time spent fixating on the novel stimulus (Jacobson et al., 1985). Lower scores on this test have been shown to correlate with lower intelligence later in life (Fagan and Montie, 1988).

At 4 years of age the children were tested on the McCarthy Scales of Children's Abilities. Higher cord serum PCB levels resulted in lower verbal and memory scale scores, primarily due to the forward and backward digit span short-term memory scores (Jacobson et al., 1990). A very interesting finding was that 17 of the 236 children refused to cooperate during at least one test. These were the children whose mothers had significantly higher PCB levels in their milk, which has been shown in a larger sample of 4-year-olds living in Michigan to be a principal source of children's exposure to PCBs and DDT (Jacobson et al., 1989). If one can assume that testing is a mildly negative experience for 4 year olds, it appears as if those children probably exposed to higher levels of toxins due to breast feeding reacted more negatively to the testing procedure.

We are currently extending this ground-breaking research. Our behavioral testing involves babies born between 1991 and 1994 in the Oswego Hospital (located on the southeastern end of Lake Ontario) whose mothers have or have not eaten Lake Ontario fish. Even though we are also measuring a large number of possible confounding variables (as did the Jacobsons), we cannot be sure that all have been accounted for. Therefore, if we find differences we will not be able to conclude that there is a cause-and-effect relationship. The results, however, can be used to *predict* behavioral differences in babies of mothers who were exposed to the toxic chemicals found in Great Lakes fish (see any research methods in behavioral sciences textbook, e.g., Rosenberg and Daly, 1993, for a discussion of prediction from correlation).

### 3.2. Adult Humans

I know of no study that tested behavioral changes in adult humans who have eaten Great Lakes fish. However, we have begun testing the parents of the babies we are studying and should complete testing by 1993–94.

### 3.3. Adult Rats

3.3.1. History

Prior to the initiation of behavioral tests, it had been established that mammals who consumed large amounts of Lake Ontario or Lake Michigan salmon had physiological changes. Female mink fed a 30% diet of whole Lake Michigan salmon for 6 or 11 months

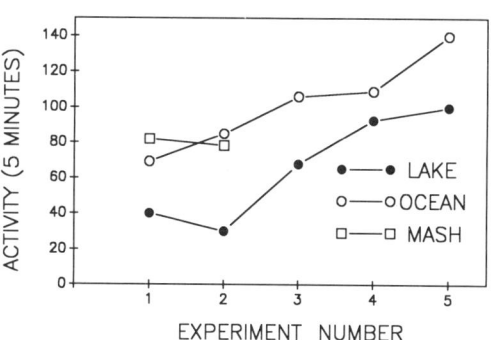

FIGURE 1. Mean activity level for the 5-min period in an "open field" on the first day of testing for five experiments. Rats were females rather than males in experiments 2 and 5; were fed as juveniles rather than as adults in experiments 1, 2, and 4; and were not food deprived in experiments 1, 2, 3, and 5. Adapted from Hertzler (1990, Fig. 4).

had no live offspring, but controls fed West Coast salmon were not affected (Aulerich et al., 1971). A 100% diet of whole Lake Ontario salmon fed to laboratory rats for 1 or 2 months resulted in dilated sinusoidal spaces in areas of the adrenal cortex and adrenal medulla compared with controls fed Pacific Ocean or no salmon (Leatherland and Sonstegard, 1980), and the epithelial cells of the thyroid gland were enlarged (Leatherland and Sonstegard, 1982). Hepatic mixed-function oxidase activity was slightly increased in the livers of laboratory rats fed Lake Ontario salmon (Villeneuve et al., 1981), especially at the higher doses (5%, 10%, or 20% diet fed for 28 days).

Martin (1983) at SUNY Oswego showed both reproductive deficits (decrease in number of young born per litter) in voles fed a 30% diet of Lake Ontario salmon for 30 days prior to being paired with the males and liver changes (increased vacuolation and swelling of parenchymal cells). Controls were fed ocean salmon or no salmon. Hertzler, also at SUNY Oswego, extended the work of Martin from voles to laboratory rats. He fed rats a 30% diet of Lake Ontario salmon (fish preparation and feeding procedures are reviewed in Section 3.3.2) for 20 days, and then tested their activity level in a novel environment (a 68 × 68 cm box with 16 3-cm holes in the floor, called an *open field*). Figure 1 shows the results of five experiments. The rats fed the Lake Ontario salmon diet had lower activity scores for the 5-min testing period than control rats fed Pacific Ocean salmon or no salmon. These effects occurred independent of sex and age of the rats, and whether they were food deprived or not during testing.

Since it is difficult to interpret why rats show decreased activity levels in novel environments, I decided to test the rats fed Lake Ontario salmon in a complicated learning task. I was fully convinced that the combination of persistent toxic chemicals found in Lake Ontario salmon would result in severe learning deficits. When the first experiment (see Section 3.3.4a) indicated that the rats were very adept at learning, I accused the person who had the subject codes hidden away that he had reversed them. I replicated the experiment under slightly different conditions and found the same results. We now know that consumption of Lake Ontario salmon does not produce a general learning deficit in rats. But is there a consistent pattern of behavioral effects? The experimental results indicate yes. The rats fed Lake Ontario salmon are hyperreactive to negative events.

3.3.2. Fish Preparation

Pacific salmon, stocked as fingerlings in Lake Ontario, were obtained as adults when they swam upstream to spawn in the Salmon River near Altmar, New York, a river on the eastern end of Lake Ontario that is heavily fished by sports fishermen. Lake Ontario salmon were also obtained in the spring from sports fishermen fishing from boats and bringing their catch to a weigh station. Identical results were obtained using salmon caught in the river or lake (Daly, 1991). The salmon were between 10 and 20 lb. They were filleted according to the guidelines of the New York State Department of Environmental Conservation, which are designed to minimize ingestion of contaminants. The fillets obtained in a given season were ground together (skin excluded) and frozen in 100- to 400-g packages. Control Pacific Ocean salmon fillets or steaks were obtained and were filleted in Oswego. They were also ground and frozen. Pacific Ocean salmon are used as controls because we have been unable to find a source of Pacific salmon from a non-polluted fresh-water lake.

The ground salmon was defrosted when needed, and a mixture of 30% salmon and 70% ground Purina laboratory rat chow was combined with tap water (75 g fish-chow mixture with 75 cc of water) to form a mash. Purina chow pellets (75 g) were combined with 85 cc of tap water overnight to form the no-salmon mash (more water was added to equate the water content of the salmon).

### 3.3.3. General Methods

Male Sprague Dawley rats bred in the Oswego colony (derived from stock obtained from the Holtzman Co., Madison, WI) were fed Purina rat chow ad libitum until the experiments were begun, typically around 80 days of age. When needed, they were removed from the colony cages, weighed, placed in individual cages, and *randomly assigned* to either the experimental (LAKE) or control groups (OCEAN and MASH). The appropriate diet was placed into their cages (75 g dry weight), and a fresh portion was given daily for 20 days. All rats readily ate the fish diets. On the 20th day they were reweighed, given Purina rat chow pellets, and were never given a fish diet again. Since we have never found weight differences among the groups, we assume that there is no major illness caused by the LAKE diet.

One to 3 days later, one experimenter brought the rats to a second experimenter, who was not told the fish diet of the rat. This person numbered the tail with magic marker, reweighed the rats, and placed them on a food deprivation schedule. *Persons involved in collecting the data were unaware of which fish condition each rat had experienced* until the end of the experiment. The rats were weighed, gentled, and fed the appropriate amount of rat chow pellets each day to maintain them at 80% of their weight on the first day of food deprivation. Seven days later they were placed in individual pre-feed cages and remained there until they ate the reward pellets to be used in the experiment (typically 37 mg P.J. Noyes, formula A pellets; 45 mg pellets for lever-press experiments). Rats (typically eight per fish diet) were given only one behavioral test, unless otherwise noted. Results reported as significant (ANOVAs) reached minimally the $p = .05$ level, but frequently reached the $p < .001$ level.

### 3.3.4. Behavioral Changes

3.3.4a. Preference for Predictable Rewards. The first two experiments involved testing the rats in a two-choice maze. Following a choice to one side (e.g., right side), one of two stimuli (black or white inserts) were presented (each was presented on half of the trials). In

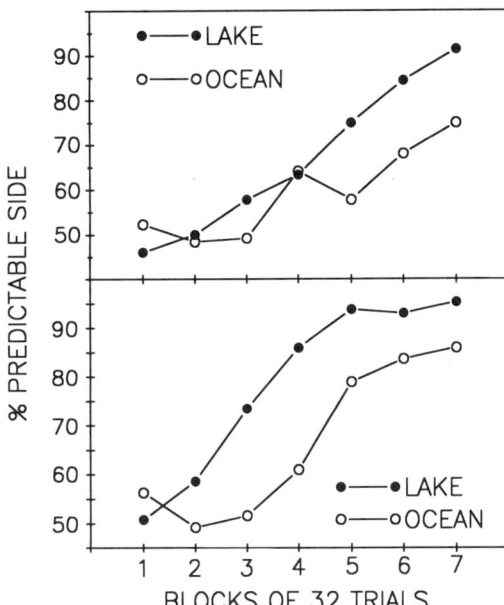

**FIGURE 2.** Mean percent preference for the predictable reward side (50% is chance responding) when the black and white stimuli were presented on both sides (upper panel) and when a gray stimulus was present on the unpredictable reward side (lower panel). Adapted from Daly et al. (1989, Fig. 1 and 2).

the presence of one color (e.g., black), a large 15-pellet food reward was given 15 sec after the choice, and in the presence of the other color, no reward was given (predictable reward side). A choice to the other side resulted in presentation of the same two stimuli, but now both were followed by the food reward in 15 sec on half of the trials (unpredictable reward side). In other words, the black insert on the right side resulted in food, the black insert on the left side resulted in food on half of the trials, the white insert on the right side resulted in no food, and the white insert on the left side resulted in food on half of the trials. The stimuli were not present until after the choice (see Daly et al., 1989 for additional details). All groups were given eight trials per day for 28 days.

Contrary to my prediction that the toxic chemicals would result in learning deficits, the rats fed Lake Ontario salmon had no trouble learning to predict when food would be given on the predictable reward side and acquiring the preference for the predictable reward side. In addition, they showed a larger preference for the predictable reward side than the control group fed Pacific Ocean salmon. Figure 2 (top panel) shows acquisition of the preference for the predictable reward side. Both groups began at chance level (50% preference) and slowly began to show a preference for the predictable reward side. Significant group differences emerged on the last three blocks of trials. We replicated the study, but made the task simpler by having a gray stimulus present on every trial on the unpredictable reward side. Figure 2 (bottom panel) shows that the group differences occurred sooner (see Daly et al., 1989, Experiments 1 and 2).

Rats normally show a preference for the predictable reward side (Daly, 1985, 1989), because unpredictable nonreward has been shown to be aversive, whereas predictable nonreward is far less aversive (Daly, 1992). Since the rats fed Lake Ontario salmon showed a larger preference for predictable reward, it occurred to me that perhaps the toxic chemicals found in Lake Ontario salmon were increasing the aversiveness of unpredictable nonreward. Computer simulations of a mathematical model (DMOD; see Daly and Daly, 1982, 1987, 1991; originally developed to account for behavior of normal subjects in over 60 learning tasks) showed a nice fit between the data and the simulation if the one parameter reflecting the intensity of the aversive reaction to nonreward is increased for the group fed Lake Ontario salmon (see Figures 1, 2, and 3 in Daly et al., 1989).

We have used DMOD to successfully predict the results obtained in all subsequent experiments. Only one assumption was made: Consumption of Lake Ontario salmon increases the reaction to negative events, such as mild shock, reward reductions, and unpredictable nonreward, but not to positive events.

3.3.4b. Mild Shock. In the next two experiments we investigated the effects of a mild electric shock. In the first experiment, the rats previously tested in the two-choice maze (Figure 2, bottom panel) were trained to run down a 180-cm long runway (a long narrow box with a Plexiglas® lid) to obtain a large 12-pellet (45 mg) food reward in the goalbox at the end of the runway (60 acquisition trials, six/day). Then an extremely mild electric shock (0.1 mA, 1 sec) was given to the feet of the rat just before he reached the goalbox (passive avoidance task). Shocks were presented on trials 3 and 5 (first shock day) and on trials 8–13 (second shock day). The rats barely flinched to the mild shock, and across the first eight trials the two shocks had very little effect. On the second day, the subjects fed Lake Ontario salmon showed a large increase in time to run down the runway, even though this behavior delayed the start of eating the food reward. The results can be seen in Figure 3, which shows the time to leave the startbox and run down the runway on the second day of the shock phase (trials 7–13). The large difference between the groups occurred even though it was 54 days since the rats had been given the salmon diet (see Daly et al., 1989, Experiment 3, for additional details).

In the second experiment rats were initially trained to press a lever to obtain a 1-pellet (45 mg) food reward on a variable interval (VI) 2-min schedule (on the average they are given a food reward every 2 min following a response). Then, while they were responding on the VI-2 min schedule, they were given a 30-sec tone followed by a foot shock (0.25 mA, 0.5 sec). Four such trials occurred in each 90-min test session (conditioned emotional response task). The influence of the shock on the rate of lever pressing was immediate and large in the group fed Lake Ontario salmon. Figure 4 shows that by the second and third test days they showed a 33% drop in the number of lever presses, even while the tone that signaled the onset of the shock was off. The control groups fed Pacific Ocean salmon or no salmon showed a 1% and 5% drop, respectively. The shock apparently conditioned a larger amount of aversiveness to the environmental chamber (context) in the rats fed Lake

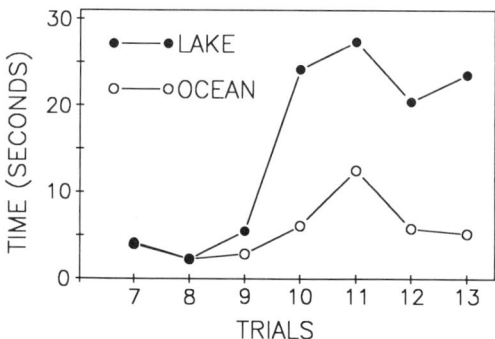

**FIGURE 3.** Time in seconds to run down a 180-cm runway to a food reward when shocks were presented on every trial. Adapted from Daly et al. (1989, Fig. 5).

**FIGURE 4.** Percent drop in lever-press responses on the second and third test days when four shocks per 90-min test session were given. Adapted from Daly et al. (1989, Fig. 6).

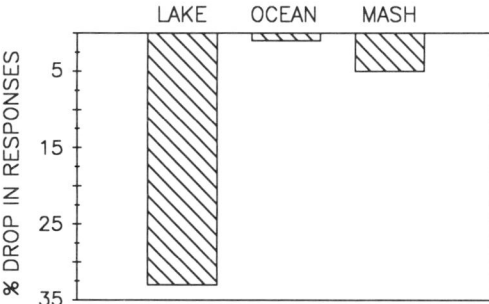

Ontario salmon, and this interfered with responding on the lever for food (see Daly et al., 1989, Experiment 4).

These experiments not only supported the hypothesis that rats fed Lake Ontario salmon would show a larger reaction to negative events, they extended the type of negative event from unpredictable omission of a food reward to mild electric shocks.

3.3.4c. *Reward Reductions.* The next two experiments were designed to test a third type of negative event: receipt of a smaller than expected food reward. Rats were trained to run down a 199-cm long runway to receive either a large 15-pellet or a small 1-pellet reward. Following 72 acquisition trials (6/day) the rats previously given 15 pellets were shifted to the 1-pellet reward. The reaction of a normal rat when shifted from 15 to 1 pellet is to stop approaching the goal and to run more slowly than a rat who had always been given the small 1-pellet reward (called a *contrast* or *depression effect*). This behavior is presumed to be due to the negative emotional response (frustration) experienced when a smaller than expected reward is given, similar to the experience you feel if your paycheck was only $50 when you expected it to be $500 (Daly & Daly, 1991). Repeated experiences with the small reward, however, should result in learning to expect the small reward. Therefore, the small reward should no longer be aversive and there should be recovery from the depression effect.

Figure 5 (top panel) shows the time taken to leave the startbox and run down the runway for the last 2 days of the acquisition phase, and the 15 days (six trials/day) of the shift phase. At the end of the acquisition phase, the groups receiving 15 pellets ran faster than the groups receiving 1 pellet (2 vs. 3–4 sec), and there was no influence of type of fish diet. The groups fed Pacific Ocean salmon or mash were influenced by the shift in reward, and took about 12 sec on the second shift day to run the 199 cm, but recovered to the level of the control groups given 1 pellet throughout training by the seventh shift day. The group fed Lake Ontario salmon, however, found the shift in reward far more aversive, taking about 22 sec to run the 199 cm on the second shift day. Even after 90 experiences with the small reward (day 15), they were still running substantially slower than all other groups, indicating that they still found the small reward aversive (see Daly, 1991).

This experiment was replicated and extended. Figure 5 (bottom panel) shows that the rats fed Lake Ontario salmon again ran more slowly following the shift to the small reward than the rats fed Pacific Ocean salmon or mash. The groups labeled 30%-20D were identical to the groups in the first experiment: They were fed a 30% diet of salmon for 20 days. The other two groups, labeled 10%-60D, were fed a 10% diet of salmon for 60

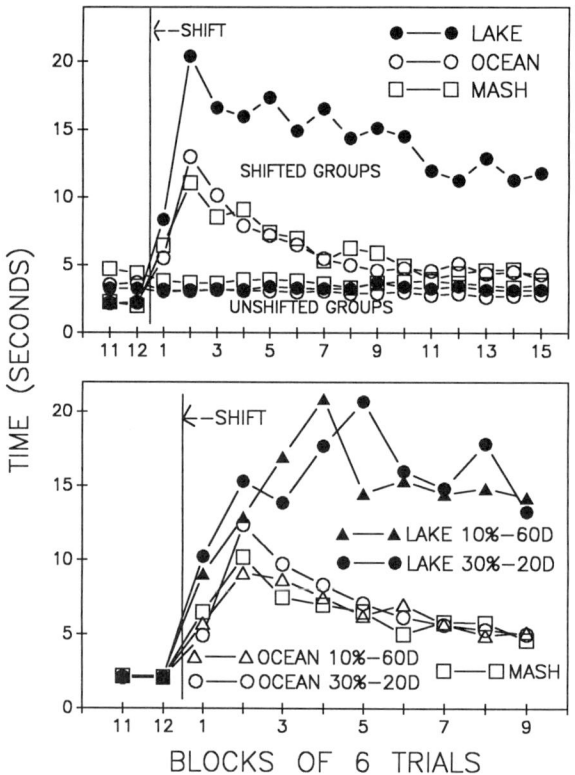

**FIGURE 5.** Time in seconds to run down a 199-cm runway when given a 15- or 1-pellet reward during the last 2 days of first phase, and 1 pellet during the shift phase. From Daly (1991, Figs. 1 and 2).

days. The total amount of fish intake was the same, but a smaller amount of fish was fed each day for a greater number of days. There were no differences between the 30%-10D or 10%-60D groups (Daly, 1991). If these results can be generalized to humans, the implication is that people who eat small amounts of Lake Ontario salmon throughout the year would show the same changes in behavior as those who eat large amounts only during the height of the salmon fishing season.

In a third reward-reduction experiment subjects were given runway training to a large reward, just as was done in the first two experiments, but instead of shifting them to a small reward, they were shifted to no reward (extinction). This too is a negative event (like a broken candy machine, see Daly and Daly, 1991). The group fed Lake Ontario salmon should find no reward more aversive than the control groups and should extinguish more quickly (run more slowly down the runway). Figure 6 shows that this prediction was upheld: The group labeled LAKE CRF ran more slowly during extinction than the OCEAN CRF and MASH CRF groups. The hypothesis that rats fed Lake Ontario salmon would react more to aversive events was again supported.

Three additional groups were included. Instead of being given the large reward on every trial during the first phase (called *continuous reinforcement,* CRF), these groups were given the food reward on a random half of the trials and no reward on the other half of the trials (called *partial reinforcement,* PRF). It is well documented that rats given PRF training run more quickly during the extinction phase than those given CRF training (see Daly and Daly, 1982 for an analysis of this result). Should rats fed Lake Ontario salmon

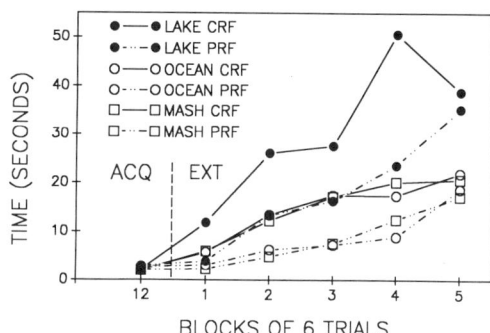

FIGURE 6. Time in seconds to run down a 199-cm runway when shifted from continuous reinforcement (CRF) or partial reinforcement (PRF) during acquisition to extinction.

also extinguish more slowly following PRF than CRF acquisition, but more quickly than rats fed the control diets? Computer simulations of DMOD, again assuming that the Lake Ontario fish increased only the reaction to negative events, such as unexpected nonreward, indicated yes, and predicted the exact pattern of results seen in Figure 6.

The rats fed Lake Ontario salmon presumably extinguished more quickly following both PRF and CRF acquisition because unpredictable nonreward was more aversive than for the groups fed the control diets. These results, therefore, support the interpretation of the preference for predictable reward results (Section 3.3.4.a). I had assumed that the rats fed Lake Ontario salmon preferred the predictable reward side because of the heightened aversiveness of unpredictable nonreward. The runway extinction experiment provided evidence for this interpretation.

3.3.4d. *Counterintuitive Predictions: Reacquisition and Progressive Ratio Schedules.* If rats fed Lake Ontario salmon are more reactive to negative events, one would not expect that they would reacquire the response of running down the runway more quickly after being shifted from a large to a small and back up to the large reward than rats fed the control diets. One would also not expect them to respond more on a progressive ratio schedule, where the amount of work required to obtain the same food reward increases, e.g., rats must press a lever two times, then four times, then six times, etc., increasing the number of responses by two each time to obtain the next reward (called a progressive ratio 2 [PR2] schedule). DMOD, however, made these two counterintuitive predictions, primarily because the more aversive small rewards and nonreward are, the greater is the positive effect of a subsequent large reward (see Appendix).

After 15 days (six trials/day) of being shifted from 15 to 1 pellets (see Figure 5, upper panel) all groups were given the large 15-pellet reward for nine trials. Figure 7 shows the time in seconds taken to leave the startbox on the last three reacquisition trials. As predicted, the group fed Lake Ontario salmon and previously shifted from 15 to 1 pellets (labeled 15-LAKE) reacquired the response more quickly than the other groups (shorter time to leave the startbox). Although the differences were small and variable, if one reduces the variability by using replications as a factor, the differences are significant. The time to enter the goalbox did not differ among the groups, as had been predicted by DMOD (see Appendix).

The rats from the second contrast effect study (Figure 5, bottom panel) were trained to press a lever for a 1-pellet food reward and then given 2 days of PR2 training (36–37

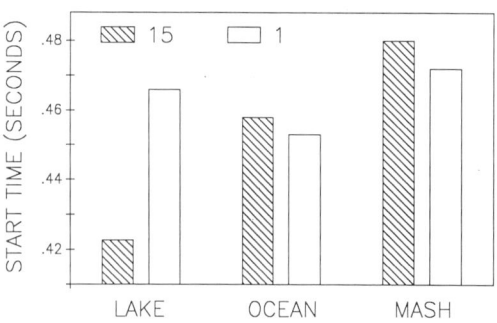

**FIGURE 7.** Time in seconds to leave the start-box of a runway on the last three trials (trials 7–9) when shifted from 1 to 15 pellets (group 1), or back up to 15 pellets (group 15).

days since the last fish meal). Training was continued each day until the rat did not respond for 2 min. It was then removed from the training box, and the schedule was restarted the next day. Figure 8 (left panel) shows the results. The top portion of the figure shows the number of minutes of work, and the lower panel shows the number of responses. The rats fed Lake Ontario salmon worked harder and longer than the two control groups. In a second study, naive rats were given 2 days of PR2 (11–12 days since the last fish meal) and 4 days of progressive ratio 5 training (PR5; rat is reinforced after 5, then 10, then 15 responses, an increase in 5 responses after each reinforcement). The results appear in the right panel of Figure 8. The group differences are large. For example, on the PR2 schedule, the rats fed Pacific Ocean salmon worked for about 30 min, and the rats fed Lake Ontario salmon worked for about 90 min, a threefold increase due to the Lake Ontario salmon diet.

3.3.4e. *Novel Environments: First Day in a Runway and Open Field.* One would expect that the combination of the novelty of being picked up and placed into an unfamiliar place such as a runway or the "open field" would be aversive. The more aversive this experience, the slower the rats should move. If, however, subjects had been handled prior to training and/or trained in a similar apparatus, then the experience may be less

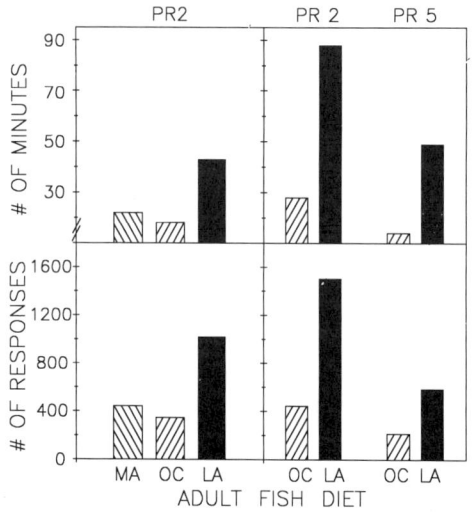

**FIGURE 8.** Mean number of minutes and number of responses on a progressive ratio 2 (PR2) or progressive ratio 5 (PR5) schedule. LA = LAKE; OC = OCEAN; MA = MASH.

aversive. We have run four runway experiments. In the first one, the subjects had previously been trained in a two-choice maze (see Figure 2, lower panel), and there were no group differences during CRF acquisition (Daly et al., 1989, Figure 4). In the second one, the rats had not been previously tested (were naive) and had been given very little handling or gentling prior to the first day in the runway. The rats fed Lake Ontario salmon ran more slowly than the two control groups on the first 12 trials only (29, 12, and 12 sec, for LAKE, OCEAN, and MASH, respectively; see Daly, 1991). By the third block of six trials there were no group differences. In the third and fourth runway experiments the rats were naive, but all had been given extra gentling during the 7-day food deprivation period. There were no group differences. This pattern of results is precisely what would be predicted if the Lake Ontario salmon diet results in hyper-reactivity to negative events: They should run more slowly when first placed into a runway, but only if they were naive and not given prior handling.

Naive rats previously fed Lake Ontario salmon should also show less activity when placed for the first time in an open field. The open-field data have already been presented (see Figure 1), and in all five experiments the rats fed Lake Ontario salmon had lower activity levels. With continued testing, the differences among the groups disappeared (see Hertzler, 1990, Figures 1 and 2), just as one would expect if the novelty of being picked up and placed into the open field diminished with repeated exposure.

3.3.4f. Responding under "Pleasant" Conditions. Although we have not tested behavior under many "pleasant" conditions, the four runway experiments that included groups given rewards on every trial (CRF condition) showed no differences between the rats fed Lake Ontario salmon and the control group(s), except as previously noted in the one experiment on the first 2 days of training. In fact, the overlap between the groups is always quite remarkable. For example, the CRF groups seen in Figure 6 had mean asymptotic response times of 2.2, 2.1, and 2.0 sec (last 5 days of training; see also Daly et al., 1989, Figure 4). We have also not found differences in the Skinner box under the CRF schedule (unpublished); however, we have not given extensive training.

3.3.4g. Dose-Response Effects. The second reward reduction experiment (see Figure 5, bottom panel) showed that the total amount of Lake Ontario fish eaten was important, and not whether they ate a 10% diet for 60 days or a 30% diet for 20 days (Daly, 1991). Hertzler (1990) varied the percentage of fish in the diet mixture, and found that activity in the open field was lower the higher the dose (30% < 15% < 8%, fed for 20 days). The 8% group did not differ from the OCEAN and MASH controls. The open-field measure may not be very sensitive. Therefore, we plan to test several dose levels in the reward shift (contrast effect) and progressive ratio tasks.

## 3.4. Rat Offspring

The Jacobsons' data indicate that the toxic chemicals found in Lake Michigan fish are transferred to the baby from the mother and resulted in behavioral changes measured at birth, 7 months, and 4 years (see Section 3.1). If this result also occurs in rats, then the correlational results obtained by the Jacobsons may reflect a cause-and-effect relationship.

I have begun to test the behavioral changes in the offspring of rats fed Lake Ontario salmon. Results indicate that the same behavioral changes occur in the offspring as occur in the adults fed Lake Ontario salmon, even when the offspring are tested as adults and were never fed the fish diet.

### 3.4.1. General Methods

Female and male rats were fed the 30% mixture of Lake Ontario salmon, Pacific Ocean salmon, or the mash diet from the day they were placed together (3–4 days before conception) until the pups were 7 days old. The pups continued nursing until they were 21 days old. The offspring never ate fish, but could obtain the toxic chemicals from the mother while in utero and through the milk. After weaning they were group housed until testing, which occurred either as juveniles (around 45 days old) or as adults (between 80 and 120 days old).

The mothers were not fed the fish prior to mating to try to avoid the reproductive outcome problems that occurred in mink (see Section 3.3.1). We were apparently successful, since the number of days until birth, successful births, pups per litter, sex ratio, and the weight of the pups at 1, 7, and 21 days of age did not differ among the groups.

When placed on the food deprivation schedule, the juvenile rats dropped quickly to 80% of their ad libitum weight and were food deprived for only 24 hr prior to testing. They were fed increasing amounts of food each day to maintain their weights at approximately 80% of what they would have weighed if not deprived. All other aspects of training were identical to those used with the adult rats.

### 3.4.2. Behavioral Changes

3.4.2a. Progressive Ratio Schedules. We originally pilot tested just four 48-day-old rats (previously been tested in a runway) on the PR2 and PR5 schedule (2 days each). There were large differences, especially on the last PR5 day: the two LAKE subjects worked for more minutes and made more responses than the two OCEAN subjects (89 and 84 min. vs. 45 and 8 min; 920 and 657 responses vs. 323 and 69 responses). We then trained 44-day-old rats not previously tested and found no difference on the first 2 days of PR2 testing and first 3 days of PR5 testing. On the last 2 days of PR5 testing (days 6–7), there were significant differences (e.g., 57, 34, and 33 min of work for the LAKE, OCEAN, and MASH groups, respectively).

These same rats were retested when they reached adulthood (81 days old), and the results are presented in the left panel of Figure 9. Group differences occurred immediately. Another group of rats who had not been tested as juveniles on the progressive ratio task were tested as adults (128 days old), and these results are presented in the right panel. The data from both studies clearly show that the offspring of mother rats fed Lake Ontario salmon worked longer and harder than the offspring of mothers fed Pacific Ocean salmon when tested as adults, even though they had never been given fish to eat.

3.4.2b. Reward Reductions. We have run only one two-group pilot study in the runway, where we shifted from a large 15-pellet reward to a small 1-pellet reward when the rats were 59 days old. Only 48 acquisition trials were given, which could decrease the size of

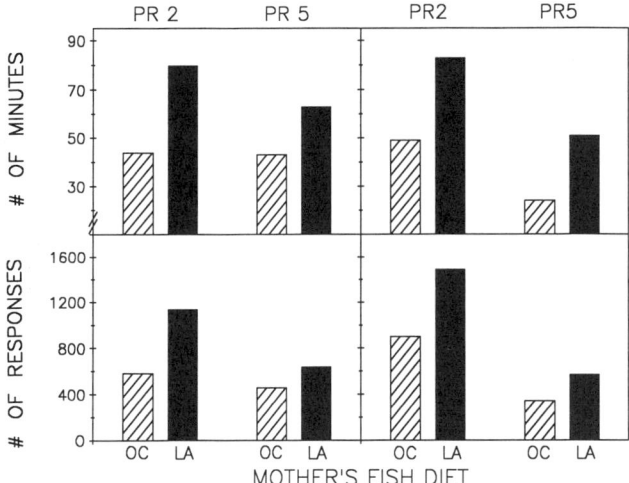

**FIGURE 9.** Mean number of minutes and number of responses on a progressive ratio 2 (PR2) or progressive ratio (PR5) schedule. Subjects were offspring of rats fed the fish diets. LA = LAKE; OC = OCEAN.

the contrast effect. Figure 10 shows that the differences were smaller and less persistent than when adults were fed the fish diets, but on the fourth shift day the differences were large and significant, with all but one subject in the LAKE group running more slowly than the slowest subject in the OCEAN group. We will be testing additional subjects on this task, but will use the same procedures as we did with the adult rats and will also test them in adulthood. Given the greater ease of obtaining differences on the progressive ratio schedule when the rats reached adulthood (previous section), we anticipate larger and more prolonged group differences when the offspring of mothers fed Lake Ontario salmon are tested in adulthood.

3.4.2c. Preliminary Conclusions. This first set of studies raises many questions. Would the effects be larger if the mother were given the fish diet for a longer period prior to conception? How much of the effect occurs by transmitting the chemicals during nursing?

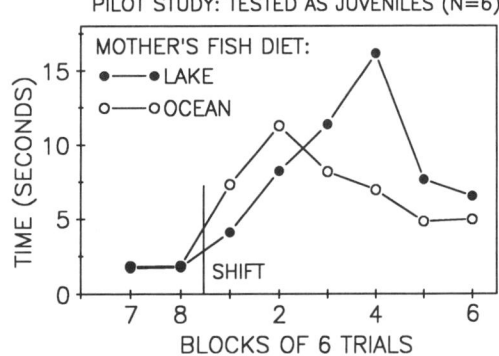

**FIGURE 10.** Time in seconds to run down a 199-cm runway when shifted from 15 to 1 pellet during the last 2 acquisition days and the shift phase. Subjects were offspring of rats fed the fish diets.

Are the behavioral effects larger when tested in adulthood, or are motivational and/or procedural differences making the effects appear larger when the rats reach adulthood?

These preliminary studies indicate that the behavior of the offspring can be influenced by the mother's consumption of Lake Ontario salmon. Because the differences occur even when the rats were tested as adults, we can speculate that the children in the Jacobson study will show behavioral differences when they reach adulthood.

## 4. INTERPRETATIONS

One consistent pattern of findings has emerged from the data: Rats fed Lake Ontario salmon were hyper-reactive to negative events when life was made unpleasant, but showed no behavioral differences when life was pleasant. We have shown that they react more when mild shocks were given (Figures 3 and 4), when food rewards were reduced or presented in an unpredictable situation (Figures 2, 5, 6, and 10), or when they were placed in a novel environment and had not been previously gentled (Figure 1 and first day in runway). They also reacquired the running response more quickly when shifted back up to a large reward (Figure 7), and worked harder and longer on a progressive ratio schedule (Figure 8). When there were no aversive events, there were no group differences: no differences in time to run down a runway when rewarded on a CRF schedule, or in a lever-press task, and no differences after repeated placements into the open field. All results were predicted by DMOD given just one assumption: The effect of the Lake Ontario salmon diet is to increase the reaction to negative events such as reductions in reward, omission of rewards, and mild shocks.

A large number of alternative explanations can be rejected. (1) Decreased activity level: Since rats fed Lake Ontario salmon responded more on a progressive ratio schedule, reacquired responses more quickly, showed no difference on a CRF schedule (runway and lever-press tasks), and showed differences in choice behavior (typically thought of as independent of activity level), the results cannot be accounted for by assuming a decrease in activity level. (2) Increased activity level: Since rats fed Lake Ontario salmon showed larger passive avoidance and CER suppression, a larger contrast effect, more rapid extinction, longer time in the runway on the first day, lower activity in the open field, no differences on the CRF schedule, and differences in choice behavior, the results cannot be accounted for by assuming an increase in activity level. (3) Major physical illness: Since there were no differences in weight gain in the adults fed the fish diets, and no differences in successful births or weight of the pups, it is unlikely that the results are due to a major observable physical illness. (4) Taste aversion: The lack of differences on the CRF schedule and faster reacquisition indicate that food has not become aversive (no conditioned taste aversion). (5) Sensory impairments: Rats fed Lake Ontario salmon acquired the discrimination between the black and white inserts and preference for the predictable reward side in the two-choice maze more quickly than controls, indicating no visual impairment. (6) Sensory enhancement: Although it is possible that they have heightened pain sensitivity, this interpretation cannot explain why the rats fed Lake Ontario salmon were also more reactive to nonpainful negative events (reward reductions, novel environments). (7) Memory changes: There were no differences on the CRF schedule, and since the differences in open-field activity are probably not memory related, the Lake Ontario salmon diet probably does not result in a general memory enhancement. (8) Deprivation level: There were no differences on the CRF schedule, which indicates that the rats fed Lake Ontario salmon are not hungrier. Since there are activity differences in the open field when the rats are not food deprived, the behavioral changes are not dependent on being food deprived.

It appears that the most plausible interpretation of the set of results we have obtained is that the rats fed Lake Ontario salmon are hyper-reactive to negative events. Whether this hyper-reactivity results in an increase or decrease in behavior is determined by the task involved and was successfully predicted by DMOD.

## 5. WHICH CHEMICALS ARE RESPONSIBLE? WE DO NOT KNOW

A large number of toxic chemicals have been released into the Great Lakes basin (estimates range as high as 2800) (Chu et al., 1984), but a complete characterization of the chemicals found in Lake Ontario fish fillets has not been done. Research in the early 1980s (Villeneuve et al., 1981) indicated that of the 15 organochlorine contaminants measured, the Lake Ontario salmon had higher levels of PCBs, p,p'-DDT, p,p'-DDE, p,p'-DDD, mirex, photomirex, *cis*-chlordane, *trans*-chlordane, and dieldrin than Pacific Ocean salmon. Of the 24 inorganic contaminants measured, 17 were higher in diets prepared from Lake Ontario than Pacific Ocean salmon (e.g., mercury), O'Keefe et al. (1983) showed higher levels of 2,3,7,8-tetrachlorodibenzo-p-dioxin (TCDD) in Lake Ontario salmon than in other Great Lakes fish. Hertzler (1990) reported that PCBs and mirex (the only two chemicals tested) were higher in the brains of rats fed Lake Ontario salmon than the control rats fed Pacific Ocean salmon or no salmon. Researchers at the Wadsworth laboratories in Albany, New York are currently measuring the concentrations of a large number of the chemicals in Lake Ontario salmon fillets and in the brains of the rats fed the LAKE or OCEAN salmon diet.

Which chemical, or combination of chemicals, is (are) responsible for the behavioral changes is a difficult question to answer. One approach is to test each chemical individually, and in combinations of two, three, four, etc., to determine which chemicals are producing the effect and if the effects are additive or synergistic. One could also remove one chemical at a time and measure the decrease in the size of the effect. Both of these techniques are time consuming, especially since measuring behavioral changes is very labor intensive. Therefore, Seegal and Shain have begun using simpler preparations (PC-12 rat cells) to measure neurotransmitter changes (e.g., dopamine) due to the chemicals found in Lake Ontario salmon (see Seegal et al., 1989). They are attempting to isolate the mixture of chemicals that gives the largest reaction, and we will then test the behavioral effects of this mixture in the live rat.

Although one could speculate about which chemicals are responsible for the behavioral changes, this may be harmful. Even if research shows a correlation between PCB level in umbilical cord blood and behavioral changes, it is only a correlation, and other chemicals that correlate with PCB levels may be the real cause of the behavioral change. Hopefully, research with combinations of chemicals tested in simpler preparations will provide us with preliminary answers soon.

## 6. SUMMARY AND CONCLUSIONS

A large number of persistent toxic chemicals (e.g., PCBs, DDT, dioxin, mercury) have been, and continue to be, released into the environment all around the world. They have become concentrated in fish, even in bodies of water as large as the Great Lakes. Consumption of Lake Michigan fish by human mothers results in both high levels of PCBs in umbilical cord blood and behavioral differences in their babies compared with controls who had not eaten Lake Michigan fish (see Section 3.1). It is difficult, if not impossible, to prove that the toxic chemicals in the fish *caused* the behavioral differences, because the mothers chose whether to eat the fish or not (correlational model). Therefore, one cannot rule out other variables as the cause. However, to prove a cause-and-effect relationship, the experimental method was used with animals. We randomly assigned laboratory rats to the experimental group and gave them a 30% diet of Lake Ontario salmon for 20 days, or to the control groups, which received a 30% diet of Pacific Ocean salmon or a no-salmon diet, both containing far lower quantities of the toxic chemicals (Hertzler, 1990; Villeneuve *et al.*, 1981).

Results from all experiments testing rats fed Lake Ontario salmon indicate a consistent pattern of results. When there are no aversive events, there is no effect of the Lake Ontario salmon diet. If, however, even a mildly negative event is introduced (reward reductions, mild shocks, or novel environments), the rats fed Lake Ontario salmon show a greater reaction to this event than the controls. The behavioral effects are not subtle, but are impressively large (see Figures 3, 4, 5, and 8).

I have been able to predict and integrate the results with a mathematical model (DMOD), using the assumption that the combination of chemicals found in the fish results in hyper-reactivity to negative events. The model made two counterintuitive predictions given the same assumption: The rats fed Lake Ontario salmon should reacquire a response more quickly when shifted back up to a large reward, and should work harder and longer on a progressive ratio schedule (see Appendix). These predictions were supported.

Are there similarities between the behavioral changes found in rats and humans? Novel stimuli are presented to the subject in both the Fagan Infant Test of Intelligence for human babies and the open-field test for rats. In both cases the subjects exposed to the Great Lakes fish showed a greater reaction to the novelty as if it were aversive; the babies did not look as much at the novel picture, and the rats were less active. Based on the results with rats, we would also expect the children to try to avoid unpleasant situations. Therefore, it was of no surprise that the Jacobsons found that the children with high exposures to the chemicals were the ones who refused to be tested at 4 years of age on the McCarthy tests.

We are currently extending the research of the Jacobsons to babies whose mothers ate Lake Ontario fish. The results from the rat work are currently guiding our selection of tests with humans to determine if they too are hyper-reactive to negative events. If we extend the Jacobsons' results to Lake Ontario, then one might want to recommend early testing of all babies whose mothers have consumed large quantities of Great Lakes fish. The unfortunate finding is that the Jacobsons' results showed changes in the Fagan test. This test has been shown to correlate (r values between 0.33 and 0.66) with later psychometric intelligence (Fagan and Montie, 1988), which could have serious implications for the babies of mothers who have consumed contaminated fish. Weiss (1990) has analyzed that a 5% drop in intelligence test scores would, for every 100 million people, decrease the number of persons with IQs above 130 from 2.3 million to 990,000. Once it is determined which chemical(s) is (are) causing the behavioral changes, then babies of mothers exposed to these chemicals by any means (workplace, accidental spill, release from a toxic waste dump) should probably be tested.

Will the fish in the Great Lakes remain contaminated? Many of the potentially harmful chemicals are still being released, both legally, illegally, and from landfills, so that it does not appear that restrictions on consumption of environmentally contaminated fish from our lakes and rivers will be able to be lifted any time soon. Even if there were no more persistent toxic chemicals released into the environment, it will probably take a number of decades for the lakes around the world to reach levels considered to be acceptable by current standards. If we find that doses far smaller than those that result in physical illnesses cause behavioral changes, then the acceptable levels of exposure to these chemicals may have to be reduced, and it would take even longer until the fish reach levels acceptable for consumption.

## APPENDIX

DMOD (Daly MODification of the Rescorla/Wagner model) is a mathematical/computer simulation model developed to account for the behavior of normal subjects in a large variety of learning tasks (see Daly and Daly, 1991 for a review). One basic equation is used to calculate the trial-by-trial changes in learning, as well as asymptotic values

$$\Delta V = \alpha\beta (\lambda - \bar{V}),$$

where $V$ = learning, $\bar{V}$ = total amount of learning to all stimuli present, $\alpha$ = salience of the stimulus, $\beta$ = learning rate, and $\lambda$ = size of the goal event. There are, however, a number of different goal events possible, such as food reward, omission of the reward, reintroduction of the reward, shock, etc. Each goal event conditions a different V value, with the $\lambda$ value in the equation determined by the type of goal event (Daly and Daly, 1982, 1987, 1991).

DMOD not only predicted a larger contrast effect, more rapid extinction, and greater response suppression following shock in rats fed Lake Ontario salmon (intuitive results), it also predicted two counterintuitive results. The first prediction was that rats fed Lake Ontario salmon would reacquire the running response more quickly than control rats when shifted back up to a large reward. This result should occur only far from the aversiveness of the goal, such as the time to leave the startbox of the runway, and the differences should be small. The reason for this counterintuitive prediction is that it is not only assumed that organisms learn to approach positive goal events (condition Vap) and learn to avoid negative goal events (Vav), but also learn "courage" to approach a place where they have experienced negative events if now positive events occur (Vcc, also called *counterconditioning*). Behavior (Vt) is determined by the sum of the three V values (Vt = $\bar{V}$ap + $\bar{V}$av + $\bar{V}$cc). The amount of courage (Vcc) conditioned is greater the larger the aversiveness (Vav) expected (Daly and Daly, 1991). Therefore, if rats fed Lake Ontario salmon condition more aversiveness (larger Vav) when shifted from a large to a small reward, more courage (Vcc) should be conditioned when they are shifted back to the large reward. The higher the Vcc value, the faster subjects run down the alley. The impact of Vav on behavior is assumed to be less the further the subject is spatially from the goal (Daly and Daly, 1982, p. 447). DMOD simulations show that Vcc should be large enough to counteract Vav far from the goal only, and therefore the rats fed Lake Ontario salmon should reacquire the response more quickly only on the start measure.

Since the control groups given 1 pellet on every trial prior to this last phase should have no Vav, no Vcc is conditioned, and Vt is based on the Vap value. The rats fed Pacific Ocean salmon or no salmon and shifted from 15 to 1 pellet had learned to expect the 1-pellet reward and no longer found it aversive. Therefore, their Vav had extinguished, Vcc should not be conditioned, and they should reacquire the response at the same rate as the 1-pellet control groups. The group fed Lake Ontario salmon was still showing a depression effect following 15 days of training with the small reward (see Figure 5, top panel), indicating that Vav was still present. Therefore, Vcc should be conditioned when they were shifted back up to the large reward and should reacquire the response more quickly.

A larger Vcc value is also one of the reasons DMOD made the second counterintuitive prediction: Rats fed Lake Ontario salmon should work harder and longer on a progressive ratio schedule than control rats. Vav should be larger due to the nonreinforced trials, which should condition a larger Vcc value when the reward is eventually received. The larger Vcc value counteracts the larger Vav value in the lever-press task (the manuscript on the extension of DMOD to the free-operant lever-press task is in preparation). In addition, preliminary simulations indicated that the rats fed Lake Ontario salmon should also show more bursting (a rapid series of responses), which should increase the number of responses. Notes on the data sheets indicated that the rats who showed bursting were typically those who we then found out had been fed a Lake Ontario salmon diet, but no exact measurements of bursting were taken.

ACKNOWLEDGMENTS. The research was supported in part by a Significant Research Advance Award from the State University of New York Central Office and a grant from the Great Lakes Research Consortium.

## REFERENCES

Aulerich, R.J., Ringer, R.K., Seagran, H.L., and Youatt, W.G., 1971, Effects of feeding coho salmon and other Great Lakes fish on mink reproduction, *Can. J. Zool.* 49:611–616.

Chu, I., Villeneuve, D.C., Valli, V.E., Ritter, L., Norstrom, R.J., Ryan, J.J., and Becking, G.C., 1984, Toxicological response and its reversibility in rats fed Lake Ontario or Pacific coho salmon for 13 weeks, *J. Environ. Sci. Health* B19:713–731.

Colborn, T.E., Davidson, A., Green, S.N., Hodge, R.A., Jackson, C.I., and Liroff, R.A., 1990, *Great Lakes, Great Legacy?* The Conservation Foundation, Washington, D.C.

Daly, H.B., 1985, Observing response acquisition: Preference for unpredictable appetitive rewards obtained under conditions predicted by DMOD, *J. Exp. Psychol. [Anim. Behav.]* 11:294–316.

Daly, H.B., 1989, Preference for unpredictable rewards occurs with high proportion of reinforced trials or alcohol injections when rewards are not delayed, *J. Exp. Psychol. [Anim. Behav.]* 15:3–13.

Daly, H.B., 1991, Reward reductions found more aversive by rats fed environmentally contaminated salmon, *Neurotoxicol. Teratol.* 13:449–453.

Daly, H.B., 1992, Preference for unpredictability is reversed when unpredictable nonreward is aversive, in: *Learning and Memory: The Behavioral and Biological Substrates*, (I. Gormezano and E. Wasserman, eds.), Erlbaum, Hillsdale, NJ, pp. 84–104.

Daly, H.B., and Daly, J.T., 1982, A mathematical model of reward and aversive nonreward: Its application in over 30 appetitive learning situations, *J. Exp. Psychol. [Gen.]* 111:441–448.

Daly, H.B., and Daly, J.T., 1987, A computer simulation/mathematical model of learning: Extension of DMOD from appetitive to aversive situations, *Behav. Res. Meth. Instrum. Comput.* 16:38–52.

Daly, H.B., and Daly, J.T., 1991, Value of mathematical modeling in appetitive and aversive learning: Review and extension of DMOD, in: *Fear, Avoidance, and Phobias: A Fundamental Analysis* (M.R. Denny, ed.), Erlbaum, Hillsdale, NJ, pp. 165–197.

Daly, H.B., Hertzler, D.R., and Sargent, D.M., 1989, Ingestion of environmentally contaminated Lake Ontario salmon by laboratory rats increases avoidance of unpredictable aversive nonreward and mild electric shock, *Behav. Neurosci.* 103:1356–1365.

Dawson, C.P., and Brown, T.L., 1989, Characteristics of 1987–88 Oswego County Fishing License Purchasers and Snaggers on the Salmon River. New York Sea Grant Program, Cornell Cooperative Extension and SUNY Oswego, NY.

Fagan, J.F., and Montie, J.E., 1988, The behavioral assessment of cognitive well being in the infant, in: *Understanding Mental Retardation: Research Accomplishments and New Frontiers* (J. Kavanagh, ed.), Paul H. Brookes, Baltimore.

Fein, G.G., Jacobson, J.L., Jacobson, S.W., Schwartz, P.M., and Dowler, J.K., 1984, Prenatal exposure to polychlorinated biphenyls: Effects of birth size and gestational age, *J. Pediatr.* 106:315–320.

Glenn, B.S., and Foran, J.A., 1989, Lake Michigan sport fish consumption advisory project: Technical support document, National Wildlife Federation.

Hertzler, D.R., 1990, Neurotoxic behavioral effects of Lake Ontario salmon diets in rats. *Neurotoxicol. Teratol.* 12:139–143.

Jacobson, J.L., Humphrey, H.E.B., Jacobson, S.W., Schantz, S.L., Mullin, M.D., and Welch, R.W., 1989, Determinants of polychlorinated biphenyls (PCBs), polybrominated biphenyls (PBBs), and dichlorodiphenyl trichloroethane (DDT) levels in the sera of young children, *Am. J. Public Health* 79:1401–1404.

Jacobson, J.L., Jacobson, S.W., Fein, G.G., Schwartz, P.M., and Dowler, J.K., 1984, Prenatal exposure to an environmental toxin: A test of the multiple effects model. *Dev. Psychol.* 20:525–532.

Jacobson, J.L., Jacobson, S.W., and Humphrey, H.E.B., 1990, Effects of in utero exposure to polychlorinated biphenyls and related contaminants on cognitive functioning in young children, *J. Pediatr.* 116:38–45.

Jacobson, S.W., Fein, G.G., Jacobson, J.L., Schwartz, P.M., and Dowler, J.K., 1985, The effect of intrauterine PCB exposure on visual recognition memory, *Child Dev.* 56:853–860.

Kubiak, T.J., Harris, H.J., Smith, L.M., Schwartz, T.R., Stalling, D.L., Trick, J.A., Sileo, L., Docherty, D.E., and Erdman, T.C., 1989, Microcontaminants and reproductive impairment of the Forster's tern on Green Bay, Lake Michigan—1983, *Arch. Environ. Contam. Toxicol.* 18:706–727.

Leatherland, J.F., and Sonstegard, R.A., 1980, Structure of thyroid and adrenal glands in rats fed diets of Great Lakes coho salmon, *Environ. Res.* 23:77–86.

Leatherland, J.F., and Sonstegard, R.A., 1982, Thyroid responses in rats fed diets formulated with Great Lakes coho salmon, *Bull. Environ. Contam. Toxicol.* 29:341–346.

Martin, K.H., 1983, Effects of a Lake Ontario Fish diet on reproduction in voles, in: *Proceedings of the 26th Conference on Great Lakes Research*, International Association for Great Lakes Research, Oswego, New York.

O'Keefe, P., Meyer, C., Hilker, D., Aldous, K., Jelus-Tyror, B., Dillon, K., and Donnelly, R. 1983, Analysis of 2,3,7,8-tetrachlorodibenzo-p-dioxin in Great Lakes fish, *Chemosphere* 12:325–332.

Rosenberg, K., and Daly, H.B., 1993, *Foundations of Behavioral Research: A Basic Question Approach*, Harcourt Brace Jovanovich, Fort Worth, Texas.

Seegal, R.F., Brosch, K., Bush, B., Ritz, M., and Shain, W., 1989, Effects of arochlor 1254 on dopamine and norepinephrine concentrations in pheochromocytoma (PC-12) cells, *Neurotoxicology* 10:757–764.

Villeneuve, D.C., Valli, V.E., Norstrom, R.J., Freeman, H., Sanglang, G.B., Ritter, L., and Becking, G.C., 1981, Toxicological response of rats fed Lake Ontario or Pacific coho salmon for 28 days, *J. Environ. Sci. Health* B16:649–689.

Weiss, B., 1990, The scope and promise of behavioral toxicology, in: *Behavioral Measures of Neurotoxicity* (R.W. Russell, P.E. Flattau, and A.M. Pope, eds.), National Academy Press, Washington DC, pp. 395–413.

# Chapter 8

# Neurotoxicants and Limbic Kindling

*M. E. Gilbert*

## 1. TOXICANTS AND NEUROLOGICAL DISEASE

Potentially neurotoxic chemicals occur naturally in the environment; are used in industry; appear as residues of pesticides, herbicides, and fungicides applied to our food supply; are added to foods to enhance and preserve their flavor or appearance; are used in cosmetic products; or are taken therapeutically or as drugs of abuse (OTA, 1990). Recently the contribution of toxicants to the pathogenesis of several neurological disease states has come under scrutiny. The direct link between people exhibiting the classic symptoms of Parkinson's disease and exposure to MPTP (a chemical produced during the illicit manufacture of synthetic heroin) provided dramatic evidence of how a chemical can poison the nervous system (Langston *et al.*, 1983). A link between the early onset of such disease states as Alzheimer's, amyotrophic lateral sclerosis, and Parkinsonism and environmental neurotoxicant exposure has been suggested (OTA, 1990; Rajput *et al.*, 1987). Our study of the convulsive properties of neurotoxicants also suggests that long-lasting functional changes in the central nervous system (CNS) occur in animals repeatedly exposed to pesticides. In laboratory studies this has been linked with a persistent increase in the susceptibility of animals to develop seizure disorders. This chapter will deal with the kindling epilepsy model and its utility in the identification and characterization of the excitatory CNS effects of environmental toxicants.

The manuscript has been reviewed by the Health Effects Research Laboratory, U.S. Environmental Protection Agency, and approved for publication. Approval does not signify that the contents necessarily reflect the views and policies of the Agency nor does mention of trade names or commercial products constitute endorsement or recommendation for use.

---

*M. E. Gilbert* • Mantech Environmental Technology Inc., Research Triangle Park, North Carolina 277
*The Vulnerable Brain and Environmental Risks, Volume 1: Malnutrition and Hazard Assessment,* edite Robert L. Isaacson and Karl F. Jensen. Plenum Press, New York, 1992.

## 2. TOXICANTS AND CONVULSIONS

There are many toxicants that produce convulsions in humans and animals in response to acute high-dose exposure. A summary of neurotoxicity of more than 760 industrial chemicals comprised by Anger and Johnson (1985) revealed that convulsions were the second most commonly reported effect of exposure and comprised the primary neurotoxic effect of approximately 25% of the chemicals included on the list (M. Gage, unpublished observations). Pesticides appear to be among the most prominent convulsant agents among the groups of neurotoxicants (Morgan, 1989), and several instances of human poisonings by pesticides that lead to convulsive attacks have been reported (Aleksandrowicz, 1979; Demeter and Heyndrickx, 1978; Goldman et al., 1990; Gupta, 1975; Hayes, 1957; Morgan, 1989; Rowley et al., 1987).

Three syndromes of human neurotoxicity have been recognized by Hayes (1963) for members of the chlorinated hydrocarbon class of pesticides. These are outlined in Figure 1 (an adaptation of the scheme presented in Jager, 1970). The first syndrome depicts an acute, high-dose exposure that leads to an increasing stimulation of the CNS to culminate in one or more convulsions. The second syndrome results from a larger number of moderately sized doses that accumulate in the body until the convulsive threshold is surpassed. The third syndrome results from low-level chronic exposure in which many relatively small doses produce one or a few convulsions, but with fewer accompanying symptoms. Convulsive attacks, however, may recur even in the absence of continued exposure.

Jager (1970) interprets this final category as a manifestation of an acute convulsive intoxication superimposed upon a subclinical accumulative intoxication. Such an interpretation is reasonable, considering the persistence of many of the chlorinated hydrocarbon pesticides (Hayes and Laws, 1991). However, recent advances in our understanding of the neurobiology of epilepsy caution against attributing all instances of persistent neurological effects following prolonged exposure to an accumulation of the toxicant in the body. The following section will describe a model of neuroplasticity known as kindling. Kindling results in a permanent alteration in the function of the CNS in response to repeated subthreshold exposure to a variety of treatments. The most prominent outcome is the development of an epileptic disorder, although other subtle adverse effects on behavior also accompany the development of kindling. These include alterations in affective behavior (Adamec, 1990) and disruptions of cognition (Boast and McIntyre, 1977; Leung et al., 1990; Peele and Gilbert, 1992; Robinson et al., 1989) which may appear before, and persist long after, the onset of behavioral signs of motor seizure. As discussed below, consideration of the kindling phenomenon suggests the inclusion of two additional categories of intoxication to the scheme depicted in Figure 1.

## 3. ELECTRICAL KINDLING

Kindling is an epilepsy model in which seizures are gradually induced with repeated electrical stimulation of the brain (Goddard et al., 1969). The convulsive motor response develops over time and is accompanied by the enhancement of electrographic seizure activity at the stimulation site (the seizure focus) and subsequent propagation of epileptiform activity throughout the brain. The resulting change in brain is a permanently

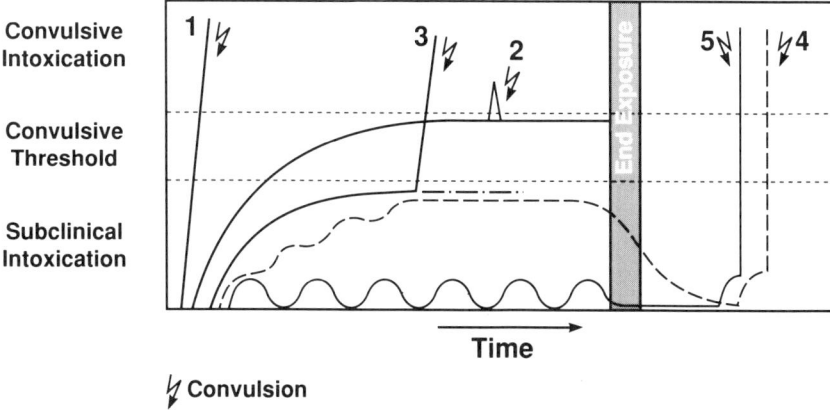

**FIGURE 1.** Three types of convulsive intoxication of chlorinated hydrocarbon insecticides. Type 1 results from an acute, high-dose exposure that is well above the threshold convulsive dose. Type 2 results from a larger number of moderately sized dosages that accumulate until the next exposure exceeds the convulsive threshold. Type 3 convulsive intoxication results from many small dosages that may accumulate, but produce convulsions at body and brain burdens below the convulsive threshold. Chemical kindling is most analogous to type 3 intoxication, but may occur in the absence of significant accumulation of the compound. Types 4 and 5 represent progressive enhancement of seizure responsiveness with repeated exposure in the absence of significant body burden, as is seen with PTZ (type 4), or be superimposed upon some degree of accumulation of toxicant, as with endosulfan and dieldrin (type 5). Adapted from Hayes (1963) and Jager (1970).

enhanced sensitivity to the electrical stimulus that initially had provoked no clinical response and only brief focal electrographic disruptions. The model is thought to best represent the human epileptic condition because of its progressive nature, its permanence, and its responsiveness to classic anticonvulsant therapies (Sato et al., 1990). In addition, the interictal electroencephalogram (EEG recorded between discrete seizure events) is characterized by paroxysmal spikes, and if stimulation is continued for an extracted period of time, spontaneous convulsions occur in the absence of the electrical triggering stimulus (Pinel et al., 1975).

The induction of a focal epileptogenic event (an afterdischarge, AD) is requisite for kindling to develop (Racine, 1972a). However, repeated stimulation at a level that is below the threshold for inducing a focal AD gradually lowers the threshold for evoking an AD. Once an AD is triggered, the threshold continues to decrease, and the kindling process is set in motion (Racine, 1972a, 1972b). Limbic structures seem to be particularly prone to seizure induction, and the amygdala/pyriform area is among the fastest areas to kindle (Racine, 1978). Properties of neurons within this region suggest that they represent a critical neural substrate for the initiation and spread of seizures (McIntyre, 1986; Racine and Burnham, 1984; Racine et al., 1986).

Independent manipulation of a number of different neurotransmitter systems can delay or enhance the development of kindling (Table 1). Cholinergic, glutaminergic, GABAergic, noradrenergic, and serotonergic neurotransmission have all been implicated in the kindling process (see reviews by McNamara et al., 1980; Peterson and Albertse 1982; Racine, 1978). Agonists and antagonists of these systems modulate, in an oppo fashion, the characteristic rate and pattern of electrographic indices (AD duration

TABLE 1. Effects of Chemicals on Electrical and Chemical Kindling Development

| Compound | Electrical Kindling | | Chemical Kindling | |
|---|---|---|---|---|
| | Effect | Citation | Effect | Citation |

**Pharmacological Agents: Proconvulsants**

| Compound | Effect | Citation | Effect | Citation |
|---|---|---|---|---|
| Aspartate | NT | — | ↑ | Bradford and Croucher, 1989; Mori and Wada, 1987 |
| Beta-endorphin | NT | — | ↑ | Cain and Corcoran, 1984 |
| Bicuculline | ↑ | Kalichman et al., 1981 | ↑ | Uemura and Kimura, 1988; 1990; Nutt et al., 1982 |
| c-AMP | NT | — | ↑ | Yokoyama et al., 1989 |
| Carbacol | NT | — | ↑ | Cain, 1983; Wasterlain and Fairchild, 1985 |
| Cocaine | ↑ | Stripling et al., 1989 | ↑ | Weiss et al., 1990; Kilbey et al., 1979 |
| Corticotropin RF | NT | — | ↑ | Weiss et al., 1986 |
| FG-7142 | NT | — | ↑ | Corda et al., 1990; Little et al., 1987 |
| Flurothyl | NT | — | ↑ | Pritchard et al., 1969 |
| Glutamate | NT | — | ↑ | Bradford and Croucher, 1989; Mori and Wada, 1987 |
| Lidocaine | ↑ | Gilbert and Mack, 1989; Stripling et al., 1989 | ↑ | Lekic, 1988; Post et al., 1975 |
| Mercaptopropionic | ↑ | Kalichman et al., 1981 | NT | — |
| Metenkephalin | NT | — | ↑ | Cain and Corcoran, 1984 |
| Muscarine | ↑ | Jonec and Wasterlain, 1981 | NT | — |
| Pentylenetetrazol | ↑ | Bowyers and Albertson, 1982 | ↑ | Cain 1981; Mason and Cooper, 1972; Nutt et al., 1982 |
| Phenytoin | ↑ | Racine et al., 1975 | NT | — |
| Physostigmine | NT | — | ↑ | Girgis, 1981 |
| Picrotoxin | O[a] | Kalichman et al., 1981 | ↑ | Cain, 1984; Corda et al., 1990 |
| Procaine | ↑ | Racine et al., 1975 | NT | — |
| Strychnine | O | Bowyer and Albertson, 1982 | NT | — |

**Pharmacological Agents: CNS Depressants**

| Compound | Effect | Citation | Effect | Citation |
|---|---|---|---|---|
| Atropine | ↓ | Arnold et al., 1973 | — | — |
| Clonidine | ↓ | Gilbert and Mack, 1989; McIntyre and Guigno, 1988 | — | — |
| Diazepam | ↓ | Peterson et al., 1981; Racine et al., 1975 | — | — |

| Chemical | Effect | Reference |
|---|---|---|
| Fluzinamide | ↓ | Albertson et al., 1984 |
| MK-801 | ↓ | Gilbert, 1988 |
| Pentobarbital | ↓ | Kalichman et al., 1981 |
| Scopolamine | ↓ | Cain et al., 1989 |
| SKandF-89976-A | ↓ | Schwark and Haluska, 1987 |

**Pesticides**

| Chemical | Effect | Reference |
|---|---|---|
| Amitraz | ↑ | Gilbert, 1988 |
| Chlordimeform | ↑ | Gilbert, 1988 |
| Cismethrin | ↑ | Gilbert et al., 1990 |
| Deltamethrin | ↑ | Gilbert et al., 1990 |
| Dieldrin | ↑ | Joy et al., 1980 |
| Endosulfan | ↑ | Gilbert, 1992b |
| Lindane | ↑ | Joy et al., 1982, 1983 |
| Parathion | O | Joy et al., 1981 |

**Other Toxicants**

| Chemical | Effect | Reference |
|---|---|---|
| Delta-9-THC | ↑/↓[c] | Karer et al., 1984 |
| IDPN[b] | ↓ | Gilbert, unpublished observation |
| Kainic acid[b] | ↑ | Feldman and Ackerman, 1987 |
| Phenylenediamine | O | Gilbert, unpublished observations |
| Triadimefon | O | Gilbert, unpublished observations |
| Trimethyl tin[b] | ↑ | Dyer et al., 1983 |
| Soman | NT | — |

| | Shih et al., 1990 |

Chemicals were administered acutely, prior to each daily stimulation of the amygdala in the electrical kindling paradigm. Chemical kindling was induced by repeated administration over a number of days to weeks.

[a] Only a single low dose (1 mg/kg) of picrotoxin was used.
[b] Single administration prior to commencement of kindling.
[c] Low dosages of delta-9-THC facilitate, and high dosages retard, kindling.

↑ = facilitates electrical kindling, produces chemical kindling; ↓ = retards electrical kindling; O = no effect on electrical or chemical kindling; NT = not tested.

threshold) and behavioral development of the kindled response (latency, duration of clonic seizure activity, rate of development of generalized motor symptoms).

## 4. KINDLING AS A MODEL OF PLASTICITY

Apart from its obvious tie to seizure disorders, kindling is also studied as a model of neuroplasticity (Racine, 1978). Plasticity refers to any long-lasting change in the functional properties of neurons, the most robust examples of which are development and learning. Several investigators have argued that the physiological alterations induced by kindling may be similar to those that underlie processes such as learning and memory (Goddard and Douglas, 1975; Goddard et al., 1969; Joy, 1985; Racine, 1972a). Focal ADs that fail to result in behavioral signs of seizure promote potentiation of synaptic responses at a number of limbic sites (Racine et al., 1983). Increases in synaptic efficacy that accompany kindling are similar to those observed in long-term potentiation (LTP), an electrophysiological model of learning and memory (deJonge and Racine, 1987; Sutula and Steward, 1987). Antagonists of the N-methyl-d-aspartate receptor subtype disrupt learning, block LTP, retard kindling, and suppress kindling-induced potentiation (Cain et al., 1988; Collingridge, 1986; Gilbert and Mack, 1990; Morris et al., 1986; Robinson et al., 1989a; Wozniak et al., 1990). Kindling-induced potentiation may depend on the same biochemical mechanisms as LTP (Burdette et al., 1989; Cain, 1989; deJonge and Racine, 1987; Gilbert and Mack, 1990). Thus, toxicants that disrupt the development of kindling may also interfere with the neurobiological substrates and processes that subserve learning and memory.

## 5. ACUTE GENERALIZED SEIZURE TESTS AND ELECTRICAL KINDLING

Convulsions that follow acute high-dose chemical exposure may result from direct CNS actions of the compound or be secondary to the peripheral effects of the toxicant on other organ systems. Kainic acid is a highly neurotoxic chemical and produces convulsions by directly exciting a class of glutaminergic receptors in the brain, particularly the hippocampus (Olney, 1980). Other toxicants may lead to convulsions that are unrelated to any direct CNS stimulant effects of the compound itself. This may be the case in seizures resulting from ischemic or hypoxic episodes induced by exposure to tris(2-chloroethyl)-phosphate, a chemical used for its flame-retardant properties (Matthews et al., 1990; Tilson et al., 1990). Similarly, high dosages of toxicants such as phenylenediamine, an ingredient of some cosmetic products, produce an abrupt increase in motor activity and "thrashing about the cage" in what has been described as convulsive behavior (R. MacPhail, unpublished observations). The behavioral pattern may result from respiratory distress, which, if severe enough, may produce a cyanosis and possibly seizure activity. Behavioral criteria alone, however, are insufficient to support the convulsive nature of this compound. Further testing of phenylenediamine failed to reveal a facilitation in electrical kindling or augmentation of pentylenetetrazol-induced seizures in pretreated animals (M. Gilbert and R. Dyer, unpublished observations). Severe tremors, choreoathetosis, or barrel-rolling produced by high dosages of some toxicants have also been described as convulsive behavior. It is unwise to designate a compound as a chemoconvulsant in the absence of electrographic verification of seizure activity. Furthermore, electrographic seizure activity may be present in the absence of behavioral seizure manifestations (Racine, 1972a, 1972b).

Lower dosages of some chemicals may not lead to overt convulsions, but direct CNS effects on neuronal excitability can be revealed by challenging animals with a convulsant treatment. Convulsions induced by electroshock (MES) or high doses of convulsant drugs such as pentylenetetrazol (PTZ) are two examples of acute generalized seizure (GS) tests. These tests were primarily developed and refined by the pharmaceutical industry, and a battery of them are typically used to screen for the therapeutic efficacy of new antiepileptic drugs (Loscher and Schmidt, 1986; Santucci et al., 1985). Anticonvulsant candidates are screened for their ability to increase thresholds, decrease severity, or increase the latency to onset of tonic seizures. Tonic seizures induced by MES and high dosages of PTZ involve a tonic whole-body flexion with forelimb extension, followed by hindlimb extension and hindlimb clonus (Browning, 1985). Clonic seizures entail a maintained rhythmic twitching of the face and forelimbs with rearing (Racine, 1972b). Tonic seizures are of brainstem origin, whereas clonic seizures emanate from forebrain regions (Browning, 1985).

Since neurotoxicants can have either stimulative or depressive effects on the CNS (Anger and Johnson, 1985), both increases and decreases in severity, latency, or thresholds for convulsive response may represent evidence of direct effects of the toxicant on the nervous system. To identify neurotoxicant-induced alterations in both CNS excitability and depression, a GS model employing a lower dose of PTZ has been described by Dyer (1987). Lower dosages, however, lead to increased variability in the responsiveness of control animals to PTZ, creating significant obstacles for data analysis and interpretation (M. Gilbert, unpublished observations). Furthermore, the direct interaction of the toxicant under study with the chemoconvulsant can occur. The use of electroshock models overcomes the difficulty of interactions between chemicals, but MES seizures are notoriously variable (Fox and Doctor, 1983) and often lead to broken vertebrae when applied to rodents larger than mice (Dyer, 1987).

Over the past several years, we (Gilbert, 1988a; Gilbert and Mack, 1989; Gilbert et al., 1990) and others (Joy et al., 1982, 1983, 1985) have utilized the electrical kindling model to identify and characterize the action of a variety of neurotoxicants on the CNS. In this paradigm, animals are implanted with chronic indwelling electrodes and stimulated once daily following drug administration. Excitatory or depressant properties of toxicants can be indicated by appropriate changes in the threshold for inducing a focal afterdischarge (AD), durations of ADs in response to focal stimulation, seizure severity, or the number of daily stimulation sessions required to produce a generalized seizure. The advantages of the kindling model over acute GS tests include the greater control over the site and time of application of the stimulus. Unlike chemoconvulsants, the stimulus is under control of the experimenter, and the frequency, duration, and intensity of stimulation can be graded precisely. The stability and reliability of the phenomenon makes it extremely useful for the analysis of excitatory and depressant properties of neurotoxicants. It is also possible to study effects on the development of seizures as well as the fully developed convulsive response (Gilbert, 1988b; Joy, 1985; Peterson and Albertson, 1982).

The development of amygdala kindling is sensitive to both increases and decreases in seizure responsiveness at dosages of neurotoxicants well below the lethal or convulsive dose ($LD_{50}$ and $CD_{50}$ are doses required to produce lethality or convulsions in 50% of the animals, respectively) and below those detectable with acute GS models. We observed

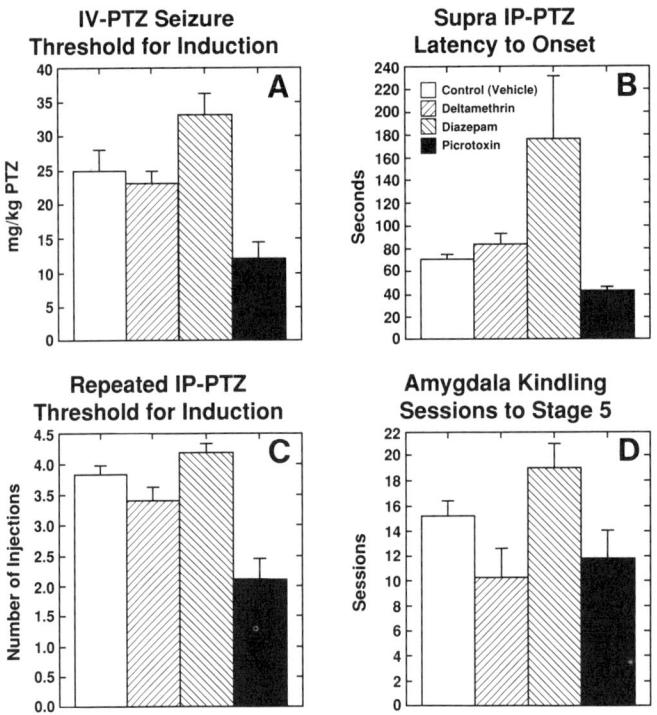

**FIGURE 2.** Electrical kindling but not PTZ detected proconvulsant effects of the pyrethroid, deltamethrin. Seizure susceptibility to acute administration of deltamethrin, diazepam, and picrotoxin following i.v. PTZ administration (A), a single i.p. injection of 60 mg/kg of PTZ (B), or a series of i.p. PTZ injections of 15 mg/kg every 15 min until the onset of generalized seizures (C). In all cases (n = 10–12/group) diazepam increased, picrotoxin decreased, and deltamethrin failed to reduce PTZ thresholds (A and C) or GS onset latency (B) relative to vehicle-treated controls (pooled controls n = 19–25). The mean number of stimulations required to evoke stage 5 seizures in amygdala kindling with prior treatment with deltamethrin, diazepam (taken from Racine *et al.*, 1975), and picrotoxin (taken from Kalichman *et al.*, 1981) are shown in D. Diazepam protected against PTZ-induced seizures, whereas picrotoxin enhanced the seizure response evoked by PTZ. Deltamethrin was without effect. (A–C) Proconvulsant effects of deltamethrin were revealed, however, by amygdala kindling (D).

subtle alterations in the rate of seizure spread in electrical kindling of the amygdala when pyrethroid insecticides (cismethrin and deltamethrin) were administered prior to each stimulation session (Gilbert *et al.*, 1990). Conventional measures of PTZ-induced seizures (i.e., thresholds, severity, latency) were not altered by prior pyrethroid administration. In an attempt to develop a more sensitive GS test for use in a neurotoxicity screening battery, PTZ was administered in a variety of ways (single i.p. injection of either 60 or 75 mg/kg, repeated i.p. or s.c. injections of 15 mg/kg PTZ every 15 min, or i.v. administration of PTZ via the tail vein) 60 min following administration of two different pyrethroids. Apart from deltamethrin inducing a higher incidence of tonic seizures following i.p. administration of 60 mg/kg of PTZ (Gilbert *et al.*, 1990), none of the PTZ protocols revealed convulsant-promoting properties of these insecticides. The PTZ tests were positive, however, for the proconvulsive action of picrotoxin (3.0 mg/kg i.p.) and the anticonvulsant action of diazepam (1.0 mg/kg i.p.). Representative data for deltamehtrin, diazepam, and picrotoxin are summarized in Figure 2. Figure 2D presents kindling rates for control and deltamethrin-treated animals from our laboratory, data from Racine *et al.* (1975) for diazepam, and data from Kalichman *et al.* (1981) for picrotoxin.

Repeated i.p. or i.v. PTZ tests resulted in fewer failures to convulse under control conditions (0% and 8.7%, respectively) than a single i.p. administration of 60 mg/kg of PTZ (23.1%). Similarly, repeated i.p. and i.v. administration of PTZ resulted in a lower incidence of tonic seizures and death in control animals (0% and 4.3%, respectively), relative to single i.p. injection of 60 mg/kg (7.7%) or 75 mg/kg (100%). Both repeated i.p. and i.v. PTZ tests, however, require significantly more time to administer.

Kindling is also sensitive to persistent toxicant-induced alterations in the plasticity of the nervous system. Administration of imino-diproprionitrile (IDPN) to rats and mice produces a syndrome of dyskinesia, characterized by hyperactivity, circling, and enhanced startle response (Cadet and Karoum, 1988). Reports of hearing loss, motor dys-

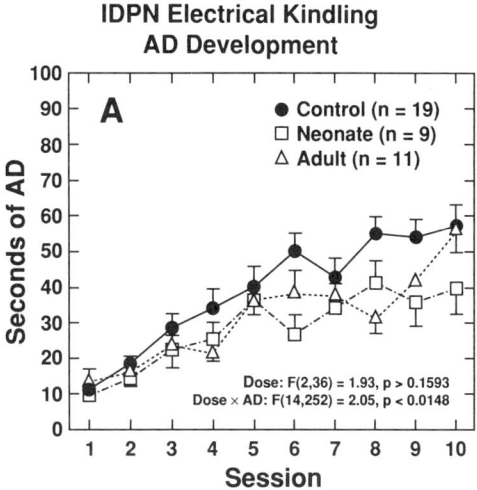

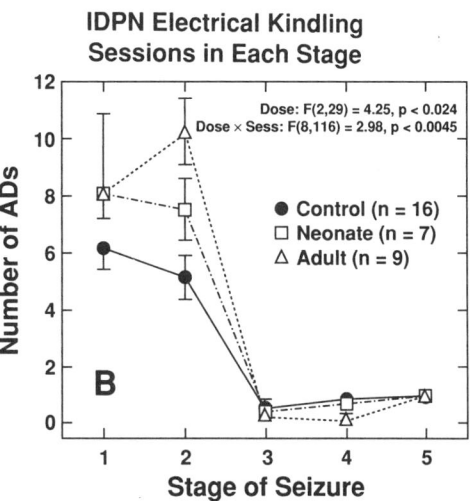

**FIGURE 3.** Amygdala kindling development animals treated with immino-diproprionitrile (IDPN) as neonates or adults. Animals were dosed for 3 consecutive days (200–225 mg/kg, i.p. IDPN) and were electrically kindled 1–3 months later. IDPN resulted in (A) shorter afterdischarges (AD) and (B) slightly slower kindling rates.

function (Crofton and Knight, 1991; Llorens and Crofton, 1991), and pronounced cognitive deficits (Peele *et al.*, 1990) weeks to months after IDPN exposure have recently appeared. Increases in the levels of glial fibrillary acidic protein (GFAP) in the olfactory bulb, cortex, midbrain, and pons/medulla have also been reported after treatment with IDPN (Lorens *et al.*, 1991). Persistent alterations in plasticity as measured by amygdala kindling were evident following moderate doses of IDPN to adult (200 mg/kg for 3 consecutive days) and neonatal rats (250 mg/kg on postnatal days 5, 6, and 7). An increase the number of stimulations required to induce kindled seizures was accompanied by a retardation in the development of AD duration in both neonatal- and adult-treated rats (Figure 3). These changes were observed 5–8 weeks after adult dosing and 3 months after neonatal exposure. As we had seen with the pyrethroids, PTZ (60 mg/kg, i.p.) failed to detect the effects of IDPN (data not shown).

## 6. PROCONVULSANT KINDLING STUDIES

Administration of a low dose of a neurotoxicant just prior to focal brain stimulation in the kindling paradigm may be used to study the acute chemical-related alterations in CNS excitability that either prolong or curtail seizure activity. Toxicant disruption of kindling development may reflect a chemical's action on processes underlying the dynamic phase of neuroplasticity, whereas effects on seizures evoked in a fully kindled animal may be more analogous to acute GS models.

Extensive study of the kindling plasticity model has resulted in a large scientific literature base. Such a literature, encompassing manipulations of transmitter systems by lesions, chemical depletions, or acute drug-induced alterations (Table 1), in addition to biochemical, anatomical, and electrophysiological consequences of kindling, provides a means to characterize the effects of a toxicant and some insight into its mechanism of action. For example, the formamidine pesticides chlordimeform and amitraz facilitate the development of amygdala and hippocampal kindling (Gilbert, 1988a). On the basis of in vitro assays, both of these pesticides were reported to possess both alpha-2 adrenergic and local anesthetic properties (see Gilbert and Mack, 1989). In vivo evidence for the alpha-2 mechanism of action in the CNS, however, was discerned from the effects of chlordimeform on the visual system (Boyes and Moser, 1988). Comparing the rate of amygdala kindling development in animals treated daily with chlordimeform; the alpha-2 adrenergic agonist clonidine; or the local anesthetic lidocaine revealed significant facilitation in development and prolonged AD durations with both chlordimeform and lidocaine. In contrast, clondine had the opposite effects (Gilbert and Mack, 1989). These findings are consistent with and provide further evidence of local anesthetic action of this class of pesticides.

## 7. CHEMICAL KINDLING

Soon after the initial report of electrical kindling by Goddard *et al.* (1969), it was discovered that a chemical stimulus could be substituted for the electrical triggering event and produce a similar long-lasting change in brain function (see review by Post, 1980). This has come to be known as reverse tolerance, pharmacological kindling, or chemical kindling. In this paradigm, a chemical that at an acute high dosage is convulsant is repeatedly administered at a concentration that is subthreshold for seizure induction. After several spaced administrations, the animal begins to demonstrate signs of seizure activity, initially subtle in nature (motor arrest, eye blinking, ear twitching), which progress to more overt symptoms (myoclonic jerks, clonic movements of forelimbs), and eventually culminate in generalized motor seizures. When challenged several weeks after the last dosage (to allow clearance and removal of any transient drug effects), the same dose of the drug that failed to produce seizure symptoms upon initial exposure now results in significant motor manifestations of seizure activity. This enhanced responsiveness is long lasting and generalizes to other convulsant treatments, most notably, electrical kindling (Table 1).

Chemical kindling has been documented for a wide variety of agents. Chemicals with agonistic activity on the cholinergic system (e.g., carbacol, physostigmine), GABAergic antagonists (e.g., bicuculline, picrotoxin, FG-7142, PTZ), local anesthetics (lidocaine, cocaine, procaine), second messengers in transmission in the monoamine system (e.g., cAMP), and excitatory amino acids (aspartate, glutamate) have all been reported to possess the ability to gradually lower thresholds and to promote seizure development and spread with repeated low-level dosing (Table 1).

In order to attribute a chemical's seizure-inducing properties to a kindling mechanism, however, it must first be determined that these effects are dependent upon "functional" as opposed to "dispositional" alterations in sensitivity (Nutt et al., 1982). For instance, a toxicant with high persistence in the body could accumulate until levels surpassed the $CD_{50}$ to result in a convulsive response (Type 2 toxicity in Figure 1). This may be the case with some persistent chemicals such as lindane or telodrin (Jager, 1970; Tusell et al., 1988). Kindling, however, requires that the enhanced susceptibility to convulsions is maintained long after the poison has cleared the body. It is also possible that repeated exposure to some chemicals may produce alterations in pharmacokinetics of the administered drug, leading to poor clearance, increased concentrations of the toxic agent in the body, or enhanced delivery to the brain. PTZ, cocaine, lidocaine, and picrotoxin, however, all chemically kindle (Cain, 1981, 1984; Kilbey et al., 1979) but have short biological half-lives and do not accumulate in the body in any appreciable amounts (Gilman et al., 1989). Furthermore, direct application of PTZ, picrotoxin, carbacol, opiate peptides, glutamate, or aspartate to the amygdala leads to a similar enhancement in behavioral and electrographic seizure responsiveness with repeated intracerebral infusions (Cain, 1982, 1987; Cain and Corcoran, 1985; Croucher and Bradford, 1989; Girgis, 1981; Mori and Wada, 1987; Wasterlain and Fairchild, 1985).

Given that convulsions are a common response to acute exposure to high doses of environmental toxicants and that some chemicals are known to possess chemical kindling potential, it remains to be determined if environmental chemicals can kindle following repeated exposures to lower dose levels. Can low-level environmental exposure to chemicals insidiously promote the permanent increase in seizure susceptibility and consequent increase in the risk of epilepsy? Apart from a single report on dieldrin (Joy et al., 1980), little to date has been discovered about the potential for environmentally relevant toxicants to act as chemical-kindling agents. This is of particular importance given the high percentage of chemicals with convulsive properties (Anger and Johnson, 1985; Morgan, 1989) and the number and quantity of such chemicals used commercially for their pesticidal efficacy. As a result, we sought to address two basic questions: (1) can environmentally relevant chemicals kindle animals and lead to a permanently enhanced predisposition to seizures, and (2) can the proconvulsant kindling properties of potential neurotoxicants be used to predict the risk of chemical kindling? A summary of proconvulsant vs. chemical kindling effects of a variety of compounds is outlined in Table 1. It is readily apparent that many chemicals can facilitate electrical kindling, and many chemicals can act as kindling agents. However, only 7 of 29 chemicals with seizuregenic potential in either paradigm have been evaluated in both (chemicals in bold type in Table 1). Six of these seven chemicals are proconvulsant in an electrical kindling paradigm and also produce chemical kindling. The one exception, picrotoxin, did not facilitate electrical kindling in a proconvulsive paradigm, but, as pointed out by the authors (Kalichman et al., 1981), only a single, low dosage was used (Table 1). A direct systematic comparison of electrical and chemical kindling has occurred for only two of these chemicals, dieldrin and endosulfan. Dieldrin administered every second day for 9–14 dosing days produced a progressive increase in seizure severity. However, all animals died during the course of treatment, preventing the incorporation of a challenge test several weeks after dosing or the transfer to electrical kindling (Joy et al., 1980). The following reports the results of a series of experiments conducted in our laboratory over the last year on the proconvulsant and chemical kindling effects of the pesticide endosulfan.

## 8. ENDOSULFAN CHEMICAL KINDLING

Endosulfan (6,7,8,9,10,10-hexachloro-1,5,5a,6,9,9,9a-hexahydro-6,9,methano-2,4,3-benzodioxathiepin 3-oxide) is a member of the cyclodiene class of chlorinated hydrocarbon pesticides (Hayes and Laws, 1991). The use of endosulfan in the United States is estimated to be 1.5–2.0 million pounds of the active ingredient annually (OTS, 1982). Unlike many of the chlorinated hydrocarbon insecticides (Hayes and Laws, 1991), endosulfan is not a persistent residue in the fat or other tissues of animals that have consumed the insecticide (Maier-Bode, 1967). With greater restrictions on the use of chlorinated insecticides that do show persistence, endosulfan is one of the few members of this group still used extensively. Many cases of human poisonings have been reported for endosulfan, all of which resulted in one or multiple convulsive episodes (Aleksandrowicz, 1979; Demeter and Heyndrickx, 1978; Ely et al., 1967; Isaeli et al., 1969; Shemesh et al., 1988). These properties lead us to our investigation of the proconvulsant and chemical kindling properties of endosulfan.

Adult male rats were treated three times a week (Monday/Wednesday/Friday) for 10–21 dosages of endosulfan (0, 5, 10 mg/kg in corn oil p.o.). Behavioral observations of seizure manifestations were performed at various times throughout the dosing regimen. Two weeks after the last dose (to permit complete metabolic clearance of endosulfan), a challenge dose (5 or 10 mg/kg to compare the response elicited on day 1 of dosing) was administered and the seizure response observed. The challenge occurred at a time, based on feeding studies of 5 and 10 mg/kg daily for 15 days, that minimal residues of endosulfan or its metabolites remained in the blood, brain, or fat tissue (Gupta and Chandra, 1977). The number of animals displaying myoclonic jerks and bouts of clonic seizure activity increased with repeated dosing, and this was more prominent in the 10 mg/kg than the 5 mg/kg dosage group.

Upon challenge, the incidence of seizure manifestations was further enhanced in the 10 mg/kg group, with more than 75% of the animals responding with myoclonic jerks

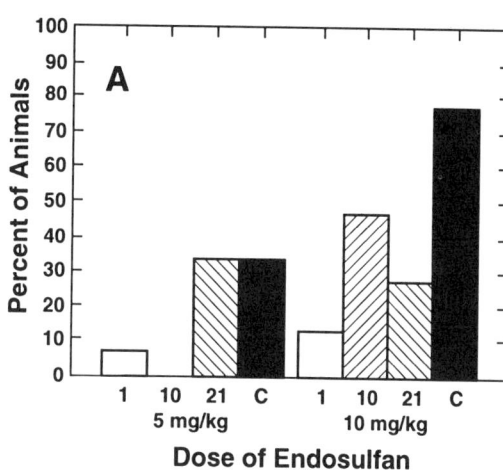

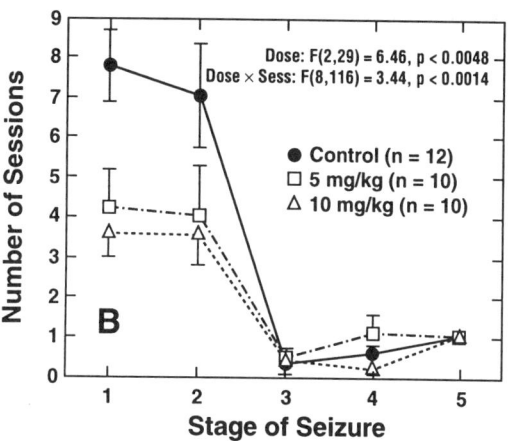

FIGURE 4. (A) Repeated administration of endosulfan three times per week resulted in an increase in the percentage of animals displaying myoclonic jerks in the 10 mg/kg, and to a lesser extent in the 5 mg/kg, dosage group. Some animals in the 10 mg/kg group also exhibited clonic seizures after 10 days of dosing (data not shown). Upon challenge (C) 2 weeks after the last dose, however, more than 75% of the animals in the 10 mg/kg group exhibited myoclonic jerks and 33% had clonic seizures. (B) Two to four weeks following the challenge dose, and with no further treatment with endosulfan, both the 5- and 10-mg/kg groups developed stage 5 seizures with fewer amygdala stimulations than corn-oil-treated controls. The facilitation was apparent primarily in the focal seizure stages (stages 1 and 2 of Racine, 1972b).

(Figure 4A). Thus, behaviorally, animals showed evidence of chemical kindling. A similar pattern of increased seizure responsiveness to the effects of low doses of PTZ (20 mg/kg) was observed in a parallel group of animals. In contrast, animals dosed for 21 days with 5 mg/kg of endosulfan (daily or triweekly schedule) did not show strong development of behavioral seizures.

Endosulfan-treated animals were subsequently prepared with electrodes in the amygdala and were stimulated (60-Hz, 1-sec train of 200 µA) once daily beginning 1–2 months after completion of the subchronic dosing regimen. Animals previously treated with endosulfan demonstrated a significant facilitation in electrical kindling relative to corn-oil-treated controls. Importantly, faster kindling was also evident in the low-dose animals (5 mg/kg) who had displayed only a slight increase in sensitivity to endosulfan. These findings are similar to those previously reported for PTZ sensitization and positive transfer to electrical kindling by Cain (1981). No differences between corn-oil- and endosulfan-treated animals were apparent in thresholds for inducing an AD, duration or latency to clonic seizures once developed, nor the growth in AD duration that occurs with each kindling stimulus. Thus a predisposition to develop seizures occurred in the apparent absence of significant amounts of endosulfan remaining in the body or the brain, was transferable to other seizure-inducing treatments (i.e., electrical kindling), and was evident in animals that had not demonstrated robust clinical seizures during chronic dosing.

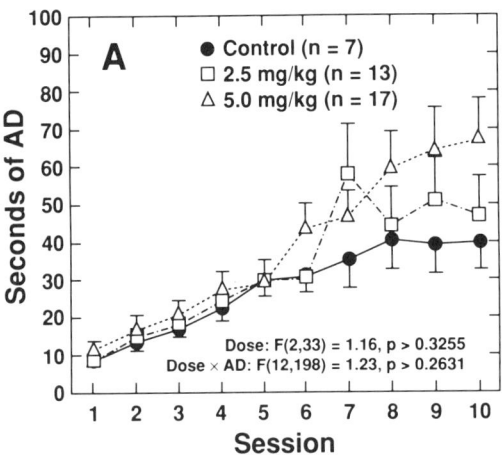

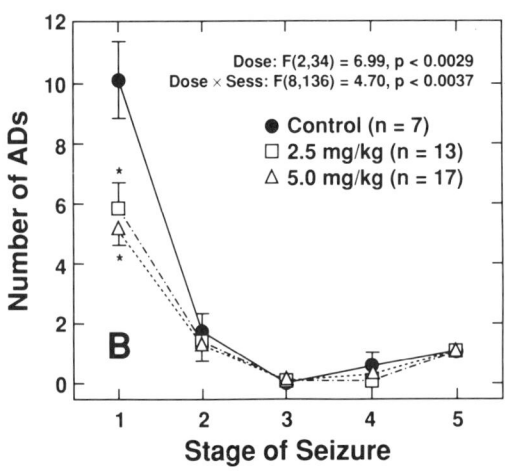

**FIGURE 5.** Low dosages of endosulfan (2.5 and 5.0 mg/kg) administered three times per week, 60 min prior to electrical stimulation of the amygdala, significantly reduced the number of sessions required to evoke stage 5 seizures (A). The degree of facilitation was equivalent in both dosage groups, (B) 5.0 mg/kg appeared to produce longer afterdischarges in later stimulation sessions, but this difference was not statistically significant.

A second series of experiments tested the proconvulsant properties of endosulfan administered acutely, 60 min prior to each stimulation. A significant facilitation in kindling development was evident in animals receiving 2.5 and 5.0 mg/kg (Figure 5B). A trend towards longer ADs was evident in the 5.0 mg/kg group, but this difference failed to reach statistically significant levels (Figure 5A).

## 9. CLINICAL RELEVANCE

Does a kindling-like phenomenon occur in humans in response to electrical stimulation or repeated chemical exposure? Electrical kindling has been described for all animal species studied thus far, ranging from frogs to baboons (Racine, 1978), so it appears likely that kindling would also occur in the human brain. A report of possible electrical kindling in humans has appeared (Sato et al., 1990). Recurrent spontaneous convulsions have developed in schizophrenic patients who have received repeated electroconvulsive shock therapy (Sato et al., 1990), and incidents of persistent seizure disorders have been reported following exposure to neurotoxicants in humans (Gupta, 1975; Hayes, 1957).

Persistent neurological disorders may occur in humans, but be manifested in symptoms more subtle than overt behavioral convulsions. Primates require many more electrical kindling stimulations to produce major motor seizures than do nonprimates. Kindling of rhesus monkeys results in the relatively easy induction of mild, focal seizures (immobility, staring, facial automatisms), but secondarily generalized clonic seizures commonly seen in rats are rare (Wada and Osawa, 1976). The predominant behavioral pattern observed in monkeys, however, is very similar to that of humans suffering from complex partial seizures. Approximately 25% of patients with partial complex epilepsy never experience a secondarily generalized convulsion, and the frequency of such attacks in the remaining 75% is low (Delgado-Escueta et al., 1982).

Functional disruption induced by kindling may also take the form of disturbances of affect or emotion. Although controversial (Adamec, 1990; Adamec and Stark-Adamec, 1983c; Flor-Henry, 1976; Hermann and Whitmann, 1984), it has been reported that epileptic patients, particularly those with partial-complex type, suffer a predisposition to psychopathology in the form of severe clinical depression and anxiety. Experimentally, heightened defensive responding toward a variety of threats has been identified in partially kindled cats (Adamec, 1990; Adamec and Stark-Adamec, 1983a). What is particularly significant about these findings is the presence of altered behavioral patterns in the absence of overt motor signs of seizure. Repeated evocation of epileptiform neural firing that has remained focal to the site of stimulation produced marked and persistent alterations in defensive behavior. The emergence of these behavioral patterns was correlated with a large increase in the monosynaptic evoked population response between the amygdala and the hypothalamus (Adamec and Stark-Adamec, 1983b). Thus a long-lasting enhancement of synaptic transmission between brain areas believed to underlie the emotive response accompanies the early phases of kindling.

Potentiation in the efficacy of synaptic transmission may therefore contribute to alterations in emotional behavior seen in kindled cats, in humans suffering from partial complex epilepsy (Adamec, 1990; Flor-Henry, 1976; Hermann and Whitman, 1984), and perhaps in humans exposed to neurotoxicants (Anger, 1990). Of the chemicals with convulsant properties compiled by Anger and Johnson (1985), 32% also result in symptoms of an emotional or affectual nature (M. Gage and M. Gilbert, unpublished observations). Enhanced irritability has been reported in rats kindled with lidocaine (Post, 1980; Post *et al.*, 1984) and electrically kindled rats display a pronounced increase in aggressive responsivity upon challenge with corticotropin releasing hormone (Weiss *et al.*, 1990). Thus, persistent neurological sequelae may follow chronic neurotoxicant exposure prior to or in the absence of overt convulsions.

Deficits in learning and memory also occur in epileptic patients (Aarts *et al.*, 1984; Gallassi *et al.*, 1988; Halgren and Wilson, 1985; Hermann *et al.*, 1987) and are well known to accompany neurotoxicant exposure (Anger, 1990; Peele and Vincent, 1989). Limbic structures, including the amygdala and hippocampus, have been shown to play a critical role in the acquisition and retention of complex behavioral tasks (Gray, 1982). Neurotoxicant interference with function of limbic brain regions may contribute to this cognitive dysfunction. Administration of acute brain stimulation or the induction of kindled seizures during task acquisition disrupts cognitive performance (Kesner, 1982; Olton and Wolfe, 1982; Peele and Gilbert, 1992). A history of kindling, in the absence of overt behavioral manifestations of seizure behavior, has also been shown to have persistent deleterious effects upon cognitive performance (Boast and McIntyre, 1974; Leung *et al.*, 1990; Lopes de Silva *et al.*, 1986; Peele and Gilbert, 1992; Robinson *et al.*, 1989b). Leung *et al.* (1990) recently demonstrated disruption of radial-arm-maze performance following hippocampal kindling that persists in the absence of EEG abnormalities.

In conclusion, long-term alterations in the functional properties of the CNS resulting from chronic low-level exposure to environmental toxicants may therefore not only take the form of overt behavioral convulsive responses in humans. This raises the possibility that the incidence of these types of poisonings, and therefore the risk to human health, may be much higher than we are currently aware and may contribute to a profile of toxicity encompassing apparently unrelated symptomatologies. The inclusion of two additional categories to Hayes' (1963) scheme of neurotoxicity syndromes (Figure 1) is warranted. An exposure scenario that may result is a reduction in threshold to induce a very brief subclinical seizure response that gradually and progressively, in the absence of any significant accumulation or high body burden, serves as a kindling stimulus. In the case of PTZ, for example, no accumulation occurs (type 4 of Figure 1). Repeated exposure to dieldrin (Joy *et al.*, 1980) or endosulfan may result in some accumulation in the brain (but not in excess of the $CD_{50}$ levels) and produce a predisposition to seizures (type 5 of Figure 1). It is clear that many chemicals (Table 1) facilitate the development of electrical kindling. Although some overlap exists between chemicals that accelerate electrical kindling and chemicals that produce kindling on their own, more research is required to determine the predictive power of proconvulsant to chemical kindling effects.

ACKNOWLEDGMENTS. The technical assistance of C.M. Mack, S.K. Acheson, E. Thompson, and C.R. Murchison is gratefully acknowledged. Special thanks to W.K. Boyes for review of an earlier version of this chapter. The research described in this chapter has been supported by the U.S. Environmental Protection Agency, through contract #68-02-4450 to Mantech Environmental Technology Services Inc.

## REFERENCES

Aarts, J.H.P., Binnie, C.D., Smit, A.M., and Wilkins, A.J., 1984, Selective cognitive impairment during focal and generalized epilepitform EEG activity, *Brain* 107:293–308.

Adamec, R.E., 1990, Does kindling model anything clinically relevant? *Biol. Psychiatry* 27:249–279.

Adamec, R.E., and Stark-Adamec, C., 1983a, Partial kindling and emotional bias in the cat: Lasting aftereffects of partial kindling of the ventral hippocampus: Behavioral changes, *Behav. Neural Biol.* 38:205-222.
Adamec, R.E., and Stark-Adamec, C., 1983b, Partial kindling and emotional bias in the cat: Lasting aftereffects of partial kindling of the ventral hippocampus: Physiological changes, *Behav. Neural Biol.* 38:223-239.
Adamec, R.E., and Stark-Adamec, C., 1983c, Limbic kindling and animal behavior—implications for human psychopathology associated with complex partial seizures, *Biol. Psychiatry* 18:269-289.
Albertson, T.E., Joy, R.M., and Stark, L.G., 1984, Anticonvulsant action of fluzinamide (AHR-8559) on kindled amygdaloid seizures, *Epilepsia* 25:511-517.
Aleksandrowicz, D.R., 1979, Endosulfan poisoning and chronic brain syndrome, *Arch. Toxicol.* 43:65-68.
Anger, W.K., 1990, Worksite behavioral research: Results, sensitive methods, test batteries and the transition from laboratory data to human health, *Neurotoxicology* 11:629-720.
Anger, W.K., and Johnson, B.L., 1985, Chemicals affecting behavior, in: *Neurotoxicity of Industrial and Commercial Chemicals* (J.L. O'Donoghue, ed), CRC Press, Boca Raton, FL, pp. 134-148.
Arnold, P.S., Racine, R.J., and Wise, R.A., 1973, Effects of atropine, resperine, 6-hydroxydopamine and handling on seizure development in the rat, *Exp. Neurol.* 40:457-470.
Boast, C.A., and McIntyre, D.C., 1977, Bilateral kindled amygdala foci and inhibitory avoidance behavior in rats: A functional lesion effect, *Physiol. Behav.* 18:25-28.
Bowyer, J.F., and Albertson, T.E., 1982, The effects of pentylenetetrazol, bicuculline and strychnine on the development of kindled seizures, *Neuropharmacology* 21:895-990.
Boyes, W.K., and Moser, V.C., 1988, An alpha-2 adrenergic mode of action of chlordimeform on rat visual function, *Toxicol. Appl. Pharmacol.* 92:402-418.
Browning, R.A., 1985, Role of the brain-stem reticular formation in tonic-clonic seizures: Lesion and pharmacological studies, *Fed. Proc.* 44:2425-2431.
Burdette, L.J., Gilbert, M.E., and O'Callaghan, J.P., 1989, Kindling induces greater protein kinase C activation than long-term potentiation, *Soc. Neurosci. Abstr.* 15:455.
Cadet, J.L., and Karoum, F., 1988, Central and peripheral effects of iminodipropionitrile on catecholamine metabolism in rats, *Synapse* 2:23-27.
Cain, D.P., 1981, Transfer of pentylenetetrazol sensitization to amygdaloid kindling, *Pharmacol. Biochem. Behav.* 15:533-536.
Cain, D.P., 1982, Bidirectional transfer of intracerebrally administered pentylenetetrazol and electrical kindling, *Pharmacol. Biochem. Behav.* 17:1111-1113.
Cain, D.P., 1983, Bidirectional transfer of electrical and carbachol kindling, *Brain Res.* 260:135-138.
Cain, D.P., 1987, Kindling by repeated intraperitoneal or intracerebral injection of picrotoxin transfers to electrical kindling, *Exp. Neurol.* 97:243-254.
Cain, D.P., 1989, Long-term potentiation and kindling: How similar are the mechanisms? *TINS* 12:6-10.
Cain, D.P., and Corcoran, M.E., 1985, Epileptiform effects of met-enkephalin, beta-endorphin and morphine: Kindling of generalized seizures and potentiation of epileptiform effects by handling, *Brain Res.* 338:327-336.
Cain, D.P., Desborough, K.A., and McKitrick, D.J., 1988, Retardation of amygdala kindling by antagonism of NMD-aspartate and muscarinic cholinergic receptors: Evidence for the summation of excitatory mechanisms of kindling, *Exp. Neurol.* 100:179-187.
Collingridge, G.L., 1987, Long-term potentiation in the hippocampus: Mechanisms of initiation and modulation by neurotransmitters, *TIPS* 6:407-411.
Corda, M.G., Giorgi, O., Orlandi, M., Longoni, B., and Biggio, G., 1990, Chronic administration of negative modulators produces chemical kindling and $GABA_A$ receptor down-regulation, in: *GABA and Benzodiazepine Receptor Subtypes*, (G. Biggio and E. Costa, eds.), Raven Press, New York, pp. 1-25.
Crofton, K.M., and Knight, T., 1991, Auditory deficits and motor dysfunction following iminodioproprionitrile administration in the rat, *Neurotoxicol. Teratol.* 13:575-581.
Croucher, M.J., and Bradford, H.F., 1989, Kindling of full limbic seizures by repeated microinjections of excitatory amino acids into rat amygdala, *Brain Res.* 501:58-65.
deJonge, M., and Racine, R.J., 1987, The development and decay of kindling-induced increases in paired-pulse depression in the dentate gyrus, *Brain Res.* 412:318-328.
Delgado-Escueta, A.V., Bacsal, F.E., and Treiman, D.M., 1982, Complex partial seizures on closed circuit television and EEG—A study of 691 attacks and 79 patients, *Ann. Neurol.* 11:292-300.
Demeter, J., and Heyndrickx, A., 1978, Two lethal endosulfan poisonings in man, *J. Anal. Toxicol.* 2:68-74.
Dyer, R.S., 1987, Evaluation of seizure models as indicators of neurotoxicity, Health Effects Research Laboratory, Office of Research and Development, Deliverable No. 2260A, US Environmental Protection Agency, Research Triangle Park, NC.
Dyer, R.S., Wonderlin, W.F., and Walsh, T.J., 1982, Increased seizure susceptibility following trimethyl tin administrations in rats, *Neurobehav. Toxicol. Teratol.* 4:203-208.
Ely, T.E., MacFarlane, J.W., Galen, W.P., and Hine, C.H., 1967, Convulsions in thiodan workers: A preliminary report, *J. Occup. Med.* 9:35-37.
Feldman, S., and Ackermann, R.F., 1987, Increased susceptibility to hippocampal and amygdala kindling following intrahippocampal kainic acid, *Exp. Neurol.* 97:255-269.
Flor-Henry, P., 1976, Epilepsy and psychopathology, in: *Recent Advances in Clinical Psychiatry* (K. Granville-Grossman, ed.), Churchill Livingstone, New York, pp. 262-294.

Fox, D.A., and Doctor, S.V., 1983, Triethyltin decreases maximal electroshock seizure severity in adult rats, *Toxicol. Appl. Pharmacol.* 68:260–267.
Gallassi, R., Morreale, A., Lorusso, S., Pazzaglia, P., and Lugaresi, E., 1988, Epilepsy presenting as memory disturbances, *Epilepsia* 29:624–629.
Gilbert, M.E., 1988a, Formamidine pesticides enhance susceptibility to kindled seizures in amygdala and hippocampus of the rat, *Neurotoxicol. Teratol.* 10:221–227.
Gilbert, M.E., 1988b, The NMDA-receptor antagonist, MK-801, suppresses limbic kindling and kindled seizures, *Brain Res.* 463:90–99.
Gilbert, M.E., 1992a, Chemical kindling with lindune, *Toxicologist* (Abstr.) 12:275.
Gilbert, M.E., 1992b, Proconvulsant activity of endosulfan in amygdala kindling, *Neurotoxicol. Teratol.* 14:143–149.
Gilbert, M.E., 1992c, A characterization of the chemical kindling properties of the pesticide endosulfan, *Neurotoxicol. Teratol.* 14:151–158.
Gilbert, M.E., and Mack, C.M., 1989, Enhanced susceptibility to kindling by chlordimeform may be mediated by a local anesthetic action, *Psychopharmacology* 99:163–167.
Gilbert, M.E., and Mack, C.M., 1990, The NMDA blocker, MK-801, suppresses long term potentiation and kindling of the perforant path in the unanesthetized rat, *Brain Res.* 519:89–96.
Gilbert, M.E., Acheson, S.K., Mack, C.M., and Crofton, K.M., 1990, An examination of the proconvulsant actions of pyrethroid insecticides using pentylenetetrazol and amygdala kindling seizure models, *Neuro Toxicology* 11:73–86.
Gilman, A., Goodman, L.S., and Goodman, A., 1989, *Goodman and Gilman's The Pharmacological Basis of Therapeutics*, 6th ed., MacMillan, New York.
Girgis, M., 1981, Electrical versus cholinergic kindling, *Electroencephalog. Clin. Neurophysiol.* 51:417–425.
Goddard, G.V., and Douglas, R.M., 1975, Does the engram of kindling model the engram of normal long term memory?, *Can. J. Neurol. Sci.* 4:385–394.
Goddard, G.V., McIntyre, D.C., and Leech, C.K., 1969, A permanent change in brain function resulting from daily electrical stimulation, *Exp. Neurol.* 25:295–330.
Goldman, L.R., Smith, D.F., Neutra, R.R., Saunders, L.D., Pond, E.M., Stratton, J., Waller, K., Jackson, R.J., and Kizer, K.W., 1990, Pesticide food poisoning from contaminated watermelons in California, 1985, *Arch. Environ. Health* 45:229–236.
Gray, J.A., 1982, *The Neurophysiology of Anxiety: An Enquiry into the Functions of the Septo-Hippocampal System*, Oxford University Press, New York.
Gupta, P.C., 1975, Neurotoxicity of chronic chlorinated hydrocarbon insecticide poisoning—A clinical and electroencephalographic study in man, *Indian J. Med. Res.* 4:601–606.
Gupta, P.C., and Chandra, S.V., 1977, Toxicity of endosulfan after repeated oral administration to rats, *Bull. Environ. Contamin. Toxicol.* 18:378–384.
Halgren, E., and Wilson, C.L., 1985, Recall deficits produced by afterdischarges in the human hippocampal formation and amygdala, *Electroencephalog. Clin. Neurophysiol.* 61:375–380.
Hayes, W.J., 1957, Dieldrin poisoning in man, *Public Health Report,* 72:1087–1091.
Hayes, W.J., 1963, *Clinical Handbook of Economic Poisons,* U.S. Dept. Health, Education and Welfare, Atlanta, GA.
Hayes, W.J., and Laws, E.R., 1991, *Handbook of Pesticide Toxicology,* Vol. 2, Academic Press, New York.
Hermann, B.P., and Whitman, S., 1984, Behavioral and personality correlates of epilepsy: A review, methodological critique, and conceptual model, *Psychol. Bull.* 95:451–497.
Hermann, B.P., Wyler, A.R., Richey, E.T., and Rea, J.M., 1987, Memory function and verbal learning ability in patients with complex partial seizures of temporal lobe origin, *Epilepsia* 28:547–554.
Israeli, R., Kristal, N., and Tiberin, P., 1969, Endosulfan poisoning: Three cases, *Zentralbl Arbeitsmed Arbeitsschutz. Prophyl Ergonomic* 19:193–195.
Jager, K.W., 1970, *Aldrin, Dieldrin, Endrin and Telodrin: An Epidemiological and Toxicological Study of Long-Term Occupational Exposure,* Elsevier Publishing, New York.
Joy, R.M., 1982, Mode of action of lindane, dieldrin and related insecticides in the central nervous system, *Neurobehav. Toxicol. Teratol.* 4:813–822.
Joy, R.M., 1985, The effects of neurotoxicants on kindling and kindled seizures, *Fundam. Appl. Toxicol.* 5:41–65.
Joy, R.M., Stark, L.G., Peterson, S.L., Bowyer, J.F., and Albertson, T.E., 1980, The kindled seizure: Production of and modification by dieldrin in rats, *Neurobehav. Toxicol.* 2:117–124.
Joy, R.M., Stark, L.G., Gordon, L.S., Peterson, L.S., and Albertson, T.E., 1981, Chronic cholinesterase inhibition does not modify amygdaloid kindling, *Exp. Neurol.* 73:588–594.
Joy, R.M., Stark, L.G., and Albertson, T.E., 1983, Proconvulsant actions of lindane: Effects on afterdischarge thresholds and durations during amygdaloid kindling in rats, *NeuroToxicology* 2:211–220.
Kalichman, M.W., Livingston, K.E., and Burnham, W.M., 1981, Pharmacological investigation of gamma-aminobutyric acid (GABA) and the development of amygdala-kindled seizures in rats. *Exp. Neurol.* 74:829–836.
Karler, R., Calder, L.D., Sangdee, P., and Turkanis, S.A., 1984, Interaction between delta-9-tetrahydrocannabinol and kindling by electrical and chemical stimuli in mice, *Neuropharmacology* 23:1315–1320.
Kilbey, M.M., Ellinwood, E.H., and Easler, M.E., 1979, The effects of chronic cocaine pretreatment on kindled seizures and behavioral stereotypies, *Exp. Neurol.* 64:306–314.
Kesner, R.P., 1982, Brain stimulation: Effects on memory, *Behav. Neural Biol.* 36:315–367.
Langston, J.W., Ballarad, P., Tetrud, J.W., and Erwin, I., 1983, Chronic parkinsonism in humans due to a product of meperidine-analog synthesis, *Science* 219:979–980.

Lekic, D.M., 1988, Facilitation and antagonism of lidocaine-kindled seizures: The behavioral feature, *Physiol. Behav.* 42:83–85.
Leung, L.S., Boon, K.A., Kaibara, T., and Innis, N.K., 1990, Radial maze performance following hippocampal kindling, *Behav. Brain Res.* 40:119–129.
Little, H.J., Nutt, D.J., and Taylor, S.C., 1987, Selective changes in the in vivo effects of benzodiazepine receptor ligands after chemical kindling with FG 7142, *Neuropharmacology* 26:25–31.
Llorens, J., and Crofton, K.M., 1991, Enhanced neurotoxicity of 3,3'-iminodiproprionitrile following carbon tetrachloride pretreatment in the rat, *Neurotoxicology* 12:301–312.
Llorens, J., Crofton, K.M., and O'Callaghan, J.D., 1991, Iminodiprioprionitrile-induced increases in brain regional glial fibrillary acidic protein concentrations in the rat, *Neurotoxicology* (Abstr.) 12:136–137.
Lopes da Silva, F.H., Gorter, J.A., and Wadman, W.J., 1986, Kindling of the hippocampus induces spatial memory deficits in the rat, *Neurosci. Lett.* 63:115–120.
Loscher, W., and Schmidt, D., 1986, Which animal models should be used in the search for new antiepileptic drugs? A proposal based on experimental and clinical considerations, *Epilepsy Res.* 2:145–181.
Maier-Bode, H., 1968, Properties, effects, residues and analytics of the insecticide endosulfan, *Residue Rev.* 22:1–44.
Mason, C.R., and Cooper, R.M., 1972, A permanent change in convulsive threshold in normal and brain-damaged rats with repeated small doses of pentylenetetrazol, *Epilepsia* 13:663–674.
Matthews, H.B., Dixon, D., Herr, D.W., and Tilson, H.A., 1990, Subchronic toxicity studies indicate that tris(2-chloroethyl)-phosphate administration results in lesions in the rat hippocampus, *Toxicol. Ind. Health* 6:1–15.
McIntyre, D.C., 1986, Kindling and the pyriform cortex, in: *Kindling 3* (J.A. Wada, ed.), Raven Press, New York, pp. 249–262.
McIntyre, D.C., and Guigno, L., 1988, Effect of clonidine in amygdala kindling in normal and 6-OHDA-pretreated rats. *Exp. Neurol.* 99:96–106.
McNamara, J.O., Byrne, M.C., Dasheiff, R.M., and Fitz, J.G., 1980, The kindling model of epilepsy: A review, *Prog. Neurobiol.* 15:139–159.
McNamara, J.O., Russell, R.D., Rigsbee, L., and Bonhaus, D.W., 1988, Anticonvulsant and antiepileptogenic actions of MK-801 in the kindling and electroshock models, *Neuropharmacology* 94:563–568.
Morgan, D.P., 1989, *Recognition and Management of Pesticide Poisonings*, 4th ed., US EPA, Washington DC.
Mori, N., and Wada, J.A., 1987, Bidirectional transfer between kindling induced by excitatory amino acids and electrical stimulation, *Brain Res.* 425:45–48.
Morris, R.G.M., Anderson, E., Lynch, G.S, and Baudry, M., 1986, Selective impairment of learning and blockade of long-term potentiation by an N-methyl-D-aspartate receptor antagonist, AP5, *Nature* 319:774–776.
Nutt, D.J., Cowen, P.J., Batts, C.C., Grahame-Smith, D.G., and Green, A.R., 1982, Repeated administration of subconvulsant doses of GABA antagonist drugs. I. Effects on seizure threshold (kindling), *Psychopharmacology* 76:84–87.
Office of Pesticides and Toxic Substances, 1982, *Pesticide Registration Standard:* Hexachlorohexahydromethano-2,4,3-benzodioxathiepin 3-oxide (Endosulfan), U.S. Environmental Protection Agency, Washington, DC.
Office of Technology Assessment, U.S. Congress, 1990, *Neurotoxicity: Identifying and Controlling Poisons of the Nervous System*, OTA-BA-436, U.S. Government Printing Office, Washington, DC.
Olney, J.W., 1980, Excitatory neurotoxins as food additives: An evaluation of risk, *Neurotoxicology* 2:163–192.
Olton, D.S., and Wolf, W.A., 1981, Hippocampal seizures produce retrograde amnesia without a temporal gradient when they reset working memory, *Behav. Neural Biol.* 33:437–452.
Peele, D.B., and Gilbert, M.E., 1992, Functional dissociation of acute and persistent cognitive deficits accompanying amygdala kindled seizures, *Behav. Brain Res.* 48:65–76.
Peele, D.B., and Vincent, A., 1989, Strategies for assessing learning and memory, 1978–1987: A comparison of behavioral toxicology, phychopharmacology, and neurobiology. *Neurosci. Biobehav. Rev.* 13:317–322.
Peterson, S.L., and Albertson, T.E., 1982, Neurotransmitter and neuromodulator function in kindled seizure and state, *Prog. Neurobiol.* 19:237–270.
Peterson, S.L., Albertson, T.E., Stark, L.G., Joy, R.M., and Gordon, L.S., 1981, Cumulative afterdischarge as the principle factor in acquisition of kindled seizures, *Electroencephalog. Clin. Neurophysiol.* 51:192–200.
Pinel, J.L., Mucha, R.F., and Phillips, A.G., 1975, Spontaneous seizures generated in rats by kindling: A preliminary report, *Physiol. Psychol.* 3:127–127.
Post, R.M., 1980, Minireview: Intermittent versus continuous stimulations: Effect of time interval on the development of sensitization and tolerance, *Life Sci.* 26:1275–1282.
Post, R.M., and Kopanda, R.T., 1976, Cocaine, kindling and psychosis, *Am. J. Psychiatry* 133:627–634.
Post, R.M., Kopanda, R.T., and Lee, A., 1975, Progressive behavioral changes during chronic lidocaine administration: Relationship to kindling, *Life Sci.* 17:943–950.
Post, R.M., Kennedy, C., Shinohara, M., Squillace, K., Miyaoka, M., Suda, S., Ingva, D.H., and Sololoff, L., 1984, Metabolic and behavioral consequences of lidocaine-kindled seizures, *Brain Res.* 324:295–303.
Pritchard, J.W., Gallagher, B.B., and Glaser, G.H., 1969, Experimental seizure-threshold testing with flurothyl, *J. Pharmacol. Exp. Ther.* 166:170–178.
Racine, R.J., 1972a, Modification of seizure activity by electrical stimulation. I. Afterdischarges, *Electroencephalog. Clin. Neurophysiol.* 32:281–294.
Racine, R.J., 1972b, Modification of seizure activity by electrical stimulation. II. Motor seizures, *Electroencephalog. Clin. Neurophysiol.* 32:281–294.
Racine, R.J., 1978, Kindling, the first decade, *Neurosurgery* 3:234–252.

Racine, R.J., and Burnham, W.M., 1984, The kindling model, in: *Electrophysiology of Epilepsy* (P. Schwartzkroin and H. Wheal, eds.), Academic Press, New York, pp. 153–157.

Racine, R.J., Livingston, K., and Joaquin, A., 1975, Effects of procaine hydrochloride, diazepam, and diphenylhydantoin on seizure development in cortical and subcortical structures in rats, *Electroencephalog. Clin. Neurophysiol.* 88:355–365.

Racine, R.J., Milgram, N.W., and Hafner, S., 1983, Long-term potentiation phenomena in the rat limbic forebrain, *Brain Res.* 260:217–231.

Racine, R.J., Burnham, W.M., Gilbert, M.E., and Kairiss, E.W., 1986, Kindling mechanisms: I. Electrophysiological studies, in: *Kindling 3* (J.A. Wada, ed.), Raven Press, New York, pp. 263–282.

Rajput, A.H., Uitti, R.J., Stern, W., Laverty, W., O'Donnell, K., O'Donnell, D., Yuen, W.K., and Dua, A., 1987, Geography, drinking water chemistry, pesticides and herbicides and the etiology of Parkinson's disease, *Can. J. Neurol. Sci.* 14:414–418.

Robinson, G.S., Crooks, G.B., Shinkman, P.G., and Gallagher, M., 1989a, Behavioral effects of MK-801 mimic deficits associated with hippocampal damage, *Psychobiology* 17:156–164.

Robinson, G.B., Port, R.L., and Berger, T.W., 1989b, Kindling facilitates acquisition of discriminative responding but disrupts reversal learning of the rabbit nictitating membrane response, *Behav. Brain Res.* 31:279–283.

Rowley, D.L., Rab, M.A., Hardjotanojo, W., Liddle, J., Burse, V.W., Saleem, M., Sokal, D., Falk, H., and Head, S.L., 1987, Convulsions caused by endrin poisoning in Pakistan, *Pediatrics* 6:928–934.

Santucci, V., Fournier, M., Keane, P., Simiand, J., Michaud, J.-C., Morre, M., and Biziere, K., 1985, EEG effects of IV infusion of pentylenetetrazol in rats: A model for screening and classifying antiepileptic compounds, *Psychopharmacology* 84:337–343.

Sato, M., Racine, R.J., and McIntyre, D.C., 1990, Kindling: Basic mechanisms and clinical validity, *Electroencepalog. Clin. Neurophysio.* 76:459–472.

Shemesh, Y., Bourvine, A., Gold, D., and Bracha, P., 1988, Survival after acute endosulfan intoxication, *Clin. Toxicol.* 26:265–268.

Shih, T.M., Lenz, D.E., and Maxwell, D.M., 1990, Effects of repeated injection of sublethal doses of soman on behavior and on brain acetylcholine and choline concentrations in the rat, *Psychopharmacology* 101:489–496.

Stripling, J.S., Gramlich, C.A., and Cunningham, M.G., 1989, Effect of cocaine and lidocaine on the development of kindled seizures, *Pharmacol. Biochem. Behav.* 32:463–468.

Sutula, T., and Steward, O., 1987, Facilitation of kindling by prior induction of long-term potentiation in the perforant path, *Brain Res.* 420:109–117.

Tilson, H.A., Veronesi, B., McLamb, R.L., and Matthews, H.B., 1991, Acute exposure to tris(2-chloroethyl)phosphate produces hippocampal neuronal loss and impairs learning in rats, *Toxicol. Appl. Pharmacol.* 106:254–269.

Tusell, J.M., Sunol, E., Gelpi, E., and Rodriguez-Farre, E., 1988, Effect of lindane at repeated low doses, *Toxicology* 49:375–379.

Uemura, S., and Kimura, H., 1988, Amygdaloid kindling with bicuculline methiodide in rats, *Exp. Neurol.* 102:346–353.

Uemura, S., and Kimura, H., 1990, Common epileptic pathway in amygdaloid bicuculline and electrical kindling demonstrated by transferability, *Brain Res.* 537:315–317.

Wada, J.A., Mizoguchi,T., and Osawa, T., 1978, Secondary generalized convulsive seizures induced by daily amygdaloid stimulation in rhesus monkeys, *Neurology* 28:1026–1036.

Wasterlain, C.G., and Fairchild, M.D., 1985, Transfer between chemical and electrical kindling in the septal-hippocampal system, *Brain Res.* 331:261–266.

Wasterlain, C.G., Morin, A.M., and Jonec, V., 1982, Interactions between chemical and electrical kindling of the rat amygdala, *Brain Res.* 247:341–346.

Weiss, S.R.B., Post, R.M., Gold, P.W., Chrousos, G., Sullivan, T.L., Walker, D., and Pert, A. 1986, CRF-induced seizures and behavior: Interaction with amygdala kindling, *Brain Res.* 372:345–351.

Weiss, S.R.B., Post, R.M., Costello, M., Nutt, D.J., and Tandeciarz, S., 1990, Carbamazepine retards the development of cocaine-kindled seizures but not sensitization to cocaine-induced hyperactivity, *Neuropsychopharmacology* 3:273–279.

Wozniak, D.F., Olney, J.W., Kettinger, L. III, Price, M., and Miller, J.P., 1990, Behavioral effects of MK-801 in the rat, *Psychopharmacology* 101:47–56.

Yokoyama, N., Mori, N., and Kumashiro, H., 1989, Chemical kindling induced by cAMP and transfer to electrical kindling, *Brain Res.* 492:158–162.

Chapter 9

# Testing Visual System Toxicity Using Evoked Potential Technology

*William K. Boyes*

## 1. INTRODUCTION

Neurotoxicity is a frequent component of the toxicity profile of many compounds. Approximately 65,000 compounds used in commerce are regulated under the Toxic Substances Control Act (TSCA), but very few have been tested for neurotoxicity. A range of estimates is available regarding the proportion of compounds that are neurotoxic. The Congressional Office of Technology Assessment (OTA) estimates that about 25% of the compounds for which an adequate database exists have significant neurotoxicity (OTA, 1984). Of the approximately 1400 active pesticide ingredients registered by the Environmental Protection Agency (EPA) under the Federal Insecticide Fungicide and Rodenticide Act (FIFRA), OTA (1990) states that the majority are specifically designed to be neurotoxic.

Potential neurotoxic substances in food are regulated in the United States by at least three federal agencies. The EPA registers and approves pesticides for use under FIFRA and establishes the maximum amount of residues permissible in food. The Food and Drug Administration (FDA) is responsible for enforcing tolerance levels for pesticides and other compounds in foods, with the exception of meat, poultry, and certain egg products, for

---

This manuscript has been reviewed by the Health Effects Research Laboratory, U.S. Environmental Protection Agency, and approved for publication. Mention of trade names and commercial products does not constitute endorsement or recommendation for use.

---

*William K. Boyes* • Neurophysiological Toxicology Branch, Neurotoxicology Division, Health Effects Research Laboratory, U.S. Environmental Protection Agency, Research Triangle Park, North Carolina 27711.
*The Vulnerable Brain and Environmental Risks, Volume 1: Malnutrition and Hazard Assessment,* edited by Robert L. Isaacson and Karl F. Jensen. Plenum Press, New York, 1992.

which the U.S. Department of Agriculture is responsible. With the exception of pesticides, FDA is responsible under the Federal Food, Drug, and Cosmetic Act for identifying and regulating potential neurotoxic substances in food, which may include naturally occurring substances, food additives, and contaminants. Hattan *et al.* (1983) have reviewed FDA's activities in the regulation of potential neurotoxic substances in food. In random food samples for cases in which specific contamination was not suspected, pesticide residue levels exceeded the established tolerance levels in less than 1% of the domestic and 3% of imported food samples (FDA, 1990). This suggests that the neurotoxic threat from pesticide residues in food is typically low, given that the residue tolerance levels have been set appropriately. A scientific challenge, therefore, is to establish the best procedures for establishing appropriate exposure limits.

## 1.1. Need for Tests of Visual Function

Given that prevention of neurotoxicity is a regulatory and scientific challenge, of what importance are visual problems as a component of neurotoxicity? In its simplest conception, the nervous system receives sensory input, performs integration functions on that information, and then emits a motor response. Thus, sensory function is a prerequisite for proper nervous system function. Certainly, blindness, deafness, or loss of peripheral sensation are personal handicaps worthy of regulatory concern.

Are sensory deficits likely to result from exposure to neurotoxic compounds? One source of material convenient for examining this question is a list of purported neurotoxic compounds compiled by Anger and Johnson (1985). The Anger and Johnson list was compiled from books and review articles dealing with neurotoxic compounds, and comprised 764 compounds or compound classes that were reported to have neurotoxic effects. This data set has been entered into a computerized database that is available for certain types of analyses (Gage, 1987, 1991). Crofton and Sheets (1989) employed this database to examine the frequency of reported sensory effects for neurotoxic compounds and found that approximately 44% of the neurotoxic compounds produced sensory toxicity. A breakdown of this data by sensory modality is presented in Figure 1. Damage to the visual system was the most prevalent of the sensory effects. In addition, it is important to consider that the list compiled by Anger and Johnson was derived from reference sources on neurotoxic compounds, and therefore may under-represent the number of substances that produce visual dysfunction. For example, Grant (1986) lists over 2800 compounds that produce toxic effects on the eye or vision. It is apparent that visual changes may often occur after overexposure to chemical compounds.

The compounds reported by Anger and Johnson to have effects on vision or visual structures are presented in Table 1. The table also includes a description of the visual effects, the duration of exposure, and whether the effects were reported in laboratory animals or humans. For some compounds, the visual system effects are a result of direct ocular toxicity, as opposed to neurotoxic damage to the neural elements of the central nervous system. In comparing the frequency and type of effects reported in humans to those that were based on animal studies, it is apparent that many more reports occurred in humans and that they were different in character from those reported in animals. The predominance of human reports may reflect a bias for including human effects in review articles that were the source material for the original table, but more likely this reflects the difficulty of assessing the functional status of the visual system of laboratory animals. The

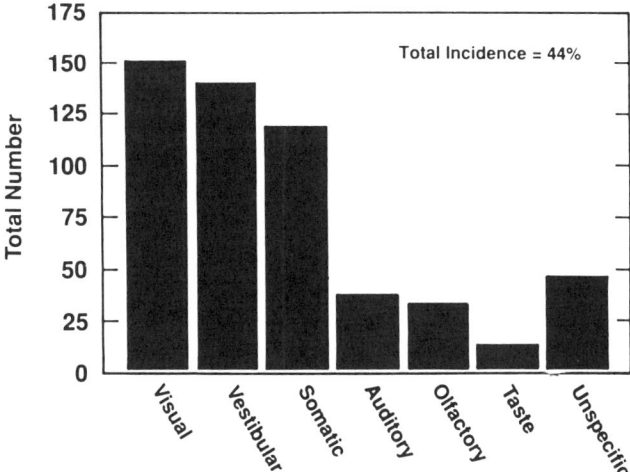

**FIGURE 1.** Number of compounds having sensory toxicity from a list of 764 neurotoxic compounds. From an analysis of the data of Anger and Johnson (1985) performed by Crofton and Sheets (1989). Reproduced from Crofton and Sheets (1989).

latter conclusion is supported by the types of effects reported for animals and humans. The reports in animals tend to be effects on the eye that are readily observable, such as changes in the pupil or lens, or that are easily inferred, such as eye pain. In contrast, the reports from humans are predominantly subjective observations, such as visual-field constriction, blurring, or dimming. Thus, a large proportion of compounds of regulatory interest may affect vision, but visual effects typically reported in laboratory animals are qualitatively different and quantitatively fewer than those reported in humans. It follows that adequate assessment of visual function in laboratory animals should be a matter of concern in toxicity testing.

## 1.2. Examples of Visually Toxic Compounds

Before discussing the testing of visual function, it may be useful to consider briefly some specific toxicants known to alter vision. A number of excellent reviews exist regarding toxicants affecting the eye or vision (Bron, 1979; Chan and Hayes, 1985; Grant, 1980, 1986; Gehring, 1971; Heywood, 1974; 1982, 1985, 1986; Heywood and Gopinath, 1990; McLaren, 1982; Meier-Ruge, 1972; Merigan, 1979; Merigan and Weiss, 1980; Plestina and Piukovic-Plestina, 1978). The classic agents that alter vision include methanol, methylmercury, carbon disulfide, and lead. At high dose levels, acrylamide given to adult animals and postnatally administered monosodium glutamate will also damage visual structures and produce loss of vision. More controversial are reports that low levels of carbon monoxide and chronic exposure to organophosphates produce visual loss.

Blindness produced by drinking wood alcohol is a matter of popular knowledge. Humans who ingest large quantities of methanol have experienced optic disk edema, optic nerve degeneration, visual loss, and blindness (Grant, 1986). The metabolism of methanol is critical to its toxicity. Sequential oxidative steps from methanol serve to form formalde-

**TABLE 1.** Compounds Having Visual Effects

| Chemical | Effects | Exposure | Species |
| --- | --- | --- | --- |
| Acrylamide | Hallucinations | Acute/subchronic | Human |
| Adiponitrile | Pupil response loss | Acute | Unspecified |
| Alcohols | Color threshold increase | Unspecified | Unspecified |
| | Visual acuity decrease | Unspecified | Unspecified |
| | Peripheral visual field constriction | Unspecified | Unspecified |
| Alkyl mercuric chlorides | Visual field constriction | Unspecified | Unspecified |
| Allyl alcohol | Vision blurring | Acute | Human |
| Aluminum | EEG, visual evoked potential shifts | Unspecified | Animal |
| Ammonia | Pupil reflex loss | Acute | Human |
| Amyl alcohols | Vision disturbances | Acute | Human |
| | Double vision | Acute | Human |
| Aspidium | Vision disturbances | Unspecified | Unspecified |
| | Blindness | Unspecified | Unspecified |
| Atrazine (2-chloro-4-ethylamino-6-isopropylamino-s-triazine) | Ptosis | Acute | Animal |
| Benzene | Visual disturbances | Acute/chronic | Human/unspecified |
| Benzyl alcohol/ benzenemethanol | Nystagmus | Acute | Animal |
| Butadiene | Vision blurring | Acute | Human |
| 1-Butanol | Vision blurring | Acute | Human |
| Butylene glycol mono-N-butylether | Eye pain | Acute (contact) | Animal |
| | Iritis | Acute (contact) | Animal |
| Butylene glycol monoethylether | Eye pain | Acute (contact) | Animal |
| | Iritis | Acute (contact) | Animal |
| Butylene glycols | Pupil constriction | Acute | Animal |
| | Eye stinging | Acute (contact) | Human |
| p-t-Butylphenol | Pupil irregularity | Unspecified | Unspecified |
| | Oculomotor paresis | Unspecified | Unspecified |
| *3-Butyn-2-one | Eye pain | Acute (contact) | Animal |
| Carbon disulfide | Eye disorders | Subchronic/chronic | Human |
| | Retinopathy | Subchronic/chronic | Human |
| | Optic neuritis | Unspecified | Unspecified |
| | Eye movement, pupil reaction fundus, cornea sensitivity changes | Unspecified | Human |
| Carbon monoxide | Vision failure | Acute | Human |
| | Blindness | Acute | Animal |
| | Visual function decrement | Acute | Human |
| Chenopodium oil American wormseed | Diplopia | Unspecified | Unspecified |
| | Blindness | Unspecified | Unspecified |
| Chlordane (1,2,4,5,6,7,8,8-Octachloro-3a,4,7,7a-tetrahydro-4,7-methanoindan) | Visual disorders | Chronic | Human |

*(continued)*

**TABLE 1.** (*Continued*)

| Chemical | Effects | Exposure | Species |
|---|---|---|---|
| Chlordecone | Opsoclonus | Acute | Animal |
| kepone | Visual hallucinations | Subchronic/chronic | Human |
| | Vision disturbances | Subchronic/chronic | Human |
| 2-Chloroethanol | Vision disturbances | Acute | Human |
| Creosote | Pupil reflex loss | Acute | Human |
| | Vision disturbances | Acute | Human |
| Cyanide | Vision loss | Chronic | Human |
| | Amblyopia | Unspecified | Unspecified |
| | Optic neuritis | Unspecified | Unspecified |
| Cyclohexylamine | Pupil dilation | Acute/subchronic | Human |
| | Vision reductions | Unspecified | Human |
| Deserpidine | Ptosis | Acute | Unspecified |
| Dialkyl tin | Ptosis | Acute | Animal |
| Diazinon | Pupil constriction | Acute | Human |
| [0,0-Diethyl 0-(2-isopropyl-4-methyl-6-pyrimidyl) phosphorothiate] | Vision blurring | Acute | Human |
| Dibrom [0,0-Dimethyl 0-(1,2-dibromo-2,2-dichloroethyl) phosphate] | Nystagmus | Acute | Human |
| Dibutyl phthalate | Photophobia | Acute | Animal |
| o-Dichlorobenzene | Lens opacity | Unspecified | Unspecified |
| p-Dichlorobenzene | Nystagmus | Chronic | Animal |
| Dichlorodiphenyl-trichloroethane DDT | Vision problems | Chronic | Human |
| 1,2-Dichloroethane ethylene dichloride | Nystagmus | Unspecified | Unspecified |
| Diethaolamine | Vision impairment | Acute (contact) | Animal |
| Diethylamine | Eye disease | Unspecified | Human |
| Diethylene glycol monomethylether | Eye pain | Acute (contact) | Animal |
| Diisopropylamine | Vision haziness | Acute | Human |
| Dimefox [bis (dimethylamino) fluorophosphine oxide] | Vision blurring | Acute | Unspecified |
| Dimethylacetamide | Visual hallucinations | Unspecified | Unspecified |
| Dimethylaniline | Vision disturbances | Acute | Human |
| Dinitrobenzene | Vision loss | Unspecified | Unspecified |
| Dinitrobenzenes (o-,m-,p-) | Vision disorders | Chronic | Human |
| 2,4-Dinitrotoluene | Vision dimming | Chronic | Human |
| Diphenyl, biphenyl | Nystagmus | Chronic | Human |
| Dipropylene glycol monomethyl ether | Eye pain | Acute (contact) | Unspecified |
| Diquat | Lens opacity | Unspecified | Animal |
| Disulfiram [bis (diethyl-thiocarbamoyl) disulfide] antabuse | Optic neuritis | Unspecified | Human |

(*continued*)

**TABLE 1.** (*Continued*)

| Chemical | Effects | Exposure | Species |
|---|---|---|---|
| Ergot | Mydriasis | Unspecified | Unspecified |
| Ethylamine monoethylamine | Vision effects | Unspecified | Unspecified |
| Ethylbenzene | Eye pain | Chronic | Human |
| Ethyl bromide | Nystagmus | Unspecified | Human |
| Ethyl bromoacetate | Blindness | Acute | Unspecified |
| Ethyl glycol | Nystagmus | Acute | Human |
|  | Ipitis | Acute (contact) | Animal |
| Ethylene glycol diethyl ether | Eye pain | Acure (contact) | Animal |
| Ethylene glycol monoethyl ether | Eye pain | Acute (contact) | Animal |
| Ethylene glycol | Iritis | Acute (contact) | Animal |
| Ethylene glycol monomethyl ether | Eye pain | Acute (contact) | Unspecified |
|  | Irregular, unequal pupils | Unspecified | Unspecified |
| Ethyl iodoacetate | Eye damage | Acute | Human |
| Ethyl mercuric phosphate | Visual-field constriction | Unspecified | Unspecified |
| N-(Ethylmercuri)-p toluene sulfonanilide | Vision deficits | Unspecified | Unspecified |
| Fenthion (0,0-dimethyl)-[3-methyl-4-(methylthio)phenyl] phosphorothioate) Baytex | Ophthalmological electroretinogram changes | Unspecified | Animal |
| Fluorides, soluble | Color vision disturbances | Acute | Human |
| Formaldehyde | Vision disorders | Unspecified | Unspecified |
| Gelsemium | Ptosis | Unspecified | Unspecified |
|  | Mydriasis | Unspecified | Unspecified |
|  | Diplopia | Unspecified | Unspecified |
| Hexachlorophene | Diplopia | Unspecified | Unspecified |
| n-Hexane | Corneal, reflex loss | Acute | Animal |
|  | Color vision abnormalities | Subchronic/chronic | Human |
|  | Vision blurring | Subchronic/chronic | Human |
|  | Visual evoked potential loss | Subchronic/chronic | Human |
|  | Optic neuropathy | Subchronic/chronic | Human |
| Hexanol | Iritis | Acute (contact) | Animal |
| 1-Hexyn-3-ol | Iritis | Acute (contact) | Acute |
| Hydrazoic acid hydrogen azide | Blindness | Acute | Animal |
|  | Optic nerve lesions | Acute | Animal |
| Isobutyronitrile | Pupil dilation | Acute | Human |
| Isoniazid Isonicotinic acid hydrazine (4-pyridinecarboxylic acidhydrazine) | Pupil dilation | Acute | Human |
|  | Photophobia | Acute | Human |
|  | Vision disturbances | Unspecified | Human |
| Lead | Blindness | Subchronic/chronic | Human/animal |
|  | Optic atrophy | Chronic | Human |
|  | Night blindness | Chronic | Animal |
|  | Visual reaction time | Unspecified | Human |

(*continued*)

**TABLE 1.** (*Continued*)

| Chemical | Effects | Exposure | Species |
|---|---|---|---|
| Leptophos | Visual acuity decrease | Unspecified | Unspecified |
| Lindane | Corneal reflex weakness | Unspecified | Human |
| Lithium | Vision blurring | Chronic | Human |
| Lithium carbonate | Vision blurring | Unspecified | Unspecified |
| Lithium chloride | Vision blurring | Acute | Unspecified |
| Lysergic acid diethylamide (LSD) | Hallucinations | Acute | Unspecified |
|  | Mydriasis | Acute | Unspecified |
| Mercury | Lens coloration | Subchronic/chronic | Human |
|  | Visual field constriction | Chronic | Unspecified |
|  | Blindness | Unspecified | Human |
|  | Amblyopia | Unspecified | Unspecified |
|  | Pupil changes | Unspecified | Unspecified |
|  | Visual field constriction (tunnel vision) | Unspecified | Human |
| Mescaline | Pupil dilation | Acute | Unspecified |
| Mesidine (2,4,6-trimethyl-aniline) | Light sensitivity decrease | Unspecified | Human |
|  | Peripheral vision reduction | Unspecified | Human |
|  | Blind spot enlargement | Unspecified | Human |
| 2-Methoxyethanol | Vision blurring | Unspecified | Human |
| Methyl acetate | Eyelid tremor | Unspecified | Human |
|  | Optic nerve atrophy | Unspecified | Unspecified |
| Methyl alcohol (methanol) | Retina, optic nerve fiber degeneration | Acute | Human/animal |
|  | Pupil dilation | Acute | Human |
|  | Vision clouding | Acute | Human |
|  | Diplopia | Acute | Human |
|  | Blindness | Acute/subchronic | Human |
|  | Mydriasis | Acute | Human |
|  | Vision blurring | Acute/chronic | Human |
|  | Hallucinations (dancing spots, flashes) | Subchronic/chronic | Human |
|  | Vision disturbances (incl. blurring, photophobia), | Subchronic/chronic | Human |
|  | Retina edema | Subchronic/chronic | Human |
|  | Pupil light reflex diminution, loss | Chronic | Human |
|  | Visual acuity loss | Chronic | Human |
|  | Optic disk, retina edema | Chronic | Human |
|  | Photoreceptor, ganglion cell degeneration | Chronic | Human |
|  | Optic nerve axon enlargement, microtubule disruption, mitochondria clustering, oligodendroglia cytoplasm swelling | Unspecified | Human |
|  | Concentric color | Unspecified | Unspecified |
|  | Visual field constriction | Unspecified | Unspecified |
|  | Optic nerve pathology | Unspecified | Unspecified |
| Methyl bromide (monobromomethane) | Vision disturbances | Acute | Unspecified |
|  | Diplopia | Unspecified | Unspecified |
| Methyl n-butyl ketone (MBK) | Optic tract lesions | Unspecified | Unspecified |

(*continued*)

**TABLE 1.** (*Continued*)

| Chemical | Effects | Exposure | Species |
| --- | --- | --- | --- |
| Methyl chloride (monochloromethane) | Vision blurring | Acute/chronic | Human |
| Methylene chloride | Visual delusions, hallucinations | Subchronic | Human |
| Methyl ethly ketone (2-butanone) (MEK) | Vision losses | Acute | Human |
| Methyl formate | Amblyopia | Acute | Unspecified |
| Methyl iodide | Diplopia | Acute | Human |
| Methylpyridine | Unequal pupil sizes | Subchronic/chronic | Human |
| | diplopia | Subchronic/chronic | Human |
| Methylstyrene | Visual threshold increase | Chronic | Human |
| | Visual field constriction | Chronic | Human |
| Mevinphos [0,0-Dimethyl 0-(1-methyl-2-carbomethoxyvinyl) phosphate] (Phosdrin) | Pupil constriction | Unspecified | Human |
| | Vision blurring | Unspecified | Human |
| Morpholine | Vision effects | Unspecified | Unspecified |
| Naphthalene | Optic neuritis | Acute | Human |
| | Lens opacity | Chronic | Human |
| B-Naphthol | Lens opacity | Unspecified | Unspecified |
| | Retina changes | Unspecified | Unspecified |
| Nicotine | Vision impairment | Chronic | Unspecified |
| Organophosphates | Amblyopia | Unspecified | Unspecified |
| | Nystagmus | Unspecified | Unspecified |
| | Pupil changes | Unspecified | Unspecified |
| Ozocerite (mineral wax) | Visual hallucinations | Acute | Human |
| | Pupil irregularities | Chronic | Human |
| Ozone | Dark adaptation, visual acuity decreases | Acute | Human |
| | Peripheral vision increase | Acute | Human |
| Paraquat | Pupil reflex loss | Acute | Animal |
| | Lens opacity | Chronic | Animal |
| Pelletierine tannate | Mydriasis | Unspecified | Unspecified |
| | Optic nerve toxicity | Unspecified | Unspecified |
| Penicillin | Visual hallucinations | Acute | Human/animal |
| 1-Pentanol | Diplopia | Acute | Human |
| | Iritis | Acute (contact) | Unspecified |
| Petroleum, unrefined | Visual field constriction | Chronic | Human |
| Phenol (carbolic acid) | Pupil constriction, dilation | Acute | Human |
| p-Phenylenediamine | Blindness | Acute (contact) | Unspecified |
| Piperidine | Visual disturbances | Acute | Human |
| Polybrominated biphenyls (PBBs) | Vision blurring | Unspecified | Human |
| Polychlorinated biphenyls (Arochlor) | Vision disturbances | Chronic | Human |
| Polymethylmethacrylate | Vision disturbances | Chronic | Human |
| Potassium cyanate | Miosis | Unspecified | Unspecified |
| Propanol | Iritis | Acute (contact) | Animal |
| Propargyl alcohol | Eye pain | Acute (contact) | Unspecified |
| n-Propyl alcohol (1-propanol) | Iritis | Acute (contact) | Animal |

(*continued*)

**TABLE 1.** (*Continued*)

| Chemical | Effects | Exposure | Species |
|---|---|---|---|
| Propylamines | Vision impairment | Acute | Human |
| Propylene glycol | Transitory eye stinging | Acute (contact) | Human |
| Propytlenglycol, isobutyl ethers | Eye pain | Acute (contact) | Animal |
| Propylene glycol dinitrate | Visual evoked response disruption | Subchronic | Human |
| Propylene glycol monoacrylate | Eye pain | Acute (contact) | Animal |
| Pyridine | Flashing lights | Chronic | Human |
| Quinones | Vision disturbances | Chronic | Unspecified |
| Santonin | Vision (color) disorders | Acute | Human |
| Selenium (compounds) | Vision impairment | Acute/subchronic | Unspecified |
| Sodium azide | Blindness | Acute | Animal |
| | Optic nerve lesions | Acute | Animal |
| Solanine | Pupil dilation | Acute | Unspecified |
| Strychnine | Photophobia | Acute | Human |
| Tellurium | Visual discrimination deficits | Chronic | Unspecified |
| Tetraalkyl tin (tetramethyl tin) | Photophobia | Acute | Human |
| 2,3,7,8-tetrachloro-dibenzo-p-dioxin) | Amblyiopia | Unspecified | Unspecified |
| Tetraethylene glycol monophenyl ether | Vision impairment | Acute | Animal |
| Tretaethyl lead | Vision difficulties | Unspecified | Unspecified |
| Thallium | Optic atrophy | Acute | Unspecified |
| | Hallucinations | Acute | Human |
| | Pupil changes | Unspecified | Unspecified |
| | Optic neuritis | Unspecified | Unspecified |
| Tin (organic) (incl. triethyltin) | Photophobia | Acute/subchronic | Human |
| | Vision disturbances | Acute/subchronic | Human |
| | Visual acuity loss | Chronic | Human |
| | Optic nerve lesions | Unspecified | Unspecified |
| Toluene (methylbenzene) | Vision disturbances | Acute | Human |
| | Optic atrophy | Chronic | Unspecified |
| | Hallucinations | Unspecified | Unspecified |
| | Cornea sensitivity decrease | Chronic | Human |
| Trialkyl tin | Ptosis | Acute | Animal |
| Trichloroethylene (acetylene trichloride) | Vision disturbances | Acute | Human |
| | Visual perception loss | Acute/subchronic | Human |
| | Vision disturbances | Chronic | Unspecified |
| Triethylamine | Eye disease | Unspecified | Unspecified |
| Trimethyl phosphite | Lens opacity | Subchronic | Animal |
| Trinitrotoluene (TNT) | Vitreal, retina damage | Unspecified | Human |
| Tripropylene glycol monomethyl ether | Eye pain | Acute | Animal |
| Vanadium (and salts) | Vision blurring | Acute/subchronic | Human |
| | Blindness | Unspecified | Unspecified |
| Xylene | Vision disturbances | Acute | Human |
| Zinc pyrithione | Blindness | Chronic | Animal |

Adapted from Anger and Johnson (1985).

hyde, formic acid, and carbon dioxide. Formic acid is thought to be the toxic metabolite, and formate conversion to carbon monoxide is performed by a folic-acid-dependent enzyme, which in humans is a rate-limiting step. High levels of methanol ingestion lead to blood formate accumulation and acidosis. The acidosis, however, is not critical in the toxicity, since formate can produce optic-disk edema without acidosis (Martin-Amat *et al.*, 1978). There are large species differences in susceptibility to optic nerve damage from methanol, which can be related to metabolism. Humans and nonhuman primates are highly susceptible, but rats are more efficient in metabolizing formate and are normally not susceptible. Recently, it has been shown that rats can be made susceptible to methanol through metabolic manipulations that disrupt the folic-acid-dependent pathway of formate metabolism (Eells, 1991; Lee, 1987). This knowledge may provide more convenient animal models in which to test hypotheses regarding the mechanism of damage of formate to the optic nerve.

Methylmercury poisoning produces many neurological symptoms. Visual problems produced in exposed adult humans include constriction of the visual field (Hunter *et al.*, 1940) and a variety of other visual problems, including loss of contrast sensitivity (Mukuno *et al.*, 1984). Primates show similar visual problems (Merigan, 1979; Merigan *et al.*, 1983), and the deficits are particularly evident at low levels of illumination (Evans *et al.*, 1975). Visual problems have been attributed to damage in portions of visual cortex located deep in the calcarine fissure, which receive topographical projections of the peripheral retina (Hunter *et al.*, 1940). Prenatal and postnatal exposure to methylmercury also produces visual deficits, but these may be somewhat different from those produced in exposed adults in that loss of spatial and temporal resolution occurs without a predominant loss of peripheral vision, which hallmarks adult toxicity (Rice and Gilbert, 1981, 1990).

Carbon disulfide has been known for years to produce multiple human neurological and psychological problems. Prominent visual complaints include central visual-field defects and problems with spatial and color vision. The associated optic atrophy was once thought to result from retinal microaneurysms, but recently it has been shown that loss of spatial vision, contrast sensitivity, and retinal ganglion cell damage can result from exposure to carbon disulfide in the absence of retinal microaneurysms (Eskin *et al.*, 1988; Merigan *et al.*, 1988). These results indicate that the damage to retinal neurons resulting from carbon disulfide exposure is not a secondary consequence of vascular damage.

Lead exposure produces multiple human neurological and psychological problems, including visual deficits, particularly at low levels of illumination (Bushnell *et al.*, 1977; Fox, 1984; Fox *et al.*, 1977, 1979). Lead exposure produced selective damage to rod photoreceptors (Fox and Chu, 1988; Fox and Farber, 1988; Fox and Sillman, 1979) which may account for the difficulties of low luminance vision. Developmental lead exposure also damages the visual cortex (Reuhl *et al.*, 1989).

Postnatal exposure to high dose levels of monosodium glutamate produces a rapid degeneration of retinal ganglion cells (Lucas and Newhouse, 1957). This can lead to adult rats with little or no optic nerve, and severely disrupted flash and pattern reversal-evoked potentials (Rigdon *et al.*, 1989).

Prolonged exposure to acrylamide in nonhuman primates produces selective degeneration of a class of medium-diameter retinal ganglion cells that project to the parvocellular layer of the dorsal lateral geniculate nucleus (Eskin and Merigan, 1986; Merigan and Eskin, 1986). This neurotoxicant-induced preparation has proved a useful model for studying the functions of the parvocellular system in that the intoxicated monkeys show selective loss of contrast sensitivity to high spatial frequency and low temporal frequency targets (Eskin and Merigna, 1986; Merigan and Eskin, 1986).

Carbon monoxide has long been reported to alter vision, in particular to increase luminance thresholds during dark adaptation (McFarland *et al.,* 1944). Recent efforts, however, have failed to demonstrate effects of carbon monoxide on luminance thresholds or other visual parameters at doses producing carboxyhemoglobin levels as high as 17% (Hudnell and Benignus, 1989).

It is well known that exposure to cholinesterase-inhibiting compounds produces acute effects on the eye and vision (Harding *et al.,* 1983, 1985; Plestina and Piukovic-Plestina, 1978). A number of Japanese studies have reported that chronic exposure to organophosphate insecticides can produce a spectrum of persistent ocular effects. In the late 1960s and early 1970s, an outbreak of ocular disorders occurred in school children and adults in the Saku region and other agricultural areas of Japan. This syndrome consisted of loss of visual acuity, myopia, astigmatism, concentric constriction of the visual field, disorders of eye movements and pupil function, changes in intraocular pressure, and a variety of ophthalmological findings, including swollen optic nerves, macular discoloration, and retinochoroidal degeneration. Ishikawa and others proposed that "Saku disease" was the consequence of inadvertent overexposure to acetylcholinesterase-inhibiting organophosphorus insecticides (see review by Ishikawa and Miyata, 1980). An independent study from India reported that workers who sprayed primarily fenthion experienced macular degeneration similar to that reported in Japan (Misra *et al.,* 1985).

There is also a body of evidence that opens doubt regarding the causative role of organophosphate insecticides in producing chronic ocular disorders. Imai (1986) reported examination of nine of the same patients diagnosed by others as having organophosphorus-induced ocular disease and found that all cases could be attributed to common ocular diseases. Organophosphates have been used throughout the world for years without prompting numerous reports of visual toxicity, as might be expected. Organophosphates also have been installed directly into the eyes in the treatment of glaucoma, apparently without producing Saku-like degeneration. An extensive review of the literature, which also included original data, concluded that there was insufficient evidence to unequivocally establish the existence of chronic effects of organophosphates on the eye (Plestina and Piukovic-Plestina, 1978). Thus, although the acute visual effects of organophosphates and other inhibitors of acetyl cholinesterase are well established, the possibility of chronic ocular toxicity produced by these compounds is an issue deserving further research.

## 1.3. Current Neurotoxicity Testing

In order to test for neurotoxic effects from compounds of unknown toxicity, a number of screening strategies have been proposed (Gad, 1989). Many of the screening approaches involve simple observational tests as an initial assessment. These may be combined with other measures, such as automated assessment of motor activity and neuropathology. This strategy currently forms the basis of testing for pesticides and toxic substances under FIFRA and TSCA, respectively (USEPA, 1991). Typical pathological examinations may include examinations of the eye but generally would not include examination of other sensory end organs.

Measures that reflect sensory function in these testing schemes are typically simple observations, such as those performed in functional observational batteries (FOB; Moser, 1989). These measures, all of which are scored by a trained observer, include behavioral responses to a click, tail pinch, touch, and approach of an object, and pupil response to light. Only the last two of these measures would be indicative of visual function. Although these measures may be obtained quickly and inexpensively, they may be subject to experimenter bias and large interobserver and interlaboratory variability (WHO, 1986). Observational measures may also be less sensitive to the effects of toxicants than more sophisticated techniques (Evans, 1982; Lochry, 1987; Moody and Stebbins, 1982). The sensory stimuli employed in each case are rather primitive and do not reflect the elaborate discriminative abilities of sensory systems. These tests require a neuromuscular response in order to observe an effect, and therefore cannot distinguish sensory from neuromuscular deficits. Finally, many of these measures are mediated by sensorimotor reflex neural pathways. These pathways are relatively simple neural circuits involving primarily lower brain and spinal areas of the central nervous system. Sensory perception, in contrast, also involves important higher brain areas, including substantial portions of the cerebral cortex. Neurotoxicant-induced damage to these higher brain areas could conceivably produce loss of sensory function without altering the sensory measures included in the FOB.

## 2. VISUAL EVOKED POTENTIALS

### 2.1. Advantages of Sensory Evoked Potentials

A number of powerful electrophysiological procedures are available that may be selected based on the aims of the investigation. The electrophysiological procedures collectively known as sensory evoked potentials are recordings of electrical field potentials following the presentation of sensory stimuli. These potentials reflect neuronal responses to sensory stimulation. Averaged sensory evoked potentials were first applied in toxicology by Xintaras and coworkers (Xintaras *et al.*, 1966), who studied the acute effects of carbon monoxide. The expanding use of sensory evoked potentials in toxicology has been extensively reviewed (Arezzo *et al.*, 1985; Dyer, 1982, 1983, 1985, 1986, 1987a, 1987b; Dyer and Boyes, 1983b; Fox *et al.*, 1982; Mattsson and Albe, 1988; Mattsson *et al.*, 1989, 1990a; Otto, 1986; Otto *et al.*, 1985, 1988; Rebert, 1983; Seppalainen, 1988; Woolley, 1977). There is a substantial clinical database demonstrating the value of these techniques in the diagnosis of sensory and neurological disorders (e.g., Regan, 1989). Arezzo *et al.* (1985), Otto, (1986), Otto *et al.* (1985), and Seppalainen (1988) have reviewed the use of evoked potentials in human neurotoxicology investigations. In laboratory animals, visual, auditory, and somatosensory evoked potentials can be measured through stimulation of the appropriate sensory system (Rebert, 1983). Rebert (1983), Dyer (1985), and Mattsson and colleagues (Mattsson and Albee, 1988; Mattsson *et al.*, 1989, 1990a) have recommended that evoked potentials recorded from multiple sensory systems become part of neurotoxicology testing practice. This review will focus primarily on sensory evoked potential measures of visual function.

### 2.2. Types of Visual Evoked Potentials

2.2.1. Flash Evoked Potentials

There are several different types of visual evoked potentials, which may be classified by the type of stimulus employed. Most extensively used in experimental neurotoxicology

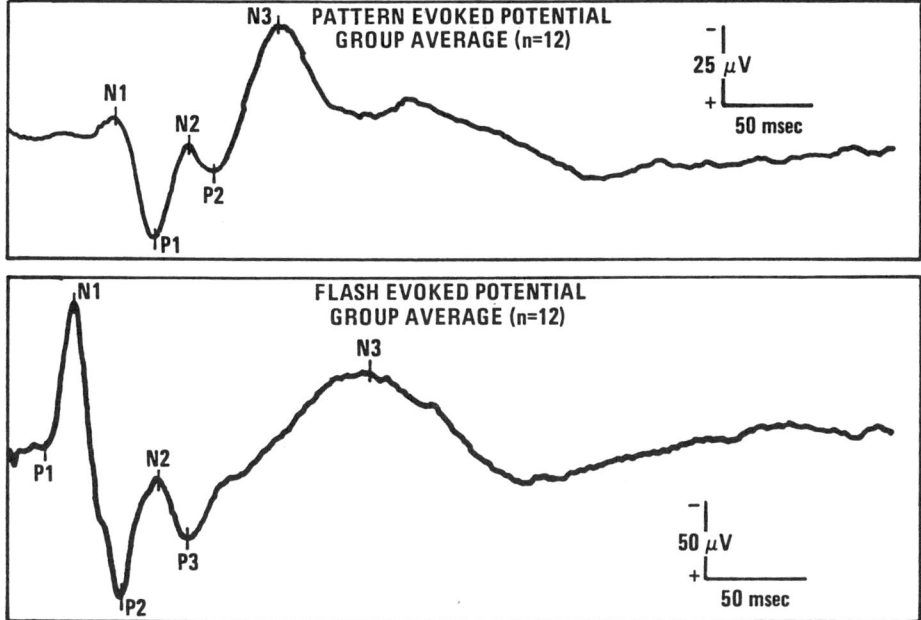

**FIGURE 2.** Pattern-reversal and flash evoked potential waveforms averaged across a group of 12 rats. The two evoked potentials differ in latency, amplitude, and shape, illustrating that they reflect different aspects of visual function. Reproduced from Boyes and Dyer (1983a).

has been the flash VEP, also known as the flash evoked potential (FEP), which is elicited by a brief flash from a strobe lamp. Procedures for recording FEPs during development have been reported (Albee and Mattsson, 1983; Rigdon and Dyer, 1987). An advantage of FEPs over other types of VEPs is that it is relatively easy to assure that the visual stimulus is properly imaged on the retina. It is possible to test rats in an awake, unrestrained fashion by simply placing the rats in a small mirrored chamber with the strobe lamp on one wall (Dyer and Annau, 1977a). In this arrangement the rat will be adequately stimulated in any position. Similarly, when testing other species, including humans, it is also relatively simple to control the adequate delivery of the flash stimulus.

The flash stimulus used to elicit FEPs is thought to elicit neural activity in most or all cells in the retina, and therefore to be the logical equivalent of a supramaximal electrical stimulus to a peripheral nerve. The massive retinal activation leads to a large and highly characteristic flash VEP waveform recorded from visual cortex (Figure 2). A typical FEP waveform consists of a series of positive and negative voltage peaks that have characteristic latencies and amplitudes depending upon the stimulation and recording parameters. Various nomenclatures have been employed for labeling these peaks, which have included successively labeling the alternate positive and negative peaks (P1, N1, P2, etc.) or labeling the peaks according to both their voltage polarity and their approximate peak latency in milliseconds (P21, N30, P45, etc.). The early latency peaks are thought to reflect the activity of primary retinal afferents arriving at the visual cortex and the subsequent depolarizations of the postsynaptic dendrites of thalamo-recipient neurons, primarily in layer IV (Kraut et al., 1985). The middle latency peaks are thought to reflect cortical-cortical circuits and cortical-thalamic loops (Dyer, 1986). Both the early and middle latency components have been repeatedly demonstrated to be sensitive to exposure

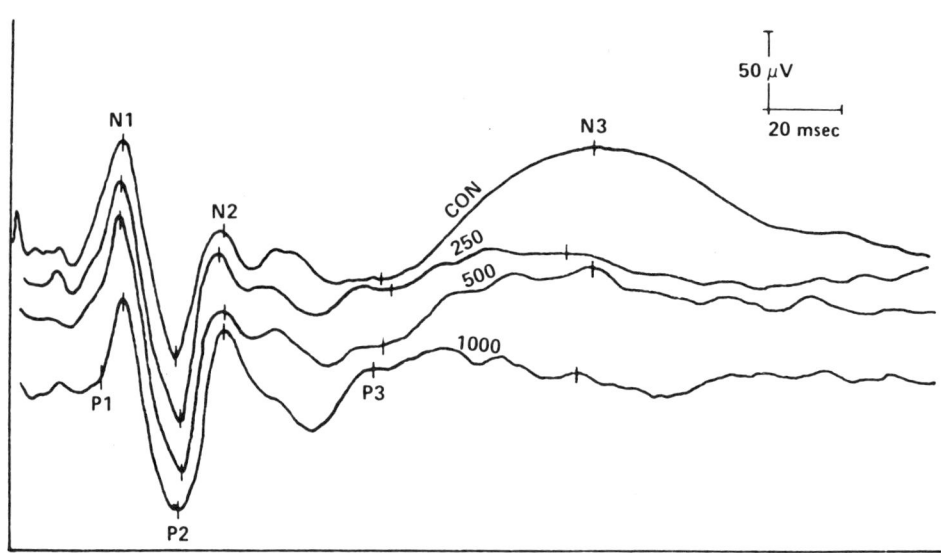

**FIGURE 3.** Flash evoked potential waveforms averaged across groups of rats that received either corn oil (CON); 250, 500, or 1000 mg/kg toluene p.o. The amplitude of the peak labeled N3 was depressed by toluene. Reproduced from Dyer *et al.* (1988).

to neurotoxic compounds (Dyer, 1986) and are good indicators of damage to the primary visual system.

Recently, the late latency components of flash evoked potentials have generated interest due to results showing that solvents, including toluene and xylene, produced a relatively selective depression of a large negative wave occurring at a latency of approximately 160 msec, as illustrated in Figure 3 (Dyer *et al.*, 1988). This peak, labeled N3, or more recently N160, represents the first cycle of the repetitive photic afterdischarge. This FEP peak has been linked to neural activity in thalamocortical loops, and has been correlated with levels of behavioral arousal and habituation. Peak amplitude grows with repeated testing (Figure 4), and the asymptotic amplitude is a function of flash intensity relative to background illumination (Herr *et al.*, 1991). These results suggest that the amplitude of this peak reflects a sensitization-like process to the flash stimulus that increases with repeated testing.

### 2.2.2. Pattern Evoked Potentials

Another class of VEPs, which can be collectively called pattern VEPs, are elicited by visually patterned stimuli. Typical pattern-reversal VEP waveforms, also known as pattern-reversal evoked potentials (PREPs) are presented in Figure 2, along with flash VEPs recorded from the same rats. The pattern-reversal VEPs occur later in time (i.e., have a longer latency), have a positive as opposed to a negative initial major component, and have a different overall structure than do flash VEPs. Flash VEPs and pattern VEPs reflect different aspects of visual function. Procedures have been developed for recording pattern VEPs in rats (Boyes and Dyer, 1983a; Onofrj *et al.*, 1982), and the effects of several stimulus manipulations have been investigated (Boyes and Dyer, 1983a; Harnois *et al.*, 1984).

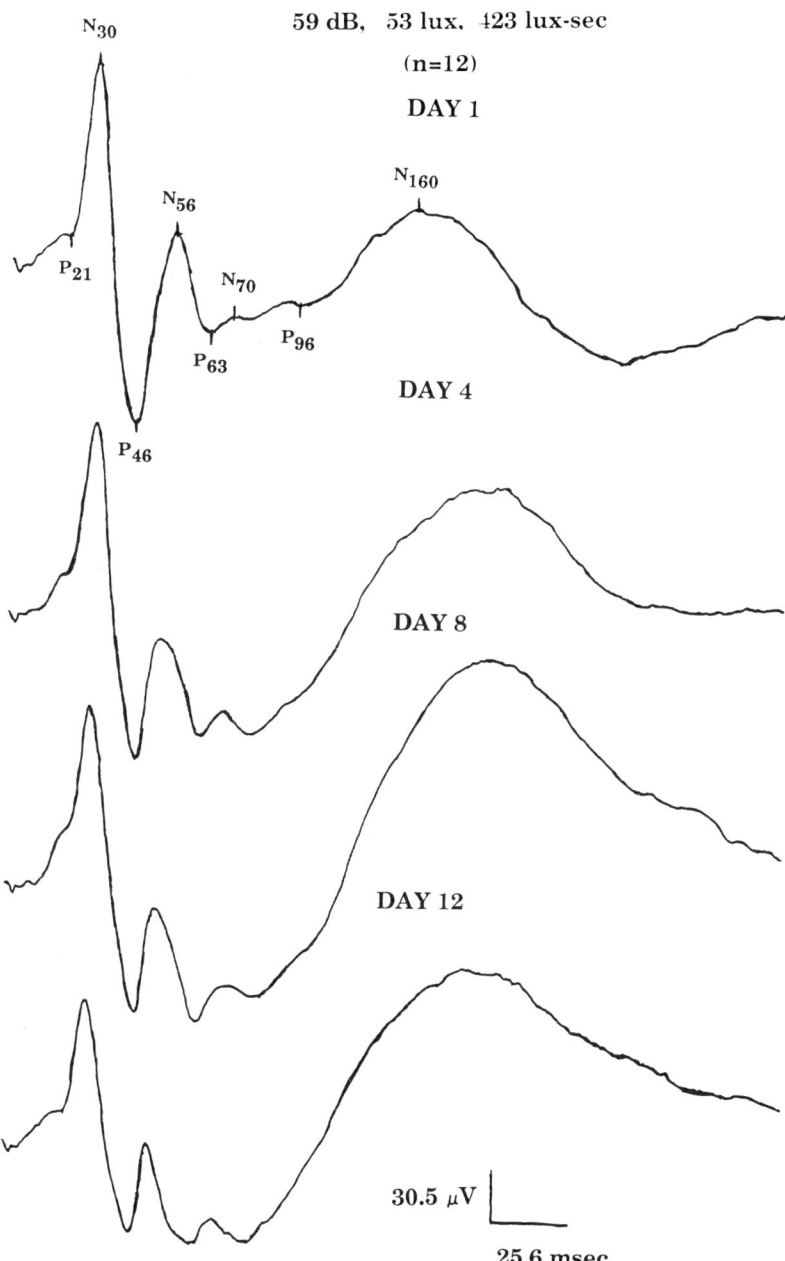

**FIGURE 4.** Flash evoked potential waveforms averaged across a group of 12 rats that were tested daily for 12 days. The amplitude of the peak labeled $N_{160}$ increased with repeated testing. Reproduced from Herr *et al.* (1991).

A variety of stimuli can be used to elicit pattern evoked potentials, including a black and white pattern such as a checkerboard, vertical or horizontal stripes, or sinusoidal gratings in which the spatial luminance profile of the stimulus forms a sinewave. In the case of a sinewave grating, the size of the pattern can be referred to as its spatial frequency and is traditionally expressed as cycles of the stimulus per degree visual angle (cpd). In addition to spatial frequency, another important parameter is contrast, which is defined as the difference in luminance between the bright and dark parts of the stimulus pattern, adjusted for the mean level.

Sinewave gratings stimuli are of interest because different spatial frequencies can be used to selectively elicit activity in subsets of visual neurons based on their receptive field sizes (Campbell, 1980; Campbell and Robson, 1968; Enroth-Cugell and Robson, 1966). The receptive fields of retinal ganglion cells vary over quite a range of sizes, and the size of the receptive field determines the size of the visual pattern to which a particular cell responds (Robson, 1975). Cells with large receptive fields respond preferentially to large patterns, and those with small receptive fields respond preferentially to small patterns. The size of retinal ganglion cell receptive fields is positively correlated with the size of the cell bodies, and also with the diameter of axons leaving the eye to form the optic nerve (Hale *et al.*, 1979). In turn, the diameter of incoming axons to the lateral geniculate nucleus, and then the visual cortex, correlates with the size of the recipient cells (Hale *et al.*, 1979). By stimulating with patterns of different spatial frequency, subpopulations of different-sized visual neurons can be selectively tested (Regan, 1982). This may be important, since cell diameter is thought to be a factor in determining the vulnerability of neurons to toxic substances (Cavanagh, 1973, 1982). Contrast is encoded neurally as the firing rate of visual cells (Enroth-Cugel and Robson, 1966), which is a major factor determining the amplitude of visual evoked potentials (Bobak *et al.*, 1988; Campbell and Maffei, 1970; Campbell and Kulikowski, 1972). Thus, spatial frequency and contrast, the critical parameters governing pattern perception, can be studied through the amplitude of evoked responses to stimuli of different pattern sizes and contrasts.

When measuring pattern VEPs, proper retinal imaging is required. For testing laboratory animals such as cats, dogs, or nonhuman primates, it is necessary to assure fixation and accommodation of the stimulus, either through behavioral training or through pharmacological immobilization and optical refraction. Fortunately, these elaborate measures are not necessary when testing rats because the rat eye is afoveal, has a large visual field, and a great focal depth of field (Hughes, 1977). Consequently, as long as the stimulus is in the rat's visual field, the visual stimulus will be adequately imaged on the retina. This can be achieved by simply restraining awake rats in a cloth harness and placing them in front of the visual display. This simple procedure allows recording of reliable pattern-VEP waveforms (Boyes and Dyer, 1983a).

In addition to the spatial structure of patterned stimuli, it is important to consider their temporal characteristics. There are also many options regarding the fashion in which the patterns are modulated over time in order to elicit evoked responses. Classically, for a stimulus condition referred to as pattern reversal, the position of the dark and light portions of the stimulus are alternated over time, while the stimulus overall maintains a constant space-averaged luminance. Alternatively, the patterned stimulus can be alternated with a blank field of the same mean luminance as the pattern, a condition referred to as *pattern appearance/disappearance* or *on/off modulation*. This can be useful for examining separately potentials generated by stimulus onset and offset, which occur simultaneously in pattern reversal (Hudnell *et al.*, 1990a). The stimulus transitions can be abrupt and regular, in which case they may be said to follow a temporal square wave, or they may be gradual and follow another function, most commonly that of a sine wave. More complex stimuli may be generated regarding both their spatial and temporal characteristics, but the use of such manipulations in toxicological applications remains relatively underdeveloped.

Steady-state procedures should be mentioned, along with the other temporal manipulations of stimuli. These procedures have often been used in conjunction with patterned stimuli, even though they can be used with other stimuli, including flashes, and somatosensory and auditory stimuli. For steady-state evoked potentials, the stimuli are modulated at a temporal rate that is fast enough, generally at least 3 Hz, that the responses to each individual evoked potential can no longer be distinguished (Fig. 5). Instead the elicited brain-wave pattern begins to take on a quasi-sinusoidal shape in which the primary response frequency is determined by the stimulus rate or its harmonics (see review by

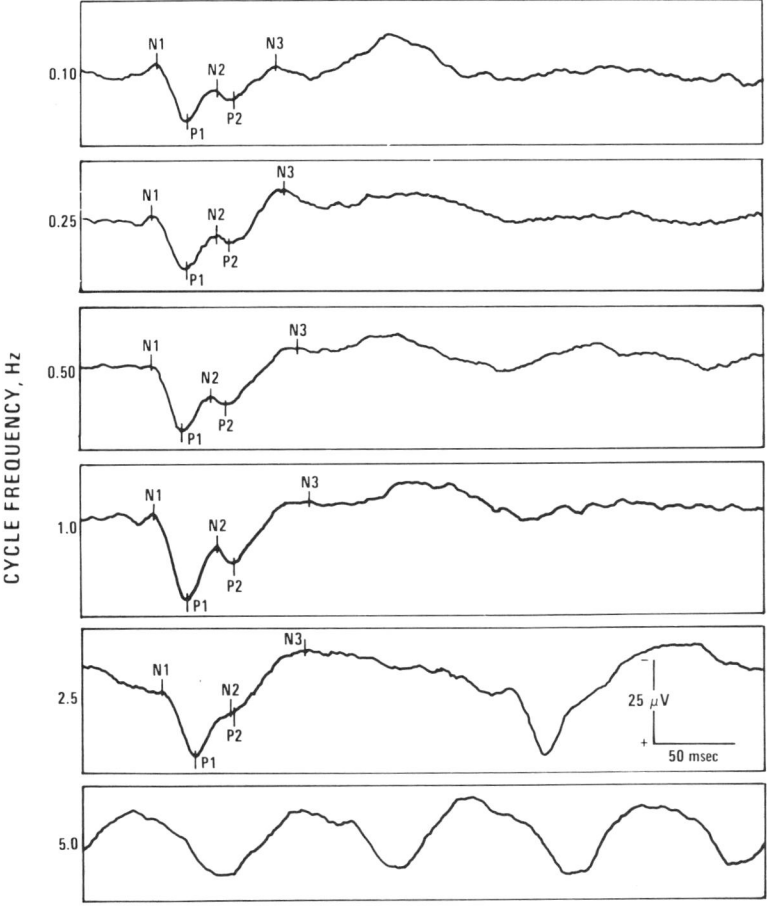

**FIGURE 5.** Pattern reversal evoked potentials averaged across nine pigmented (hooded) rats. As the stimulation frequency was increased from 2.5 to 5 Hz, the responses to individual pattern shifts were lost, and the waveform became "steady state" in character. Reproduced from Boyes and Dyer (1983a).

Regan, 1989). The results are interpretable in terms of the amount of activity in the visual cortex, which is temporally linked to the stimulus. This has both theoretical and practical advantages. Theoretically, it may be possible to link evoked potential results to what is known about single visual neurons that may respond preferentially at the stimulus rate or harmonics. Practically, the steady-state waveforms are suitable for spectral analysis using objective routines, which can eliminate the need for operator scoring of waveforms. Also, fast stimulation rates cannot be used with transient techniques, and some neurotoxicants may reduce the rate at which neurons can repetitively discharge.

Depending on how they are recorded, evoked potentials can reflect the activity of the entire sensory pathways from the receptors to the central projection areas or restricted portions of these systems. Thus, evoked potential information can be used in localization studies and in differential diagnosis (Don, 1986; Oken and Chiappa, 1986; Sherman, 1986). In the auditory and somatosensory systems, volume conducted potentials can be recorded that reflect activity along the successive stages of the ascending sensory pathways (Jewett, 1970; Wiederholt and Iragui-Madoz, 1977). In the visual system, visual evoked potential changes might be complemented with electroretinography in order to determine if the measured changes were due to lesions in the eye or brain. Additional electrophysiological procedures are available for more detailed investigation of results from sensory evoked potential or other neurotoxicological investigations (Aminoff, 1980; Fox *et al.*, 1982; Lowndes, 1987).

Through proper selection of sensory stimuli, it is possible to selectively test functional subdivisions of sensory systems (Bodis-Wollner *et al.*, 1986; Zemon *et al.*, 1986). Functional subdivisions of the visual system may be characterized by their spatial, temporal, and/or contrast response profiles. By measuring contrast sensitivity in certain neurological patients, it has been shown that visual deficits appear that were not found on more routine tests of visual function (Bodis-Wollner, 1972). Similarly, measuring contrast sensitivity functions can reveal neurotoxic lesions not apparent in other visual tests. Contrast sensitivity functions can be measured using either behavioral or VEP techniques. Evoked potential measures can correlate well with other measures of sensory function (Regan, 1989; Silveira *et al.*, 1987). In laboratory animals, the existing behavioral techniques require extensive training to perform stimulus discriminations (Evans, 1982; Moody and Stebbins, 1982). Evoked potential technology can yield a substantial time saving because lengthy training sessions are not required, as is the case for many of the behavioral procedures for measuring sensory function in animals.

## 3. STRAIN AND SPECIES CONSIDERATIONS

While a considerable amount of toxicity testing is performed using albino strains, albinism itself unfortunately produces aberrant nervous systems in general, and sensory systems in particular (Creel, 1984). Pigmentation in the retina and the cochlea is essential for normal visual and auditory function, respectively. The common misconception that rats are blind may be related to the widespread use of albino rats, who, like other albinos, have poor visual function. Pigmented rats, in comparison, have a relatively well-developed visual system. In addition to the lack of a pigmented retina, albinos have an abnormally large proportion of contralaterally projecting retinal ganglion cells (Creel and Giolli, 1972; Lund, 1965). Visually evoked potentials from albino animals differ from pigmented strains (Creel *et al.*, 1970; Dyer and Swartzwelder, 1978), and pattern-elicited

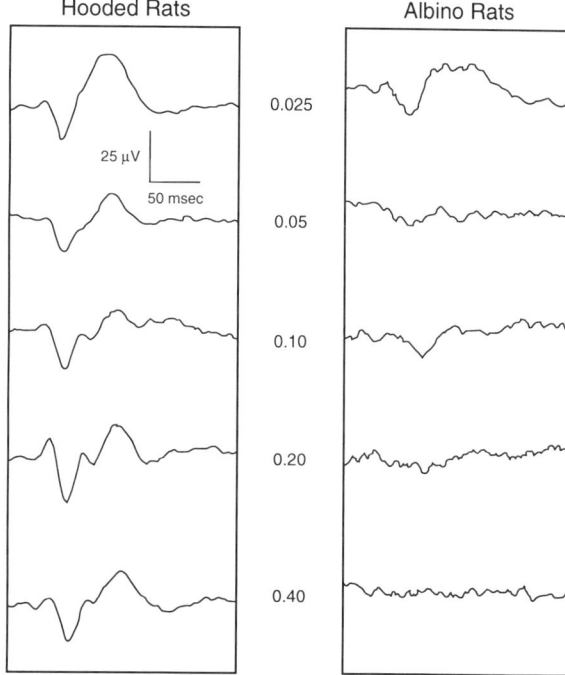

FIGURE 6. Pattern-reversal evoked potentials averaged across groups of Long Evans (pigmented or hooded) or Sprague Dawley (albino) rats when stimulated with patterns of size ranging from large to small (top to bottom). The albino rats had inferior responses, particularly at the smaller bar sizes. Reproduced from Boyes and Dyer (1983a).

visual evoked potentials are particularly poor in albinos (Figure 6; Boyes and Dyer, 1983a). In addition to the sensory systems, albino strains also differ from pigmented animals in biochemical, physiological, pharmacological, pathological, and developmental parameters (reviewed by Creel, 1980, 1984; Creel et al., 1970; Prieur, 1982). The use of albino animal models is generally considered unacceptable in visual neuroscience unless one is specifically studying albinism and should likewise be unacceptable in testing visual toxicity (Heywood and Gopinath, 1990). Toxicological data based on albino animals may be of limited value in predicting the response of normally pigmented humans to toxicant exposure.

One issue critical to the successful use of VEPs in laboratory animals as indicators of potential toxicity in humans regards the fidelity with which results in rat predict those in humans. Rats are capable of photopic vision, but they possess only one type of cone photoreceptor. Therefore, they cannot distinguish colors, a task that is dependent on the relative activity in three types of cones with different spectral sensitivities. This means that if a compound were to have effects on color vision, such as has been reported for solvents (Mergler et al., 1987), this phenomena could not be studied in rats. However, rats do discriminate visual patterns, and the extent to which pattern vision is similar in rats and humans is something that can be examined experimentally. One strategy to do so involves using parallel procedures in laboratory animals and humans. Relationships from such studies could help in predicting human health problems from animal data (Hudnell et al., 1990b; Hudnell and Boyes, 1991).

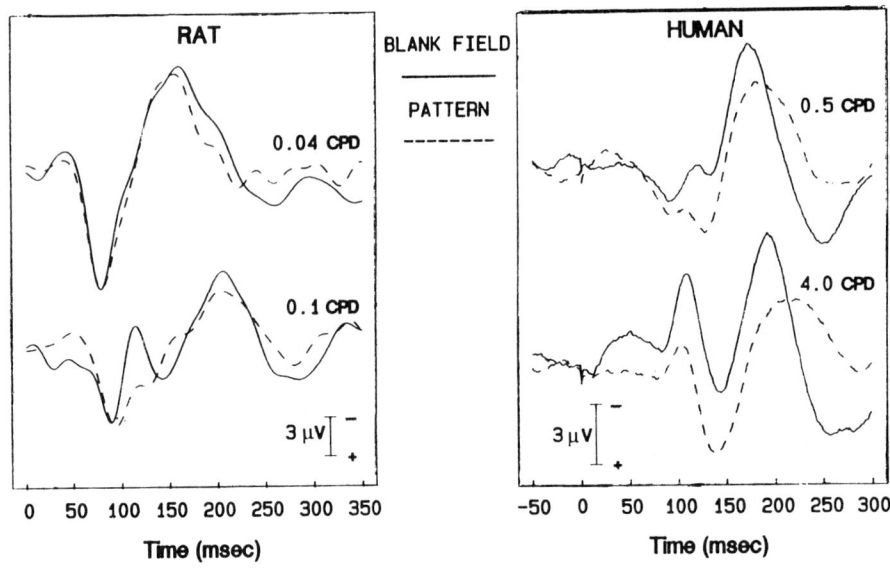

**FIGURE 7.** Pattern-onset evoked potentials, averaged across groups of rats or humans, which were recorded after 1 min of adaptation to either a blank screen or a stationary pattern of the same spatial frequency as the test stimulus. Pattern adaptation significantly attenuated the amplitude of a negative component occurring at about 110 msec in both species, but only at the higher spatial frequencies tested. Reproduced from Hudnell *et al.* (1990).

Hudnell *et al.* (1990b) have begun to establish the relationships between rat and human visual evoked potential measurements (Fig. 7). Both transient and steady-state pattern VEPs have a close correspondence in rats and humans (Hudnell *et al.*, 1990b; Hudnell and Boyes, 1991). A mathematical model that was derived to relate rat and human data showed a linear relationship between the VEP amplitudes as a function of stimulus spatial frequency (Benignus *et al.*, 1991). This linear relationship, which was a result of being able to fit the same mathematical function to the data from both species, suggests that there are substantial physiological parallels between the two species regarding the neural encoding of spatially patterned information. It follows that extrapolations from rat visual function data may be useful to predict human visual problems.

## 4. OVERVIEW OF COMPOUNDS TESTED

For VEPs to be considered as acceptable techniques for measuring toxic damage to the visual system, the data should demonstrate that they are sensitive to disruption of the visual pathways. To a large extent these data exist in the clinical literature showing that VEPs are altered in neurological disorders of the visual system (Halliday *et al.*, 1972; Regan, 1989). It is also important to show that exposure to toxic substances that disrupt vision also alter VEPs. Changes in sensory evoked potentials have been reported to antedate abnormalities of nerve conduction and behavioral signs of intoxication (Arezzo *et al.*, 1981) and to occur in the absence of related lesions detectable by neuropathological

**TABLE 2.** Effects of Neurotoxic Compounds of Visual Evoked Potentials After Acute Exposure

| Compound | Species | VEP | Lat | Amp | Reference |
|---|---|---|---|---|---|
| Metals | | | | | |
|   Tributyltin | r | f,p | n | n | U.S. EPA, unpublished |
|   Triethyltin | r | f,p | y | y | Boyes and Dyer (1983); Dyer and Howell (1982a,b) |
|   Trimethyltin | r | f | y | y | Dyer (1982); Dyer et al. (1982) |
|   Triphenyltin | r | f | n | n | U.S. EPA, unpublished |
| Solvents | | | | | |
|   Carbon disulfide | r,ra | f,p | y | y | Rudnev (1978); EPA, unpublished |
|   Ethanol | r,ra,h | f,p | y | y | * |
|   Sulfolane | r | f,p | y | y | Dyer et al. (1986) |
|   Toluene | r,h | f | y | y | Dyer et al. (1988) |
|   Xylene | r,h | f,p | y | y | Dyer et al. (1988); Seppalainen et al. (1981) |
| Pesticides | | | | | |
|   Amitraz | r | f,p | y | y | Boyes et al. 1987 |
|   Carbamates | r,c | f,p | na | y | Boyes and Hudnell (1988); Harding et al. (1983) |
|   Chlordimeform | r | f,p | y | y | Boyes and Dyer (1984); Boyes et al. (1985a,b,c) Boyes and Moser (1988) |
|   Deltamethrin | r | f | y | y | Dyer (1985) |
|   DFP | c | p | na | y | Harding et al. (1985) |
|   Dieldrin | c | f | na | y | Joy (1973) |
|   Paraoxon | r | p | na | y | U.S. EPA, unpublished |
|   Parathion | r,p | f | y | y | Woolley (1977); Woolley and Reiter (1978) |
|   Permethrin | r | f,p | n | y | U.S. EPA, unpublished |
|   Triadimefon | r | f,p | n | y | U.S. EPA, unpublished |
| Industrials | | | | | |
|   2-4-dithiobiuret | r | f,p | n | y | Crofton et al. 1991 |
|   Formaldehyde | ra | f | n | y | Rudnev et al. (1978) |
|   Phenylenediamine | r | f,p | n | n | U.S. EPA, unpublished |
|   2-methyl pyridine | r | f,p | y | n | Dyer et al. (1985) |
|   3-methyl pyridine | r | f,p | y | n | Dyer et al. (1985) |
|   4-methyl pyridine | r | f,p | n | n | Dyer et al. (1985) |
|   Pyridine | r | f,p | y | n | U.S. EPA, unpublished |
|   Styrene | r | f,p | y | y | U.S. EPA, unpublished |
| Anesthetics | | | | | |
|   Chloral hydrate | r | f | y | y | Hetzler et al. (1984) |
|   Chloralose | r | f | n | y | U.S. EPA, unpublished |
|   Chloropent | r | f | y | y | Dyer et al. (1983) |
|   Ketamine | r | f | y | y | Rigdon and Dyer (1988) |
|   Lidocaine | r | f,p | n | n | U.S. EPA, unpublished |
|   Pentobarbital | r | f,p | y | y | Creel et al. (1974); Hetzler et al. (1982); Hetzler and Norris (1988) |
|   Urethane | r | f | n | y | Dyer et al. (1987) |
| Gases | | | | | |
|   Carbon dioxide | r | f | y | y | Rebert (1987) |
|   Carbon monoxide | r,h | f | y | y | ** |
|   Hypoxic hypoxia | r | f | y | y | Dyer and Annau (1975); Rebert (1987) |
|   Ozone | r,ra | f | y | y | Berney et al. (1976); Rudnev et al. (1978) |

Species code: r = rat; ra = rabbit; c = cat; p = nonhuman primate; h = human.
VEP Code: f = flash VEP; p = pattern VEP.
Latency/amplitude code: y = yes; n = no; na = not available.
*Ethanol references: Begleiter et al. (1972); Blagova et al. (1982); Erwin and Linnoila (1981); Erwin et al. (1986); Furster et al. (1982); Goldberg et al. (1974); Hetzler et al. (1981, 1982); Lewis et al. (1970); Orbitz et al. (1977); Nakai et al. (1973); Rhodes et al. (1975); Rosadini et al. (1974); Seppalainen (1988); Simpson (1981); Zuzewicz (1981).
**References for carbon monoxide: Dyer and Annau (1975, 1977); Hosko (1970); Otto et al. (1978).
Adapted from Boyes and Dyer (1988).

examinations, which included light microscopy, perfusion fixation, and special stains (Mattsson *et al.*, 1988, 1990b).

A variety of compounds has been tested for effects on VEPs following acute or repeated exposure. The results of studies that have examined the acute effects of potentially neurotoxic compounds on VEPs are summarized in Table 2. The table indicates the compounds tested, the species used, the type of VEP used, whether effects were found on peak latencies or amplitudes, and the reference for the work. If both flash and pattern VEPs were employed, then a positive effect on either was scored as positive. In some cases multiple studies have been conducted on a single agent. Occasionally, these studies reported conflicting results, and some judgment was necessary in order to list the presence or absence of effects. Some studies reported only effects on latency or amplitude without regard to the other parameter. The compounds were grouped into six general categories: metals, solvents, pesticides, industrial compounds, anesthetics, and gases. It should be recognized that these categories, while convenient, are neither mutually exclusive nor logically consistent (e.g., some anesthetics are gases).

## 4.1. Metals

Among the metals, several (e.g., lead, methylmercury) have been tested for chronic or developmental exposure. However, the ones examined for acute effects were primarily organotin compounds. The organotins form an interesting structure-activity comparison. Trimethyltin is a potent cell body toxicant that kills hippocampal pyramidal cells and a variety of neurons in other areas, including the retina (Chang and Dyer, 1983). Triethyltin has a completely different spectrum of neurotoxic actions, damaging myelin but leaving cell bodies relatively intact. Tributyltin and triphenyltin are not known to be selectively neurotoxic to the adult organism.

## 4.2. Solvents

The solvents, as a group, can be expected to be neurotoxic. A number of different solvents have been tested, including some with substantial industrial usage: carbon disulfide, sulfolane, toluene, and xylene.

## 4.3. Pesticides

Pesticides, in particular insecticides, are designed to attack a variety of nervous system targets, depending on the class to which a compound belongs. Many of the major classes of pesticides are represented among the tested compounds, including the organophosphates, DFP, paraoxon and parathion; an organochlorine, dieldrin; the pyrethroids, deltamethrin and permethrin; the formamidines, amitraz and chlordimeform; a triazine fungicide triadimefon; and carbamates. The carbamates represented, physostigmine and neostigmine, are not actually used as pesticides, but are chemically members of the carbamates, and have anticholinesterase properties that should be characteristic of the class.

### 4.4. Industrial Compounds

The industrial compounds listed represent a heterogeneous group that have little in common regarding their potential neurotoxicity. The methyl pyridines reflect another small example of structure-activity relationships, with 2- and 3-methylpyridine being more active on VEPs than 4-methylpyridine. 2-4-Dithiobiuret was previously known to disrupt peripheral motor function, but its sensory effects were unknown (Crofton *et al.*, 1991).

### 4.5. Anesthetics

The anesthetic agents also reflect several different categories of compounds: the barbiturate, pentobarbital; Chloropent®, a mixture of a barbiturate and chloral hydrate; chloral hydrate and chloralose; a local anesthetic, lidocaine; a dissociative anesthetic, ketamine; and an agent with a poorly understood mechanism of anesthetic action, urethane (ethyl carbamate). While these agents as normally used may not be neurotoxicants, the anesthetics by definition produce acute CNS functional changes. In addition, the mechanism by which anesthetics act is relevant to the characterization of how industrial solvents may act.

### 4.6. Gases

The gases include carbon monoxide, which acts primarily through the formation of carboxyhemoglobin, thus lowering brain oxygenation. Carbon dioxide, and the irritant, ozone, have also been investigated. Finally, hypoxic hypoxia is also included, even though it is not a gas, because the effects maybe expected to resemble those of asphyxiant gases.

The general finding of Table 2 is that most of the compounds tested produced changes in VEPs. Compounds from each of the categories produced changes in VEPs. While some compounds altered both latencies and amplitudes, others effected only one or the other parameter. Only tributyltin, triphenyltin, phenylenediamine, 4-methyl pyridine, and lidocaine were completely negative. None of these compounds are known to be neurotoxic following acute treatment to adult animals. Since negative data are seldom published, more data may exist on compounds that do not effect VEPs, but these data were unavailable for the current review.

In some cases the effects of the administered compounds were similar in flash and pattern VEPs. In other cases, however, the results were not comparable. It is of considerable interest that some compounds can change flash or pattern VEP amplitudes without altering the other potential. The effects of the two formamidine insecticides, chlordimeform and amitraz, are dramatic examples of differential actions (Boyes and Dyer, 1984; Boyes and Moser, 1987). As shown in Figure 8, chlordimeform produced a severalfold increase in pattern VEP amplitude without changing the amplitude of flash VEPs recorded in the same animals. Although flash VEP latencies were increased by chlordimeform, this was found subsequently to be an indirect consequence of reduced body temperature (Boyes *et al.*, 1985c), which prolongs evoked potential amplitudes (Hetzler *et*

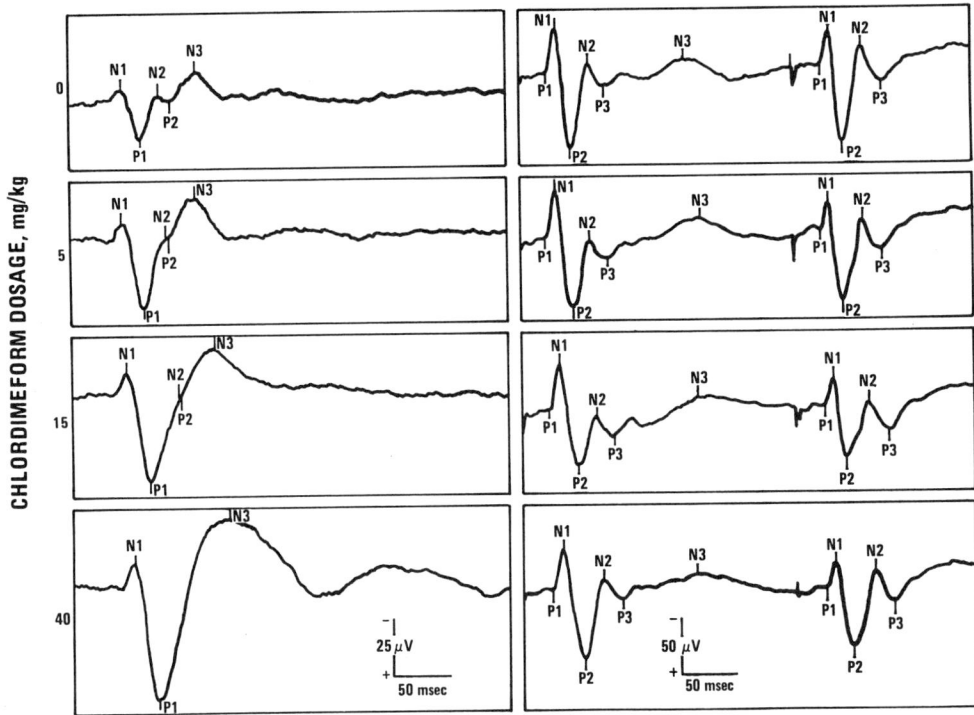

**FIGURE 8.** Pattern-reversal (left) and flash VEPs to paired stimuli (right) recorded approximately 30 min following an i.p. injection of vehicle or various doses of the formamidine insecticide/acaricide chlordimeform HC1. Pattern-reversal VEPs were increased in amplitude following treatment, but flash VEP amplitudes recorded from the same rats were unaffected. Reproduced from Boyes and Dyer (1984).

*al.*, 1988). The large effects of chlordimeform on pattern VEPs were found to be related to actions as an $\alpha_2$-adrenergic agonist (Boyes and Moser, 1988), and not to inhibition of monamine oxidase, which was once thought to be the mechanism of action for formamidine toxicity (Boyes *et al.*, 1985b). Further research demonstrated that the differing effects on pattern and flash-elicited responses was attributable to contrast-dependent actions, since the contrast was strong in the pattern-reversal stimulus, but is absent from strobe-flash stimuli (Boyes *et al.*, 1985a). A number of compounds have produced effects on flash VEPs without altering pattern VEPs. Examples of such compounds include toluene, xylene, and 2,4-dithiobiuret (Crofton *et al.*, 1991). These results illustrate that different evoked potentials reflect qualitatively different aspects of visual function that can be selectively altered by exposure to neurotoxic compounds.

## 5. CONCLUSIONS

The data show that there is a need to test compounds for potential toxic effects on sensory function, particularly vision. A substantial proportion of compounds for which toxicity data exist has produced adverse consequences on visual function. The types of deficits produced vary widely and can occur from either systemic exposure or through direct contact with the eyes. A survey of the types of visual effects reported in the literature revealed that reports of changes in visual function are likely to come from human exposures, whereas animal studies occasionally report frank blindness, but are more likely to report only observable lesions of the eyes. This finding suggests that the procedures typically used in animal toxicity testing do not provide information regarding changes in visual function, but that such changes often occur following chemical exposure.

To summarize, visual evoked potential technology can be used to obtain objective measures of the function of the visual system in laboratory animals as well as in humans. Responses recorded from laboratory animals may have properties similar to those of humans, even if they may differ in regard to some specific parameters. There are different types of visual evoked potentials, which reflect different aspects of visual function and which can be differentially sensitive to neurotoxic or neuroactive compounds. Finally, a variety of compounds, if neurotoxic or neuroactive, can produce detectable changes in visual evoked potentials.

These data demonstrate that visual evoked potentials can be useful in examining the potential of chemical compounds to alter visual function. This information can then be useful in the process of assessing and regulating exposure risks.

ACKNOWLEDGMENTS. M. Gage provided the data for Table 1. The author thanks H. K. Hudnell, D. W. Herr, and D. A. Otto for reviewing a previous version of the manuscript.

## REFERENCES

Albee, R.R., and Mattsson, J.L., 1983, Visual evoked potential testing method for neonatal rats, *Neurobehav. Toxicol. Teratol.* 5:497–501.
Aminoff, M.J. (ed.), 1980, *Electrodiagnosis in Clinical Neurology,* Churchill Livingstone, New York.
Anger, W.K., and Johnson, B.L., 1985, Chemicals affecting behavior, in: *Neurotoxicity of Industrial and Commercial Chemicals* (J.L. O'Donoghue, ed.), CRC Press, Boca Raton, FL, pp. 421–429.
Arezzo, J.C., Schaumburg, H.H., Vaughan, H.G., Spencer, S.P., and Barna, J., 1981, Hind limb somatosensory evoked potentials in the monkey: The effects of distal axonopathy, *Ann. Neurol.* 12:24–32.
Arezzo, J.C., Simson, R., and Brennan, N.E., 1985, Evoked potentials in the assessment of neurotoxicology in humans, *Neurobehav. Toxicol. Teratol.* 7:299–304.
Begleiter, H., Branchey, M.H., and Kissin, B., 1972, Effects of ethanol on evoked potentials in the rat, *Behavior. Biol.* 7:137–142.
Benignus, V.A., Boyes, W.K., and Hudnell, H.K., 1991, Quantitative methods in animal-to-human extrapolations, *Neurosci. Biobehav. Rev.* 15:165–171.
Berney, B., Dyer, R.S., and Annau, S., 1976, Ozone and visual evoked potentials in rats, *Soc. Neurosci. Abstr.* 2:1048.
Blagova, O.E., Budantsev, A.Y., Sytinsk, I.A., and Lajtha, A., 1982, Changes of neurochemical and electrophysiological indices of rat brain under ethanol intoxication, *Neurochem. Res.* 7:1335–1345.
Bobak, P., Bodis-Wollner, I., and Marx, M.S., 1988, Cortical contrast gain control in human spatial vision, *J. Physiol.* 405:421–437.
Bodis-Wollner, I., 1972, Visual acuity and contrast sensitivity in patients with cerebral lesions, *Science* 178:769–771.
Bodis-Wollner, I., Ghilardi, M.F., and Mylin, L.H., 1986, The importance of stimulus selection in VEP practice: The clinical relevance of visual physiology, in *Evoked Potentials* (R.Q. Cracco and I. Bodis-Wollner, eds.), Alan R. Liss, New York, pp. 15–27.
Boyes, W.K., and Dyer, R.S., 1983a, Pattern reversal visual evoked potentials in awake rats, *Brain Res. Bull.* 10:817–823.
Boyes, W.K., and Dyer, R.S., 1983b, Pattern reversal and flash evoked potentials following acute triethyltin exposure, *Neurobehav. Toxicol. Teratol.* 5:571–577.
Boyes, W.K., and Dyer, R.S., 1984, Chlordimeform produces profound, selective and transient changes in visual evoked potentials of hooded rats, *Exp. Neurol.* 86:434–447.
Boyes, W.K., and Dyer, R.S., 1988, Visual evoked potentials as indicators of neurotoxicity. Office of Research and Development, United States Environmental Protection Agency, Deliverable 2312A. Document number HERL0653.
Boyes, W.K., and Hudnell, H.K., 1988, Effects of acetylcholinesterase inhibition on spatial vision in rats, *Toxicologist* 8:226.
Boyes, W.K., and Moser, V.C., 1987, Investigations of amitraz neurotoxicity in rats. II. Effects on visual evoked potentials, *Fundam. Appl. Toxicol.* 9:140–153.

Boyes, W.K., and Moser, V.C., 1988, An $\alpha_2$-adrenergic mode of action of chlordimeform on rat visual function, *Toxicol. Appl. Pharmacol.* 92:402–418.

Boyes, W.K., Jenkins, D.E., and Dyer, R.S., 1985a, Chlordimeform produces contrast-dependent changes in visual evoked potentials of hooded rats, *Exp. Neurol.* 89:434–449.

Boyes, W.K., Moser, V.C., MacPhail, R.C., and Dyer, R.S., 1985b, Monoamine oxidase inhibition cannot account for visual evoked potential changes produced by chlordimeform, *Neuropharmacology* 24:853–860.

Boyes, W.K., Padilla, S., and Dyer, R.S., 1985c, Body temperature-dependent and independent actions of chlordimeform on rat visual evoked potentials and optic nerve axonal transport, *Neuropharmacology* 24:743–749.

Bron, A.J., 1979, Mechanisms of ocular toxicity, in: *Drug Toxicity* (J.W. Gorrod, ed.), Taylor and Francis, London, pp. 229–253.

Bushnell, P.J., Bowman, R.E. Allen, J.R., and Marlar, R.J. 1977, Scotopic vision deficits in young monkeys exposed to lead, *Science* 196:333–335.

Campbell, F.W., 1980, The physics of visual perception, *Phil. Trans. R. Soc. Lond.* B 290:5–9.

Campbell, F.W., and Kulikowski, J.J., 1972, The visual evoked potential as a function of contrast of a grating, *J. Physiol.* 222:345–356.

Campbell, F.W., and Maffei, L., 1970, Electrophysiological evidence for the existence of orientation and size detectors in the human visual system, *J. Physiol.* 207:635–652.

Campbell, F., and Robson, J., 1968, Application of Fourier analysis to the visibility of gratings, *J. Physiol.* 197:551–566.

Cavanagh, J.B., 1973, Peripheral neuropathy caused by chemical agents, *CRC Crit. Rev. Toxicol.* 2:365–417.

Cavanagh, J.B., 1982, The pattern of recovery of axons in the nervous system of rats following 2,5-hexanediol intoxication: A question of rheology? *Neuropathol. Appl. Neurobiol.* 8:19–34.

Chan, P.K., and Hayes, H.W., 1985, Assessment of chemically induced ocular toxicity: A survey of methods, in: *Target Organ Toxicology Series: Toxicology of the Eye, Ear, and Other Special Senses* (W. Hayes, ed.), Raven Press, New York, pp. 103–143.

Chang, L.W., and Dyer, R.S., 1983, Trimethyltin induced pathology in sensory neurons, *Neurobehav. Toxicol. Teratol.* 5:337–350.

Creel, D., 1980, Inappropriate use of albino animals in research, *Pharmacol. Biochem. Behav.* 12:969–977.

Creel, D.J., 1984, Albinism and evoked potentials: Factors in the selection of infrahuman models in predicting the human response to neurotoxic agents, *Neurobehav. Toxicol. Teratol.* 6:447–453.

Creel, D.J., and Giolli, R.A., 1972, Retinogeniculostriate projections in guinea pigs: Albino and pigmented strains compared, *Exp. Neurol.* 36:411–425.

Creel, D., Dustman, R.E., and Beck, E.C., 1970, Differences in visually evoked responses in albino versus hooded rats, *Exp. Neurol.* 29:298–309.

Creel, D.J., Shearer, D., and Wilson, C.E., 1974, Effects of increasing dose levels of pentobarbital on visually evoked responses of albino and pigmented rats, *J. Life Sci.* 4:85–92.

Crofton, K.M., and Sheets, L.P., 1989, Evaluation of sensory function using reflex modification of the startle response, *J. Am. Coll. Toxicol.* 8:199–211.

Crofton, K.M., Dean, K.F., Hamrick, R.C., and Boyes, W.K., 1991, The effects of 2,4-dithiobiuret on sensory and motor function, *Fundam. Appl. Toxicol.* 16:469–481.

Don, M., 1986, Value of ABR and cochlear potentials in differentiating cochlear from auditory nerve pathology, in: *Evoked Potentials* (R.Q. Cracco, and I. Bodis-Wollner, eds.), Alan R. Liss, New York, pp. 366–372.

Dyer, R.S., 1982, Physiological methods for assessment of trimethyltin exposure, *Neurobehav. Toxicol. Teratol.* 4:659–664.

Dyer, R.S., 1983, In vitro approaches to neurotoxicity—A physiologist's perspective, in: *In Vitro Toxicity Testing of Environmental Agents*, Part A (R. Kolber, T.K. Wong, L.D. Grant, R.S. DeWoskin, and T. J. Hughes, eds.), Plenum, New York, pp. 487–497.

Dyer, R.S., 1985, The use of sensory evoked potentials in toxicology, *Fundam. Appl. Toxicol.* 5:24–40.

Dyer, R.S., 1986, Interactions of behavior and neurophysiology, in: *Neurobehavioral Toxicology* (Z. Annau, ed.), Johns Hopkins University Press, Baltimore, pp. 193–213.

Dyer, R.S., 1987a, Macrophysiological assessment of organometal neurotoxicity, in: *Neurotoxicants and Neurobiological Function: Effects of Organoheavy Metals* (H.A. Tilson and S.B. Sparber, eds.), John Wiley, New York, pp. 137–184.

Dyer, R.S., 1987b, Somatosensory evoked potentials, in: *Electrophysiology in Neurotoxicology*, Vol. II (H.E. Lowndes, ed.), CRC Press, Boca Raton, FL, pp. 1–69.

Dyer, R.S., 1989, Peak $N_{160}$ of rat flash evoked potential: Does it reflect habituation of sensitization?, *Physiol. Behav.* 45:355–362.

Dyer, R.S., and Annau, Z., 1975, Effects of carbon monoxide and hypoxia on visual evoked potentials in the rat, *Fed. Proc.* 34:1081.

Dyer, R.S., and Annau, S., 1977a, Flash evoked potentials from rat superior colliculus, *Pharmacol. Biochem. Behav.* 6:453–459.

Dyer, R.S., and Annau, Z., 1977b, Carbon monoxide and flash evoked potentials from rat cortex and superior colliculus, *Pharmacol. Biochem. Behav.* 6:461–465.

Dyer, R.S., and Boyes, W.K., 1983a, Hypothermia and chloropent anesthesia differentially affect the flash evoked potentials of hooded rats, *Brain Res. Bull.* 10:825–831.

Dyer, R.S., and Boyes, W.K., 1983b, Use of neurophysiological challenges for the detection of toxicity, *Fed. Proc.* 42:3201–3206.

Dyer, R.S., and Howell, W.E., 1982a, Acute triethyltin exposure: Effects on the visual evoked potential and hippocampal afterdischarge, *Neurobehav. Toxicol. Teratol.* 4:259–266.

Dyer, R.S., and Howell, W.E., 1982b, Triethyltin: Ambient temperature alters visual system toxicity, *Neurobehavior. Toxicol. Teratol.* 4:267–271.

Dyer, R.S., and Rigdon, G.C., 1987, Urethane affects the rat visual system at subanesthetic doses, *Physiol. Behav.* 41:327–330.

Dyer, R.S., and Swartzwelder, H.S., 1978, Sex and strain differences in the visual evoked potentials of albino and hooded rats, *Pharmacol. Biochem. Behav.* 9:301–306.

Dyer, R.S., Howell, W.E., and Wonderlin, W.F., 1982, Visual system dysfunction following acute trimethyltin exposure in rats, *Neurobehav. Toxicol. Teratol.* 4:191–195.

Dyer, R.S., Burdette, L.J., Janssen, R., and Boyes, W.K., 1985, Neurophysiological consequences of acute exposure to methylpyridines, *Fundam. Appl. Toxicol.* 5:920–932.

Dyer, R.S., Boyes, W.K., and Hetzler, B.E., 1986, Acute sulfolane exposure produces temperature-independent and dependent changes in visual evoked potentials, *Neurobehav. Toxicol. Teratol.* 8:687–693.

Dyer, R.S., Bercegeay, M.S., and Mayo, L.M., 1988, Acute exposures to p-xylene and toluene alter visual information processing, *Neurotoxicol. Teratol.* 10:147–153.

Eells, J.T., 1991, Methanol-induced visual toxicity in the rat, *J. Pharmacol. Exp. Therap.* 257:56–63.

Enroth-Cugell, C., and Robson, J.G., 1966, The contrast sensitivity of retinal ganglion cells of the cat, *J. Physiol.* 187:517–552.

Erwin, C.W., and Linnoila, M., 1981, Effect of ethyl alcohol of visual evoked potentials, *Alcoholism: Clin. Exper. Res.* 5:49–55.

Erwin, C., Linnoila, W.M., Hartwell, J., Erwin, A., and Guthrie, S., 1986, Effects of buspirone and diazepam, alone and in combination with alcohol, on skilled performance and evoked potentials, *J. Clin. Pharmacol.* 6:199–209.

Eskin, T.A., and Merigan, W.H., 1986, Selective acrylamide-induced degeneration of color opponent ganglion cells in macaques, *Brain Res.* 378:379–384.

Eskin, T.A., Merigan, W.H., and Woods, R.W., 1988, Carbon disulfide effects on the visual system: II. Retinogeniculate degeneration, *Invest. Ophthal. Vis. Sci.* 29(4):519–527.

Evans, H.L., Laties, V.G., and Weiss, B., 1975, Behavioral effects of mercury and methyl mercury, *Fed. Proc.* 34:1858–1867.

Evans, H.L., 1982, Assessment of vision in behavioral toxicology, in: *Nervous System Toxicology* (C.L. Mitchell, ed.), Raven Press, New York, pp. 81–107.

Food and Drug Administration, 1990, Food and Drug Administration Pesticide Program-Residues in Foods—1989, *J. Assoc. Off. Anal. Chem.* 73:127A–146A.

Fox, D.A., 1984, Psychophysiologically and electrophysiologically determined spatial deficits in developmentally lead-exposed rats have a cholinergic component, in: *Cellular and Molecular Neurotoxicology* (T. Narahashi, ed.), Raven Press, New York, pp. 123–140.

Fox, D.A., and Chu, L.W.F., 1988, Rods are selectively altered by lead: II Ultrastructure and quantitative histology, *Exp. Eye Res.* 46:613–625.

Fox, D.A., and Farber, D.B., 1988, Rods are selectively altered by lead: I. Electrophysiology and biochemistry, *Exp. Eye Res.* 46:597–611.

Fox, D.A., and Sillman, A.J., 1979, Heavy metals affect rod, but not cone, photoreceptors, *Science* 206:78–80.

Fox, D.A., Lewkowski, J.P., and Cooper, G.P., 1977, Acute and chronic effects of neonatal lead exposure on the development of the visual evoked response in rats, *Toxicol. Appl. Pharmacol.* 40:449–461.

Fox, D.A., Lewkowski, J.P., and Cooper, G.P., 1979, Persistent visual cortex excitability alterations produced by neonatal lead exposure, *Neurobehav. Toxicol.* 1:101–106.

Fox, D.A., Lowndes, H.E., and Bierkamper, G.G., 1982, Electrophysiological techniques in neurotoxicology, in: *Nervous System Toxicology* (C.L. Mitchell, ed.), Raven Press, New York, pp. 299–335.

Furster, J.M., Wiley, T.J., Riley, D.M., and Ashford, J.M., 1982, Effects of ethanol on visual evoked responses in monkeys performing a memory task in *Electroencephalog Clin. Neurophysiol.* 53:621–633.

Gad, S.C., (ed.), 1989. Symposium: Screening for Neurotoxicity, Principles and Practices, *J. Am. Coll. Toxicol.* 8:5–239.

Gage, M.I., 1987, A database for computer analysis of reported neurotoxic effects, *Toxicologist* 7:257.

Gage, M.I., 1991, A catalog of neurotoxic substances: A menu driven database for computer access of neurotoxic data, *Toxicologist* 11:244.

Gehring, P.J., 1971, The cataractogenic activity of chemical agents, *Crit. Rev. Toxicol.*, 10:93–117.

Goldberg, H., Horvath, T.B., and Myers, R.A., 1974, Visual evoked potentials as a measure of drug effects on arousal in the rabbit, *Clin. Exp. Pharmacol. Physiol.* 1:147–154.

Grant, W.M., 1986, *Toxicology of the Eye*, Charles C. Thomas, Springfield, IL.

Grant, W.M., 1980, The peripheral visual system as a target, in: *Experimental and Clinical Neurotoxicology* (P.S. Spencer and H.H. Schaumburg, eds.), Williams & Wilkins, Baltimore, pp. 77–91.

Hale, P.T., Sefton, A.J., and Dreher, B., 1979, A correlation of receptive field properties with conduction velocity of cells in the rat's retino-geniculo-cortical pathway, *Exp. Brain Res.* 35:425–442.

Halliday, A.M., McDonald, W.J., and Muskin, J., 1972, Delayed visual evoked response in optic neuritis, *Lancet* 1:982–985.

Harding, T.H., Wiley, R.W., and Kirby, A.W., 1983, A cholinergic-sensitive channel in the cat visual system tuned to low spatial frequencies, *Science* 221:1076–1078.

Harding, T.H., Kirby, A.W., and Wiley, R.W., 1985, The effects of diisopropylfluorophosphate on spatial frequency responsibility in the cat visual system, *Brain Res.* 325:357–361.

Harnois, C., Bodis-Wollner, I., and Onofrj, M., 1984, The effect of contrast and spatial frequency on the visual evoked potential of the hooded rat, *Exp. Brain Res.* 57:1–8.

Hattan, D.G., Henry, S.H., Montgomery, S.B., Bleiberg, M.J., Rulis, A.M., and Bolger, P.M., 1983, Role of the Food and Drug Administration in regulation of neuroeffective food additives, in: *Nutrition and the Brain*, Vol. 6 (R.J. Wurtman and J.J. Wurtman, eds.), Raven Press, New York, pp. 31–99.

Herr, D.W., Boyes, W.K., and Dyer, R.S., 1991, Rat flash-evoked potential peak $N_{160}$ amplitude: Modulation by relative flash intensity, *Physiol. Behav.* 49:355–365.

Hetzler, B., and Dyer, R.S., 1984, Contribution of hypothermia to effects of chloral hydrate on flash evoked potentials of hooded rats, *Pharmacol. Biochem. Behavior.* 21:599–607.

Hetzler, B.E., and Oaklay, K.E., 1981, Dose effects of pentobarbital on evoked potentials in visual cortex and superior colliculus of the albino rat, *Neuropharmacology* 20:969–978.

Hetzler, B.E., Heilbronner, R.L., Griffin, J., and Griffin, G., 1981, Acute effects of alcohol on evoked potentials in visual cortex and superior colliculus of the rat, *Electroencephalog. Clin. Neurophysiol.* 51:69–79.

Hetzler, B.E., Oaklay, K.A., Heilbronner, R.L., and Vestal, T., 1982, Acute effects of alcohol on photic evoked potentials of albino rats: Visual cortex and superior colliculus, *Pharmacol. Biochem. Behav.* 17:1313–1316.

Hetzler, B., Boyes, W.K., Creason, J.P., and Dyer, R.S., 1988, Temperature-dependent changes in visual evoked potentials of rats, *Electroencephalog. Clin. Neurophysiol.* 70:137–154.

Heywood, R., 1974, Drug-induced retinopathies in the beagle dog, *Br. Vet. J.* 130:564–569.

Heywood, R., 1982, Histopathological and laboratory assessment of visual dysfunction, *Environ. Health Perspect.* 44:35–49.

Heywood, R., 1985, Clinical and laboratory assessment of visual dysfunction, in: *Toxicology of the Eye, Ear, and Other Special Senses* (W. Hayes, ed.), Raven Press, New York, pp. 61–78.

Heywood, R., 1986, The eye, in: *Target Organ Toxicity*, Vol. II (G.M. Cohen, ed.), CRC Press, Boca Raton, FL, pp. 109–124.

Heywood, R., and Gopinath, C., 1990, Morphological assessment of visual dysfunction, *Toxicol. Pathol.* 18:204–217.

Hosko, M.J., 1970, The effect of carbon monoxide on the visual evoked response in man, *Arch. Environ. Health* 21:174–180.

Hudnell, H.K., and Benignus, V.A., 1989, Carbon monoxide exposure and human detection thresholds, *Neurotoxicol. Teratol.* 11:363–371.

Hudnell, H.K., and Boyes, W.K., 1991, The comparability of rat and human visual-evoked potentials, *Neurosci. Biobehav. Rev.* 15:159–164.

Hudnell, H.K., Boyes, W.K., and Otto, D.A., 1990a, Stationary pattern adaptation and the early components in human visual evoked potentials, *Electroencephalog. Clin. Neurophysiol.* 77:190–198.

Hudnell, H.K., Boyes, W.K., and Otto, D.A., 1990b, Rat and human visual-evoked potentials recorded under comparable conditions: A preliminary analysis to address the issue of predicting human neurotoxic effects from rat data, *Neurotoxic. Teratol.* 12:391–398.

Hughes, A., 1977, The refractive state of the rat eye, *Vision Res.* 17:927–939.

Hunter, D., Bomford, R.R., and Russek, D.S., 1940, Poisoning by methylmercury compounds, *Qt. J. Med.* 9:193–213.

Imai, S., 1986, A critical evaluation of "the strange disease of Saku," *Folia Ophthalmol.* 37:1351–1354. Translated from Japanese by the Ralph McElroy Co., Austin TX, for the California Dept. Health Services.

Ishikawa, S., and Miyata, M., 1980, Development of myopia following chronic organophosphate pesticide intoxication: An epidemiological and experimental study, in: *Neurotoxicity of the Visual System*, (W. H. Merigan and B. Weiss, eds.), Raven Press, New York, pp. 233–254.

Jewett, D.L., 1970, Volume-conducted potentials in response to auditory stimuli as detected by averaging in the cat, *Electroencephalog. Clin. Neurophysiol.* 28:609–618.

Joy, R.M., 1973. Alteration of sensory and motor evoked responses by dieldrin in *Neuropharmacology* 13:93–110.

Kraut, M.A., Arezzo, J.C., and Vaughan, H.G., 1985, Intracortical generators of the flash VEP in monkeys, *Electroencephalog. Clin. Neurophysiol.* 62:300–312.

Lee, E.W., 1987, A rat model for the study of methanol visual neurotoxicity, *Toxicologist* 7:97.

Lewis, E.G., Dustman, R.E., and Beck, E.C., 1970, The effects of alcohol on visual and somato-sensory evoked responses, *Electroencephalog. Clin. Neurophysiol.* 28:202–205.

Lochry, E.A., 1987, Concurrent use of behavioral/functional testing in existing reproductive and developmental toxicity screens: Practical considerations in *J. Am. Coll. Toxicol.* 6:433–439.

Lowndes, H.E. (ed.), 1987, *Electrophysiology in Neurotoxicology*, Vols. I and II, CRC Press, Boca Raton, FL.

Lucas, D.R., and Newhouse, J.P., 1957, The toxic effect of sodium-L-glutamate on the inner layers of the retina, *AMA Arch. Ophthalmol.* 58:193–201.

Lund, R.D., 1965, Uncrossed visual pathways of hooded and albino rats, *Science* 149:1506–1507.

Martin-Amat, G., McMartin, K.E., Hayreh, S.S., Hayreh, M.S., and Tephly, T.R., 1978, Methanol poisoning: Ocular toxicity produced by formate, *Toxicol. Appl. Pharmacol.* 45:210–208.

Mattsson, J.L., and Albee, R.R., 1988, Sensory evoked potentials in neurotoxicology, *Neurotoxicol. Teratol.* 10:435–443.

Mattsson, J.L., Albee, R.R., Eisenbrandt, R.R., and Chang, L.W., 1988, Subchronic neurotoxicity in rats of the structural fumigant, sulfuryl fluoride, *Neurotoxicol. Teratol.* 10:127–133.

Mattsson, J.L., Albee, R.R., and Eisenbrandt, D.L., 1989, Neurological approach to neurotoxicological evaluation in laboratory animals, *J. Am. Col. Toxicol.* 8:271–286.

Mattsson, J.L., Eisenbrandt, D.L., and Albee, R.R., 1990a, Screening for neurotoxicity: Complementarity of functional and morphological techniques, *Toxicol. Pathol.* 18:115–127.

Mattsson, J.L., Gorzinski, S.J., Albee, R.R., and Zimmer, M.A., 1990b, Evoked potential changes from 13 weeks of simulated toluene abuse in rats in *Pharmacol. Biochem. Behav.* 36:683–689.
McFarland, R.A., Halperin, M.H., and Niven, J.I., 1944, The effects of carbon monoxide and altitude on visual thresholds, *J. Aviat. Med.* 15:381–394.
McLaren, D.S., 1982, Age-dependent changes in the effects of food toxins and other dietary factors on the eye, *Pharmac. Ther.* 16:103–142.
Mergler, D., Blain, L., and Lagace, J.-P., 1987, Solvent related colour vision loss: An indicator of neural damage?, *Int. Arch. Occup. Environ. Health* 59:313–321.
Meier-Ruge, W., 1972, Drug induced retinopathy, *CRC Crit. Rev. Toxicol.* 1:325–359.
Merigan, W.H., 1979, Effects of toxicants on visual systems, in: *Test Methods for Definition of Effects of Toxic Substances on Behavior and Neuromotor Function* (I. Geller, W.C. Stebbins, and M.J. Wayner, eds.), *Neurobehav. Toxicol.* 1 (Suppl 1):15–22.
Merigan, W.H., and Weiss, B. (eds.), 1980, *Neurotoxicity of the Visual System*, Raven Press, New York.
Merigan, W.H., and Eskin, T.A., 1986, Spatio-temporal vision of macaques with severe loss of $P_\beta$ retinal ganglion cells, *Vision Res.* 11:1751–1761.
Merigan, W.H., Maurissen, J.P., Weiss, B., Eskin, T., and Lapham, L.W., 1983, Neurotoxic actions of methylmercury on the primate visual system, *Neurobehav. Toxicol. Teratol.* 5:649–658.
Merigan, W.H., Wood, R.W., Zehl, D., and Eskin, T.A., 1988, Carbon disulfide effects on the visual system: I. Visual thresholds and ophthalmoscopy, *Invest. Ophthal. & Vis. Sci.* 29(4):512–518.
Misra, U.K., Nag, D., Misra, N.K., Mehra, M.K., and Ray, P.K., 1985, Some observations on the macula of pesticide workers, *Hum. Toxicol.* 4:135–145.
Moody, D.D., and Stebbins, W.C., 1982, Detection of the effects of toxic substances on the auditory system by behavioral methods, *Nervous System Toxicology* (C.L. Mitchell, ed.), Raven Press, New York, pp. 109–131.
Moser, V.C., 1989, Screening approaches to neurotoxicity: A functional observational battery, *J. Am. Col. Toxicol.* 8:85–93.
Mukuno, K., Ishikawa, S., and Okamura, R., 1984, Grating test of contrast sensitivity in patients with Minamata disease, *Br. J. Ophthal,* 65:284, 290.
Nakai, Y., Takeda, Y., and Takaori, S., 1973, Effects of ethanol on afferent transmission in the central visual pathway of cats, *Eur. J. Pharmacol.* 21:318–322.
Office of Technology Assessment (OTA), U.S. Congress 1984, *Impacts of Neuroscience: Background Paper,* OTA-BP-BA-24, U.S. Government Printing Office, Washington, DC.
Office of Technology Assessment (OTA), U.S. Congress, 1990, *Neurotoxicity: Identifying and Controlling Poisons of the Nervous System,* OTA-BA-436 U.S. Government Printing Office, Washington, DC.
Oken, B.S., and Chiappa, K.H., 1986, Somatosensory evoked potentials in neurological diagnosis, in: *Evoked Potentials* (R.Q. Cracco, and I. Bodis-Wollner, eds.), Alan R. Liss, New York, pp. 379–389.
Onofrj, M., Bodis-Wollner, I., and Bobak, P., 1982, Pattern visual evoked potentials in the rat, *Physiol. Behav.* 28:227–230.
Orbitz, F.W., Rhodes, L.E., and Creel, D., 1977, Effect of alcohol and monetary reward on visually evoked potentials and reaction time, *J. Studies Alcohol.* 38:2057–2064.
Otto, D., 1986, The use of sensory evoked potentials in neurotoxicity testing of workers, *Semin. Occup. Med.* 1:175–183.
Otto, D., Baumann, S., and Robinson, G., 1985, Application of a portable microprocessor-based system for electrophysiological field testing of neurotoxicity, *Neurobehav. Toxicol. Teratol.* 7:409–414.
Otto, D., Benignus, V., Prah, J., and Converse, B., 1978, Paradoxical effects of carbon monoxide on vigilance performance and event-related potentials, in: *Multidisciplinary Perspectives in Event-Related Brain Potential Research* (D. Otto, ed.), EPA-600/9-7-043, S/N 055-000-00183-9, GPO, Washington, DC, pp. 440–443.
Otto, D., Hudnell, D., Boyes, W., Janssen, R., and Dyer, R., 1988, Electrophysiological measures of visual and auditory function as indices of neurotoxicity, *Toxicology* 49:205–218.
Plestina, R., and Piukovic-Plestina, M., 1978, Effect of anticholinesterase pesticides on the eye and on vision, *CRC Crit. Rev. Toxicol.* 6(1):1–23.
Prieur, D.J., 1982, Albino animals: Their use and misuse in biomedical research, *Compar. Pathol. Bull.* 14(3):1–4.
Rebert, C.S., 1983, Multisensory evoked potentials in experimental and applied neurotoxicology, *Neurobehav. Toxicol. Teratol.* 5:659–671.
Rebert, C.S., 1987, Development and evaluation of methods for monitoring of intracellular events during hypoxia and acid-base disturbances: Nervous system. Final report for National Heart, Lung, and Blood Institute Contract No. NO1-HR-34005, Menlo Park, CA.
Regan, D., 1982, Visual information channeling in normal and disordered vision, *Psychol. Rev.* 89:407–444.
Regan, D. (ed.), 1989, *Human Brain Electrophysiology: Evoked Potentials and Evoked Magnetic Fields in Science and Medicine,* Elsevier Science, New York.
Reuhl, K.R., Rice, D.C., Gilbert, S.G., and Mallett, J., 1989, Effects of chronic developmental lead exposure on monkey neuroanatomy: Visual system, *Toxicol. Appl. Pharmacol.* 99:501–509.
Rice, D.C., and Gilbert, S.G., 1981, Early chronic low-level methylmercury poisoning in monkeys impairs spatial vision, *Science* 216:759–761.
Rice, D.C., and Gilbert, S.G., 1990, Effects of developmental exposure to methyl mercury on spatial and temporal visual function in monkeys, *Toxicol. Appl. Pharmacol.* 102:151–163.
Rigdon, G.C., and Dyer, R.S., 1987, Ontogency of flash-evoked potentials in unanesthetized rats, *Int. J. Develop. Neurosci.* 5:447–454.

Rigdon, G.C., Boyes, W.K., and Dyer, R.S., 1989, Effect of perinatal monosodium glutamate administration on visual evoked potentials of juvenile and adult rats, *Neurotoxicol. Teratol.* 11:121–128.

Rhodes, L.E., Orbitz, F.W., and Creel, D., 1975, Effect of alcohol and task on hemispheric asymmetry of visually evoked potentials in man, *Electroencephalog. Clin. Neurophysiol.* 38:561–568.

Robson, J.G., 1975, Receptive fields: Neural representation of the spatial and intensive attributes of the visual image, in: *Handbook of Perception*, (E.C. Carterette and M.P. Friedman, eds.), Academic Press, New York, pp. 80–116.

Rosadini, G., Rodriguez, G., and Siani, C., 1974, Acute alcohol poisoning in man: An experimental electrophysiological study, *Psychopharmacology* 35:273–285.

Rudnev, M., Bokina, A., Eksler, N., and Navakatikyan, M., 1978, The use of evoked potential and behavioral measures in the assessment of environmental insult, in: *Multidisciplinary Perspectives in Event-Related Brain Potential Research* (D. Otto, ed.), EPA-600/9-7-043, S/N 055-000-00183-9, Government Printing Office, Washington, DC, pp. 444–447.

Seppalainen, A.M., 1988, Neurophysiological approaches to the detection of early neurotoxicity in humans, *CRC Crit. Rev. Toxicol* 18:245–298.

Seppalainen, A.M., Savolainen, K., and Kovala, T., 1981, Changes induced by xylene and alcohol in human evoked potentials, *Electroencephalog. Clin. Neurophysiol.* 51:148–155.

Sherman, J., 1986, ERG and VEP as supplemental aids in the differential diagnosis of retinal versus optic nerve disease, in: *Evoked Potentials* (R.Q. Cracco and I. Bodis-Wollner, eds.), Alan R. Liss, New York, pp. 343–353.

Silveira, L.C.L., Heywood, C.A., and Cowey, A., 1987, Contrast sensitivity and visual acuity of the pigmented rat determined electrophysiologically, *Vision Res.* 27:1719–1731.

Simpson, D., Erwin, C.W., and Linnoila, M., 1981, Ethanol and menstrual cycle interactions in the visual evoked response, *Electroencephalog. Clin. Neurophysiol.* 52:28–35.

U.S. Environmental Protection Agency, 1991, Pesticide Assessment Guidelines, Subdivision F, Hazard Evaluation: Human and Domestic Animals, Addendum 10, Neurotoxicity, EPA 540/09-91-123, NTIS PB 91-154617, Springfield, VA, 22161.

Wiederholt, W.C., and Iragui-Madoz, 1977, Far field somatosensory potentials in the rat, *Electroencephalog. Clin. Neurophysiol.* 42:456–465.

WHO 1986, *Principles and Methods for Assessment of Neurotoxicity Associated with Exposure to Chemicals*, Environmental Criteria Document 60. World Health Organization, Geneva.

Woolley, D.E., 1977, Electrophysiological techniques in toxicology, in: *Behavioral Toxicology: An Emerging Discipline* (H. Zenick, and L.W. Reiter, eds.), EPA-600/9-77-042, U.S. Environmental Protection Agency, Research Triangle Park, NC.

Woolley, D., and Reiter, L., 1978, Dissociation between time course of acetylcholinesterase inhibition and neurophysiological effects of parathion in rat and monkey, in: *Multidisciplinary Perspectives in Event-Related Brain Potential Research* (D. Otto ed.), EPA-600/9-7-043, S/N 055-000-00183-9, Government Printing Office, Washington, DC, pp. 470–475.

Xintaras, C., Johnson, B.L., Ulrich, C.E., Terrill, R.E., and Sobecki, M.F., 1966, Application of the evoked response technique in air pollution toxicology, *Toxicol. Appl. Pharmacol.* 8:77–87.

Zemon, V., Victor, J., and Ratliff, F., 1986, Functional subsystems in the visual pathways of humans characterized using evoked potentials, in: *Evoked Potentials* (R.Q. Cracco and I. Bodis-Wollner, eds.), Alan R. Liss, New York, pp. 203–210.

Zuzewicz, W., 1981, Ethyl alcohol effect on the visual evoked potential, *Acta Physiol. Pol.* 32:93–98.

Chapter 10

# The Use of Selective Silver Degeneration Stains in Neurotoxicology

## Lessons from Studies of Selective Neurotoxicants

*Carey D. Balaban*

### 1. INTRODUCTION

A major goal of modern neurotoxicology is to elucidate cellular and subcellular targets that initiate neuronal responses to endogenous and xenobiotic neurotoxins. Cellular responses to a toxin are a dynamic process, evolving from a perturbation of cellular function to either recovery or permanent damage. Hence, a toxic effect can involve both site-specific actions and cellular or neural network attempts at recovery of function. Recognition of these factors provides the intellectual basis for classifying neurotoxins on the basis of their sites of action and sequelae. Spencer and Schaumburg (1980, 1984) pioneered this approach by classifying neurotoxins on the basis of the primary cellular and subcellular loci of action. Their first level of stratification reflected the affected cell type (Spencer and Schaumburg, 1984); thus, separate categories were proposed for toxins that act on neurons, glial cells and myelin, vasculature of the nervous system, and muscle. More specific cellular and subcellular loci of action were then nested within each of these categories.

---

*Carey D. Balaban* • Department of Otolaryngology University of Pittsburgh and the Eye and Ear Institute of Pittsburgh, Pittsburgh, Pennsylvania 15213.
*The Vulnerable Brain and Environmental Risks, Volume 1: Malnutrition and Hazard Assessment,* edited by Robert L. Isaacson and Karl F. Jensen. Plenum Press, New York, 1992.

This communication discusses issues related to the analysis of one particular class of neurotoxic effect, neuronal degeneration after neurotoxin exposure.

Modern neuroscience has revealed a remarkable morphological, connectional, and biochemical heterogeneity among neurons. This heterogeneity is thought to confer a differential susceptibility to neurotoxic degeneration. The neurobiologic literature is rife with cases of neurotoxic actions that vary in cellular specificity for neuronal populations. For example, characteristic patterns of neurotoxic degeneration have been established for neurotransmitter analogs (e.g., the excitatory amino acid analogs kainic, ibotenic, or quinolinic acid), native neurochemicals (e.g., somatostatin-14), catecholaminergic toxins [e.g., 6-hydroxydopamine and N-(2-chloroethyl)-N-ethyl-2-bromobenzylamine (DSP-4)], organometallic compounds [e.g., trimethyltin (TMT)], and pyridine derivatives [e.g., 3-acetylpyridine and 1-methyl-4-phenyl-1,2,3,4-tetrahydropyridine (MPTP)]. However, due to the biochemical and connectional complexities in the central nervous system, there is no universal paradigm for inferring the cellular bases for actions of selective neurotoxins from data documenting a selective degeneration of specific populations or portions of neurons (axons or cell somata plus axons). The identification of mechanisms of toxicity requires an integrative view of subcellular, cellular, and systems neuroscience.

The issues of a sensitive means of identification of neurotoxic degeneration, documentation of its spatial and temporal distribution, and clarification of the cellular and molecular bases of its toxic effects are interdependent. The elucidation of cellular and subcellular mechanisms of action of a particular neurotoxin requires a multidisciplinary, multitiered approach, focused on comparative analysis of susceptible and unaffected populations of neurons. Since the site(s) of toxicity and potential mechanisms of action are often unknown, the first goal is to determine (1) whether any neurons degenerate and, if so, their locations; (2) whether initial damage is dendritic, somatic, and/or axonal; and (3) the time course of toxic degeneration. This information provides important clues about cellular actions of the toxin, particularly if a toxin is selective for populations of neurons that have distinctive neurochemical properties. One prominent example is the selective toxicity of MPTP in dopaminergic neurons, which has focused mechanistic studies on MPTP metabolism and its relationship to specific neurochemical features of those cells (e.g., Sayre, 1989). More commonly, though, as in the case of trimethyltin (TMT) or 3-acetylpyridine (3-AP), neuroanatomical analyses demonstrate that a toxin has a high degree of specificity for some populations of neurons, but the neurobiologic database does not provide any clues as to whether cell death has a common biochemical basis in the affected neurons. In this case, identification of affected sites can direct investigations of cellular bases for cytotoxicity toward susceptible populations of neurons.

## 2. DISTINGUISHING PRIMARY AND SECONDARY NEURONAL DEGENERATION

The issue of the identification of cellular sites of neurotoxicity in the central nervous system is a special case of a more general issue: How can sites of neuronal degeneration be detected with high sensitivity, spatial resolution, and temporal resolution? Moreover, one is faced with the possibility that the degeneration elicited by a neurotoxin reflects multiple mechanisms, some of which may be indirect consequences of earlier primary damage. One prominent example of a secondary effect is transneuronal degeneration, which has been recognized in neurobiology for more than a century (review: Cowan, 1970). Anterograde transneuronal degeneration develops as a consequence of deafferentation of a population of neurons, while retrograde transneuronal degeneration develops as a secondary consequence of the loss of a target population of neurons. Since secondary degenerative phenomena can include transneuronal responses to injury that are not direct actions of a toxin, they are a potential confounding factor in identifying cellular and molecular bases for actions of neurotoxins in neurochemical and molecular biologic studies. These issues can be appreciated by a brief consideration of the effects of several neurotoxins. Neurotoxins such as ibotenic acid and 3-AP appear to have their effects at the level of neuronal somata; thus, the axons and somata both degenerate as a function of a direct somatic action of the toxin. Other toxins can have highly specific effects on axons while sparing somata. For example, DSP-4 destroys only noradrenergic terminals originating from the locus coeruleus; the parent somata in the locus coeruleus and other noradrenergic pathways are spared (Fritschy and Grzanna, 1989). Trimethyltin (TMT) toxicity, on the other hand, proceeds in phases, suggesting an involvement of multiple factors (Balaban *et al.*, 1988a). Clearly, the problem of deciphering a potentially multifactorial basis for toxicity requires that experiments be targeted at the susceptible sites for each toxin at times preceding cell death. Thus, the rational design of pharmacologic, physiologic, and neurochemical investigations of toxic mechanisms requires the reliable documentation of (1) the identity of degenerating neurons, including their dendritic morphology and axonal projections; (2) the relative time course of degeneration of the somatodendritic and axonal compartments of each neuronal population; and (3) the relative time course of degeneration of different populations of neurons, including whether a population degenerates after an afferent population is destroyed or damaged. Subsequent studies can then be focused on the appropriate populations of neurons and their processes.

## 3. VISUALIZING NEURONAL DEGENERATION: ORIGIN AND ROLE OF SILVER DEGENERATION STAINS

The examination of neuronal degeneration in neurobiology has focused on the pragmatic issue of using neuronal degeneration to trace pathways in the nervous system. A historical review of these studies is instructive for several reasons. First, it illustrates a logical technological progression from the use of a nonspecific method, the loss of axonal or neuronal somatic staining from Nissl, hemotoxylin-eosin, or fiber-stained preparations (*negative staining approach*), to the development of methods that selectively visualize neuronal degeneration without staining normal neuronal elements (*positive staining approach*). Secondly, it permits a discussion of the phenomena of anterograde (direct Wallerian), retrograde (indirect Wallerian), and transneuronal degeneration. All of these phenomena are essential for interpreting the time course of neuronal degeneration after intoxication. Anterograde degeneration occurs whenever an axon is separated physically from its parent soma; the terminals typically degenerate first, followed by degeneration of stem fibers (review: DeOlmos *et al.*, 1981). Anterograde degeneration can thus result when an axon is damaged physically, when anterograde axonal transport is halted, or, in the extreme case, when a neuronal soma is directly destroyed. Retrograde degeneration, on the other hand, occurs when a soma degenerates as a secondary consequence of axonal damage; the axon then degenerates in the anterograde direction from the soma to the site of injury. Transneuronal degeneration is strictly a secondary consequence of either deafferentation or a loss of target neurons. The increased susceptibility of young animals to transneuronal effects is potentially of great importance because it may be a factor in age-related differences in cell loss due to intoxication. Thus, an understanding of these factors is important for the interpretation of neurotoxicologic data obtained with morphologic methods, since they have a major impact on hypotheses concerning the cellular and subcellular loci of toxic effects.

### 3.1. Anterograde (Direct Wallerian) Degeneration: Role in Development of Selective Degeneration Stains

The problem of tracing anterograde degeneration provided the main impetus for the development of selective degeneration staining techniques. Waller (1850) first noted that after transection, the distal axonal stump of a spinal nerve degenerates while the central process survives. Subsequent confirmations of this observation resulted in the formulation of Waller's Law (reviews: Charcot, 1876; van Gehuchten, 1903), which stated that degeneration after axotomy is strictly anterograde because the distal process has a trophic dependence on the soma. Applications of this principle are found in the experimental and neurologic literature of the late 19th century, since it provided a basis for interpreting the loss of fiber staining (or sclerotic changes) after a lesion to anterograde, or direct Wallerian, degeneration of damaged axons or of axons originating from dead neuronal somata. For example, Vulpian (1866) discussed applications of the "méthode Wallérienne" to trace peripheral nerves after lesions in experimental animals, while Charcot (1876) and Pitres (1884) used this phenomenon to trace the course of the human pyramidal tract after cerebral infarcts. The development of the Marchi method (impregnation of fixed tissue with a dichromate-osmic acid solution) permitted the application of direct Wallerian degeneration to trace the course of myelinated fibers distal to a lesion in experimental animals (e.g., Marchi, 1891). The Marchi method had significant technical limitations: It only stains degenerating myelin, and its sensitivity is limited by prominent artifactual staining of normal tissue (e.g., Swank and Davenport, 1934). Although the persistence of Marchi staining up to 1 year after a lesion made this a useful technique for tracing myelinated pathways in long-term survival experiments and human autopsy material, its inability to resolve axon terminals severely limited the resolution of neuronal connectivity in experimental studies.

The technical problem of visualizing degenerating axon terminals was partially resolved by the development of the first selective silver degeneration methods in the late 1930s and early 1940s. The argyrophilia of normal neuronal somata and axons had been utilized previously in a variety of stains: The rapid Golgi method, en-bloc silver methods (e.g., Cajal method), the Bielschowsky reduced silver method, and the Bodian stain (1936) were all recognized for their capability to demonstrate normal axon morphology. After Hoff's (1932) report that it was possible to differentiate normal and degenerating terminals in silver-stained sections, a series of modifications of Bielschowsky methods were developed to stain degenerating axon terminals (Glees and Le Gros Clark, 1941; Holmes, 1943), cultimating in the Glees degeneration stain (1946). A subsequent modification of the latter method was the *unsuppressed Nauta–Gygax method* (Nauta and Gygax, 1954), which has formed the core of more recent methods. These techniques were a series of modifications of a normal reduced silver stain that involved the successive treatment of free-floating, formaldehyde-fixed frozen sections with (1) a silver nitrate solution (often containing pyridine), (2) an ammoniacal silver solution, (3) a reducing agent, and (4) a silver fixing agent (sodium thiosulfate). Thus, they required the investigator to discriminate the relatively intense argyrophilia and necrotic morphology of degenerating axons from argyrophilia of normal tissue.

The prototype of the modern suppressive silver degeneration stain was the *suppressive Nauta–Gygax method* (Nauta and Gygax, 1954). This method used pretreatment with phosphomolybdic acid, followed by oxidation with potassium permanganate and decoloration with oxalic acid and hydroquinone to suppress the argyrophilia of normal tissue. Thus, degenerating axons could be distinguished from normal tissue. Although the sensitivity of the method was compromised because the suppressive steps reduced the argyrophilia of both normal and degenerating axons, it permitted visualization of both terminals and degenerating axon shafts (Glees and Nauta, 1955). This method and its subsequent modifications (Nauta, 1957) constituted a major landmark in tract tracing technology, which served an important role in the neuroanatomic armamentarium for more than a decade.

The sensitivity and selectivity of suppressive silver stains have improved markedly since the late 1950s. The Fink–Heimer methods (1967) increased both the suppression of normal fibers and the argyrophilia of degenerating fibers by eliminating the initial phosphomolybdic acid treatment from the Nauta–Gygax method and either (1) adding uranyl nitrate to the initial silver impregnation solution (Fink–Heimer procedure I) or (2) incorporating a separate uranyl nitrate suppression step before the initial silver impregnation (Fink–Heimer procedure II). After these procedures, degenerating axons appear as black debris against a light-brown background. However, the cupric-silver methods, developed and improved continuously by De Olmos and coworkers (Carlsen and De Olmos, 1981; De Olmos, 1968; De Olmos and Ingram, 1972; unpublished protocols), appear to be the most sensitive and selective degeneration methods for demonstrating anterograde degeneration in a variety of applications (De Olmos *et al.*, 1981). Like the Fink–Heimer methods, the cupric-silver protocols are derivatives of the unsuppressed Nauta–Gygax protocol. The basic procedure involves suppression of normal staining with an initial silver impregnation solution containing cupric nitrate, allantoin, and pyridine, followed by treatment with an ammoniacal silver solution, reduction, bleaching of background staining, and fixation of the reduced silver with sodium thiosulfate and Kodak rapid fix. These procedures yield impregnation of even the finest degenerating processes against a light-yellow to transparent background. As a result, anterograde degeneration is easily detectable.

## 3.2. Axon Reaction, Retrograde Somatic Degeneration, and Indirect Wallerian Degeneration

During the final decade of the 19th century, it became clear that Waller's Law was inadequate to account for either chromatolytic reactions of neuronal somata after nerve section or, in the extreme case, the retrograde death of some neurons after axotomy (review: Soury, 1899). Following consistent descriptions of neuronal atrophy after axotomy by Gudden (1870), Monakow (1882), and Forel (1887), and Nissl's (1892) description of chromatolytic changes in central neurons after axotomy, attention was focused on the possibility the proximal portion of an axon and the soma could also be affected by a distal axonal lesion. The latter chromatolytic changes, more appropriately termed the *axon reaction,* are somatic responses to injury, probably reflecting neurochemical and metabolic changes that mediate cell repair; however, not all cells die after displaying an axon reaction (Lieberman, 1971, 1974). The seminal work of van Gehuchten (1903) established that the axon reaction proceeds to retrograde degeneration in some central structures: He concluded that after axotomy, retrograde atrophy and degeneration of the cell body produces an anterograde (indirect Wallerian) degeneration from the soma to the lesion site. This observation is germane to neurotoxologic analysis because it is a potential cause of a secondary somatodendritic degeneration of neurons after axonal damage. The phenomenon of retrograde degeneration in selected peripheral and central pathways was employed for tracing neuronal connections prior to the advent of retrograde tracer technologies in the 1970s. For example, Holmes and Stewart (1906) and Walker (1938) used retrograde degeneration to investigate the topography of olivocerebellar connections in humans and thalamocortical connections in primates, respectively. More recent work by Ito *et al.* (1980) demonstrated that inferior olivary cell death after mechanical cerebellar ablation is truly retrograde degeneration and not a transneuronal retrograde effect, because destruction of cerebellar Purkinje cells with kainic acid did not produce olivary cell loss.

Prior to the availability of suppressive silver degeneration stains, the only method for studying retrograde somatic degeneration was a Nissl technique (Cammermayer, 1963). Guillery (1959) and Powell and Cowan (1964) provided the first descriptions of the appearance of retrograde degeneration with Nauta–Gygax and Nauta–Laidlaw techniques. They reported a fine particulate argyrophilic reaction in thalamic somata undergoing retrograde degeneration after cortical lesions, which was followed by anterograde degeneration of the proximal thalamocortical axons in the thalamic radiations (Powell and Cowan, 1964). These results confirmed the earlier conclusions of van Gehuchten (1903) and motivated Grant and coworkers (Grant, 1968, 1970, 1975; Grant and Aldskogius, 1967; Grant and Westman, 1969; Grant and Walberg, 1974) to extend the analysis of the capability of Nauta–Laidlaw and Fink–Heimer methods for selectively impregnating the somata, dendrites, and axons of neurons undergoing retrograde degeneration. They noted that the time course of silver impregnation was coincident with the time course and distribution of chromatolysis at the light microscopic level and ultrastructural signs of necrosis, but reported that chromatolytic cells outnumbered silver-impregnated neurons. However, it is impossible to draw conclusions about the relative quantitative accuracy of silver stains and Nissl stains because not all chromatolytic cells degenerate (Lieberman, 1971). This issue of the quantitative accuracy of silver stains for demonstrating degenerating neurons is still unresolved.

Developmental variations in the susceptibility of the central nervous system to retrograde degeneration are an important consideration in interpreting age-related changes in neurotoxicity. The relatively high sensitivity of young animals to retrograde degeneration was well established by the end of the 19th century (Gudden, 1870; van Gehuchten, 1903), and this phenomenon was exploited by Brodal (1940) to study olivocerebellar projections with retrograde tracing methods. Quantitative studies (LaVelle and LaVelle, 1958) have confirmed that the susceptibility of neurons to retrograde degeneration appears to decrease with age in rats. Thus, retrograde degeneration after axonal damage is a potential confounding factor in comparing neurotoxic degenerative effects in the central nervous system of neonatal, juvenile, and adult animals.

## 3.3. Transneuronal Degeneration

The phenomenon of transneuronal degeneration has been observed consistently since the late 19th century (reviewed in Cowan, 1970). Anterograde transneuronal atrophy and/or degeneration has been reported at several central sites, including the dorsal and ventral lateral geniculate nuclei after optic tract damage or enucleation, the ventral cochlear nucleus and nuclei of the trapezoid body after cochlear nerve section, and the central olfactory system after peripheral or central lesions (Cowan, 1969; Heimer and Kalil, 1978). Sites displaying retrograde transneuronal degeneration include the retina after visual cortical ablation, the medial mammillary and ventral tegmental nuclei after limbic cortical ablations, and the motor cortex after limb amputations (review: Cowan, 1969). Like retrograde degeneration, these transneuronal effects tend to be most profound when young animals are subjected to lesions. Since, in many cases, the severity of transneuronal degeneration decreases with age, transneuronal effects must be considered in assessing age-dependent changes in neurotoxicity. Although silver degeneration stains have not been used widely to assess transneuronal effects, the cupric-silver method has been applied successfully to studies of anterograde transneuronal degeneration in the olfactory system (De Olmos *et al.*, 1981; Heimer and Kalil, 1978).

## 3.4. Summary: Role of Silver Stains in Demonstrating Neuronal Degeneration

Suppressive silver degeneration methods were developed to trace anterograde degeneration in the central nervous system after local chemical or mechanical destruction of either somata or axons. These methods, particularly the cupric-silver methods, have subsequently proven to be useful in detecting retrograde and transneuronal degenerative effects. Selective silver degeneration methods have the major advantage of displaying the morphology of degenerating neuronal processes (axons, dendrites, and somata), so that cell populations can be distinguished on the basis of both dendritic morphology and axonal connections. The major liability of these methods, though, is a secondary consequence of producing a lesion in the central nervous system: Fibers of passage may be damaged by an electrolytic lesion or injection cannula; thus degeneration due to interruption of other pathways can be confounded with degeneration resulting from damage of a particular site of interest. Furthermore, a second perceived liability resulted from the dynamic nature of degeneration: Survival times must be selected empirically for each fiber system under investigation so that degenerating processes could be identified. As a result, autoradiographic and molecular tracer techniques (e.g., horseradish peroxidase, lectins, and fluorescent dextrans) are most commonly employed for anterograde tract tracing at present.

## 4. INTERPRETATION OF SILVER DEGENERATION STAINS IN NEUROTOXICOLOGY

The limitations of suppressive silver degeneration stains in tract tracing studies are simply not germane to the detection of neuronal degeneration after systemic treatment with neurotoxins. The fiber-of-passage problem is a case in point: The problem is moot if the route of delivery of the toxin is the blood or CSF, or if the degeneration is secondary to effects of the neurotoxin on other neurons, glia, or vascular elements. Furthermore, the time course of neuronal degeneration is an essential dependent variable in neurotoxicologic studies; it can be used to generate hypotheses about sequences of toxic events. Thus, suppressive silver degeneration methods seem optimally suited for detecting patterns of neurotoxic degeneration.

The unique applicability of suppressive silver stains to neurotoxicology was first noted by Hedreen and Chalmers (1972) in their studies of the effects of intracerebroventricular 6-hydroxydopamine (6-OHDA) toxicity and by Desclin and Escubi (1974) in their examination of 3-AP toxicity. Both studies demonstrated that the Fink–Heimer method facilitated detection of both somatodendritic and axonal degeneration. Both Fink–Heimer and cupric–silver methods have proven to be valuable in subsequent neurotoxicologic analyses using a variety of neurotoxins (Balaban, 1985; Balaban et al., 1988a–c; Jensen et al., 1990; Ricaurte et al., 1982, 1984, 1987, 1989; Scallett et al., 1988; Switzer, 1991; Tanaka et al., 1989, 1990a, 1990b; Whittington et al., 1989). The application of silver degeneration stains to neurotoxicologic questions, though, requires a consideration of (1) the sensitivity and selectivity of silver stains in comparison with other methods and (2) criteria for interpretation of silver degeneration data to discriminate potential primary and secondary effects of neurotoxins. These issues form the focus of this section. The reader is referred to articles by Heimer (1969) and De Olmos et al. (1981) for an authoritative description of degenerating neurons and common artifacts of suppressive silver methods.

## 4.1. Identification of Neuronal Populations

Suppressive silver stains have been developed specifically to identify degenerating neuronal processes with a black precipitate, while normal neurons are unstained. In contrast to the affinity of unsuppressed reduced silver stains for bundles of 10-nm neurofilaments and fascicles of 10-nm neurofilaments and microtubules (Potter, 1975), electron microscopic studies suggest that the argyrophilic reaction of suppressive silver stains is selective for the axoplasm and degenerating mitochondria of processes showing unambiguous ultrastructural signs of necrosis (Heimer, 1969; Heimer and Peters, 1968; Walberg, 1971, 1972). This positive staining of degenerating neuronal somata and processes is a major advantage in the detection of selective effects of neurotoxins, first, by increasing the detectability of degeneration of subpopulations of neurons, and secondly, by revealing the morphology and connectivity of affected neurons (Balaban, 1985; Balaban et al., 1988a–c). This confers a distinct advantage in detectability over negative staining methods, such as Nissl stains, or immunohistochemistry for neurotypic proteins and methods assaying glial fibrillary acidic protein, which do not distinguish between areas of somatic, dendritic, and axonal (axon of passage or terminal) damage (Balaban et al., 1988). The major advantage of suppressed silver stains, then, is facilitation of correlating physiologic and behavior sequelae of intoxication with patterns of axonal, somatic, and dendritic degeneration.

Suppressive silver stains are particularly useful for detecting selective degenerative effects of neurotoxins on subpopulations of neurons in major structures on the basis of location and neuronal morphology. These data can then be compared with the existing descriptive and hodological databases in the literature to identify degeneration of specific functional groups of neurons. For example, the cupric–silver stain demonstrated that

TMT destroys a subpopulation of multipolar neurons in the deep aspect of the superficial gray of the superior colliculus; these cells were identified as wide-field collico-thalamic projection neurons (Takahashi, 1985) on the basis of their projections to the lateral posterior nucleus (Balaban et al., 1988a). Similar examples are provided by TMT-induced degeneration of layer Vb cortico-olivary and cortico-pontine projection neurons (Balaban et al., 1988a) and by the susceptibility of cerebellar cortico-vestibular and cortico-fastigial Purkinje cells in lobules I–III and IX–X to degeneration after intracerebroventricular injections of somatostatin (Balaban et al., 1988b, 1988c, 1989). These examples are indicative of the ability of suppressive silver methods to pinpoint degenerative effects to functional subpopulations of neurons.

The ability of selective silver degeneration stains to discriminate purely axonal degeneration from combined somatodendritic and axonal degeneration has been demonstrated by Ricaurte et al. (1982, 1984, 1987, 1989) in studies of the effects of amphetamine, methamphetamine, N,N-dimethylamphetamine, and MPTP on dopaminergic projections to the rat striatum. Their Fink–Heimer studies revealed that the three amphetamine derivatives produced only axonal degeneration in the striatum, which coincided with a loss of dopamine in those regions. However, both degeneration of nigral somata and axonal damage were observed in rats treated with MPTP. Since these different patterns of degeneration were associated with similar dopamine depletions in the striatum, these data suggest that silver stains facilitate the localization of toxic effects to axonal and somatic regions of neurons.

Selective silver degeneration methods clearly yield more information about the distribution and morphology of degenerating neurons than other techniques. However, morphologic methods in neurotoxicology must also be assessed on the basis of (1) sensitivity for identifying degenerating neurons and (2) lack of false-positive staining (selectivity). Although there are few objective analyses of the relative sensitivity of different methods, several results confirm the superior sensitivity and selectivity of suppressive silver methods. For example, the cupric–silver method proved to be a more sensitive detector of TMT toxicity in rats than immunohistochemistry for a neurotypic protein (protein-O-carboxylmethyltransferase) and immunoassays for glial fibrillary acidic protein (GFAP), particularly at short survival times (Balaban et al., 1988). The cupric–silver method also does not appear to be susceptible to false-positive findings: Cell loss from toxins such as 3-AP, TMT, and intracerebroventricular somatostatin has been confirmed in Nissl-stained material (Balaban, 1985; Balaban et al., 1988; Desclin and Escubi, 1974; personal observations), even at the level of subpopulations of neurons within cranial nerve nuclei (Balaban, 1985). However, the best test of the reliability of these methods is provided by ongoing studies in the literature. For example, the Fink–Heimer stain initially revealed that 3-AP damages some substantia nigra cells (Desclin and Escubi, 1974). The cupric–silver method further demonstrated that 3-AP-intoxicated substantia nigra neurons project to the dorsal and lateral aspects of the caudato-putamen in rats (Balaban, 1985). Subsequent neurochemical studies documented a slight decrease in dopamine in the whole striatum from 3-AP intoxicated rats (Deutsch et al., 1989) but showed that the loss was 40% in the dorsal and lateral regions (Deutsch et al., 1990) that displayed terminal degeneration in the previous degeneration studies (Balaban, 1985). Thus, the regional loss of striatal dopamine after 3-AP intoxication was predicted by selective degeneration data.

The patterns of argyrophilic neurons during short survival times and cell loss at long survival times are consistent for neurotoxic doses of 6-OHDA, 3-AP, TMT, and somatostatin-14 (Balaban, 1985, unpublished observations; Balaban et al., 1988a–c;

Desclin and Escubi, 1974; Hedreen and Chalmers, 1972). However, the quantitative accuracy of somatic argyrophilia for assessing cell loss has not been rigorously assessed. As a result, it is advisable to combine quantitative silver stain analyses with quantitative analyses of Nissl-stained material (from long survival times) to maximize the reliability of estimates of numbers of generated neurons.

## 4.2. Interpreting Neuronal Degeneration: Time Course and Patterns of Degeneration

From the frame of reference of a single neuron, neural degeneration after toxin exposure is a dynamic process, evolving from perturbations of subcellular components that compromise axonal and/or somatodendritic function to development of axonopathy or neuronopathy. However, in vivo studies of neuronal degeneration reveal the effects of the neurotoxin on a complex dynamic system (or neural network) that is attempting to recover from neurotoxic insult. Hence, they reveal a sequence of direct responses to a neurotoxin and indirect effects, mediated by processes that may include the generation of toxic metabolites, transneuronal degeneration, and ischemia. It is essential to recognize that morphologic screening methods cannot identify direct and indirect toxic actions at axons, dendrites, and somata per se; rather, they can help distinguish axonal and somatodendritic (1) primary effects (initial toxic effects, including direct effects on neurons) and (2) secondary effects (e.g., retrograde and transneuronal degeneration) by the relative timing and localization of degeneration. The relationship of these primary and secondary effects to cellular actions of toxins [e.g., bases for the nosology of Spencer and Schaumburg (1984)] must then be tested with other methods. The ability of silver stains to discriminate axonal and somatic damage was discussed above. This section proposes criteria for discriminating primary from secondary effects, using the spatial patterns and temporal sequences of degeneration that are revealed with suppressive silver methods.

### 4.2.1. Primary Degeneration

An essential characteristic of primary degeneration is that the timing of the degenerative changes must be prior to any other degenerative (or non-neuronal pathologic) changes in that region of the neuroaxis, either in the susceptible population of neurons or in its afferent sources or efferent targets. A site of primary degeneration may be the somatodendritic or axonal compartment of neurons. It is of interest to note that primary degeneration reflects both the *local actions* of a toxin, its metabolites, and/or related pathophysiologic processes, and the *Wallerian degeneration* of the axon distal to the damage. For example, the toxic actions of ibotenic acid are mediated by somatodendritic excitatory amino acid receptors; therefore, its toxic effects can be termed *primary somatogenic degeneration,* with the anterograde (Wallerian) degeneration of the axon resulting from damage to the soma. By contrast, DSP-4 destroys locus coeruleus axons without affecting the cell bodies; this pattern of degeneration can be termed *primary axogenic degeneration,* i.e., local and Wallerian. However, it is entirely conceivable that an axogenic pattern of degeneration can produce secondary retrograde degeneration of parent somata, followed by indirect Wallerian degeneration of the remainder of the axon. Each of these patterns, though, can be distinguished in principle by suppressive silver stains, by simply observing the temporal sequence of somatic and axonal reactions to a neurotoxin across a series of survival times.

A consistent picture of the characteristic features and time course of primary somatogenic degenerative changes has emerged from suppressive silver staining studies of the actions of 3-AP and TMT (Balaban, 1985; Balaban et al., 1988a; Desclin and Escubi, 1974). The initial changes appear as fine, spherical argyrophilic deposits in the dendrites and somata of affected neurons. The argyrophilic changes evolve over a period of about 1 day, resulting in dense silver deposits outlining large portions of the somata and punctate dendritic staining. This acute degenerative phase is typically best for displaying somato-dendritic morphology of affected neurons, since Golgi-like silver impregnations of degenerating neurons are most frequently encountered at this stage. Fine axon terminal degeneration typically accompanies the development of somatodendritic degeneration, and the axonal argyrophilia progresses to include the main axonal shaft within about 1 day of the maximum somatodendritic reaction. The argyrophilic deposits typically become more punctate in both the somatodendritic and axonal regions after the acute degenerative phase; silver staining usually disappears within 10 days of the initial degenerative changes.

It is important to note that the absolute time course of suppressive silver staining of somatogenic degeneration seems to vary with both the neurotoxin employed and the cell populations involved. The differences in the relative time courses of degeneration after 3-AP and TMT intoxication are examples of this phenomenon. The toxic effects of 3-AP are detectable within 6–7 hr of intoxication with silver staining methods, and climbing fiber degeneration in the cerebellar cortex disappears within 48 hr of toxin administration (Balaban, 1985; Desclin and Escubi, 1974). Since deoxyglucose uptake studies suggest that the metabolic effects of 3-AP are manifest in the inferior olive within 1.25 hr of intoxication (Bardin et al., 1983), this implies a temporal resolution of at least 5 hr for the cupric–silver method. By contrast, the first effects of TMT appear in the septum 1 day after intoxication; additional populations of degenerating neurons appear 2–4 days after treatment. Furthermore, the period of appearance to degenerating axon terminals varies with the pathway involved; for example, colliculo-thalamic degeneration persists through at least day 7, showing an expansion to the ventral lateral geniculate body (Balaban et al., 1988a). This variability in the absolute time course of primary degeneration probably reflects both factors associated with the toxin (e.g., distribution, metabolism, and intracellular mechanisms of action) and the well-established observation that Wallerian degenerations of different neuronal pathways proceed at different rates (De Olmos et al., 1981; Heimer, 1969). Thus, it is critical to utilize a wide range of survival times in studies of neurotoxicity to span the temporal range of action of the compound in question.

Amphetamine, methamphetamine, and N,N-dimethylamphetamine are examples of neurotoxins that appear to induce primary axogenic degeneration. Evidence for primary axogenic degeneration is twofold: (1) Only axons degenerate and (2) the degeneration appears at either early survival times or prior to degeneration of structures or pathways related to the axons. Ricaurte et al. (1982, 1984, 1989) reported only terminal degeneration in the striatum at short survival times in rats exposed to these toxins. This was in sharp contrast to the effects of MPTP (Ricaurte et al., 1987) and 6-OHDA (Hedreen and Chalmers, 1972), which produced concomitant somatic and axonal degeneration. Silver stains should also identify primary axogenic degeneration in the phenomenon termed *central-peripheral distal axonopathy* (Spencer and Schaumburg, 1984), since axons degenerate and cell bodies are spared.

## 4.2.2. Secondary Degeneration

Secondary degeneration can be defined as any neuronal degeneration that does not develop strictly as a direct action of a toxin; i.e., it develops as a secondary consequence of a direct action at another site. Since retrograde and transneuronal degenerative reactions to primary cell loss are the major potential source of secondary degeneration after exposure to neurotoxins, the possibility of confounding secondary effects of toxins cannot be overlooked. This is particularly true in neural circuits where transneuronal degeneration has been documented, such as the retinogeniculocortical system, the central auditory system, the piriform lobe, and limbic circuits (Cowan, 1970; Heimer and Kalil, 1978). Given the increased severity of transneuronal degeneration in young animals (Brodal, 1940; Cowan, 1970; Gudden, 1870), these effects are also a major concern in interpreting age-related changes in cell death after toxin exposure. It is important to note that, in contrast to primary degeneration reflecting anterograde (Wallerian) degenerative phenomena, secondary effects result from retrograde (indirect Wallerian) and transneuronal degenerative phenomena. Thus, potential secondary effects can be identified by criteria developed in basic studies of retrograde and transneuronal degeneration.

Retrograde degeneration is characterized by the criteria discussed by van Gehuchten (1903) and Cowan and Powell (1964): Distal regions of the axon will generate initially, followed in sequence by degeneration of the soma, and finally, by degeneration of the intervening axonal process. To our knowledge, there is no unequivocal example of retrograde degeneration in the neurotoxicologic studies employing silver staining methods. However, since it is a clearly documented consequence of axonal damage in selected cell populations (e.g., inferior olive, lateral geniculate nucleus, dorsomedial thalamic nucleus, ventral tier nuclei of the thalamus), it must be considered as a possible factor in neurotoxic degeneration studies if axonal degeneration precedes somatic damage.

Criteria for identifying transneuronal effects of neurotoxins are also straightforward. The hallmark of anterograde transneuronal degeneration is the appearance of afferent terminal degeneration around cell bodies prior to the initial signs of somatic degeneration. It is important to emphasize that the relative time frame of appearance is the essential criterion, for example, anterograde transneuronal degeneration develops in the olfactory cortex 1 day after olfactory bulb section (Heimer and Kalil, 1978). By contrast, retrograde transneuronal degeneration is suspected if a population of neurons degenerates after its efferent target cells die. Inspection of the TMT data reveals at least three potential sites for transneuronal effects: the central auditory system, amygdala, and dorsal division of the lateral septal nucleus. In the auditory system, degenerating neurons were observed only in the pericentral, dorsal, and external cortical nuclei of the inferior colliculus on days 2–4 after TMT administration, followed on days 5–7 by development of both terminal and somatic degeneration in the medial geniculate nucleus and cellular degeneration in the dorsal cochlear nucleus (Balaban *et al.*, 1988a). This is suggestive of transneuronal degeneration in the latter regions. Similarly, degeneration in the basolateral, anterior cortical, and posterolateral cortical amygdaloid nuclei developed on days 5–7, after dense terminal degeneration appeared in those regions; this is consistent with a transneuronal effect. Finally, in the septum, the probable primary degenerative events were observed on day 1 in the ventral and intermediate divisions of the lateral septal nucleus. Hippocampal and septal degeneration intensified on days 2–4, and by day 5 a dense terminal field containing degenerating somata developed in the dorsal division of the lateral septal nucleus. These findings raise the possibility that transneuronal degeneration is a factor in the effects of neurotoxins. In particular, they demonstrate the value of suppressive silver stains in identifying potential sites of secondary degeneration after neurotoxin treatment.

The prolonged time course of TMT-induced degeneration in the entorhinal cortex and hippocampal formation is an example of a phenomenon that cannot be resolved into a series of primary and secondary events by morphologic methods. The evolution of massive somatodendritic and axonal degeneration in the entorhinal cortex, septum, CA fields, hippocampus, subiculum, and postsubiculum was described previously in detail (Balaban *et al.*, 1988a). When faced with this type of massive progressive cell death over a period of 7 days after intoxication, it is impossible to distinguish the effects of the toxin alone, transneuronal degenerative factors alone, secondary responses to massive local necrosis, and interactions between these factors. The potential involvement of transneuronal degeneration is of particular concern because administration of TMT during the early postnatal period in rats (postnatal day 5) results in greater degeneration and gross atrophy of the hippocampal formation than in adult animals (Miller and O'Callaghan, 1984); this is consistent with the higher susceptibility of young animals to transneuronal atrophy and degeneration (Cowan, 1970; Gudden, 1870). Despite these limitations in data interpretation, it is noteworthy that the morphologic data establish the appropriate cell populations, experimental context, and hypotheses for applying in vitro and in vivo preparations to identify primary and secondary effects that produce massive, progressive degeneration.

## 5. SUMMARY: THE ROLE OF SUPPRESSIVE SILVER STAINS IN TOXIN ASSESSMENT

Suppressive silver degeneration stains (such as the cupric–silver stain) are particularly suitable as a first-line screening procedure for identifying the time course and location of degenerating neuronal somata, dendrites, and axons in the central nervous system. The primary advantage of these methods is the positive visualization of all processes of degenerating neurons. Since these methods simultaneously display somatic, dendritic, and axonal degeneration, one can determine whether an effect is restricted to axons or involves the somatodendritic compartment as well. These morphologic data also provide a positive identification of affected cells on the basis of morphology and connectivity. By utilizing a wide range of survival times, the spatio-temporal distribution of degeneration can both pinpoint affected neuronal populations and, in many cases, can discriminate potential primary and secondary effects of the neurotoxin. This has proven useful in assessing both dose-response effects and the efficacy of countermeasures that attenuate or prevent toxicity (Balaban, 1985; Balaban *et al.*, 1988b,c, 1990; Ricaurte *et al.*, 1982, 1984, 1987, 1989). Thus, studies with silver degeneration stains provide the framework for quantitative and mechanistic studies by identifying the appropriate time frame(s), neural site(s), and potential primary and secondary sequelae for detailed investigation with morphometric and biochemical methods.

In addition to traditional neurochemical and morphometric investigations (Deutsch *et al.*, 1989, 1990), first-line screening with the cupric–silver method has been useful in the application of subtractive hybridization technology to identify mRNAs that distinguish neurons destroyed by selective neurotoxins. Krady *et al.* (1990) isolated rare mRNAs that are characteristic of TMT-intoxicated neurons by subtracting mRNAs from TMT-treated rats (survival time: 7 days) from a normal rat-brain cDNA library. There was a close correspondence between the patterns of in situ hybridization of two unique cDNA clones in normal rat brain and the distribution of degenerating neurons in cupric–silver-stained sections, which suggested that specific mRNAs may be characteristic of neurons susceptible to TMT intoxication. Thus, suppressive silver stains can also provide a benchmark for identifying gene products that characterize neuronal populations affected by particular neurotoxins.

## REFERENCES

Balaban, C.D., 1985, Central neurotoxic effects of intraperitoneally administered 3-acetylpyridine, harmaline and niacinamide in Sprague-Dawley and Long-Evans rats: A critical review of central 3-acetylpyridine neurotoxicity, *Brain Res. Rev.* 9:21–42.

Balaban, C.D., O'Callaghan, J.P., and Billingsley, M.L., 1988a, Trimethyltin-induced neuronal damage in the rat brain: Comparative studies using silver degeneration stains, immunocytochemistry and immunoassay for neuronotypic and gliotypic proteins, *Neuroscience* 26:337–361.

Balaban, C.D., Fredericks, D.A., Wurpel, J.N.D., and Severs, W.B., 1988b, Motor disturbances and neurotoxicity induced by centrally administered somatostatin and vasopressin in conscious rats: Interactive effects of two neuropeptides, *Brain Res.* 445:117–129.

Balaban, C.D., Roskams, A.-J., and Severs, W.B., 1988c, Diazepam attenuation of somatostatin-induced motor disturbances and neurotoxicity, *Brain Res.* 458:91–96.

Bardin, J.M., Batini, C., Billiard, J.M., Buisseret-Delmas, C., Conrath-Verrier, M., and Corvaja, N., 1983, Cerebellar output regulation by the climbing and mossy fibers with and without the inferior olive, *J. Comp. Neurol.* 213:464–477.

Bodian, D.A., 1936, New method for staining nerve fibers and nerve endings in mounted paraffin sections, *Anat. Rec.* 65:89–97.

Brodal, A. 1940, Modification of Gudden method for study of cerebral localization, *AMA Arch. Neurol. Psychiatr.* 43:46–58.

Cammermeyer, J., 1963, Peripheral chromatolysis after transection of mouse facial nerve, *Acta Neuropathol.* 2:213–236.

Carlsen, J., and De Olmos, J.S., 1981, A modified cupric-silver technique for the impregnation of degenerating neurons and their processes, *Brain Res.* 208:426–431.

Charcot, J.M., 1876, *Leçons sur les Localisations dan les Maladies du Cerveau*, Adrian Delahaye, Paris.

Cowan, W.M., 1970, Anterograde and retrograde transneuronal degeneration in the central and peripheral nervous system, in: *Contemporary Research Methods in Neuroanatomy* (W.J.H. Nauta, S.O.E. Ebbesson, eds.), Springer, Berlin, pp. 217–251.

De Olmos, J.S., 1972, A cupric-silver method for impregnation of terminal axon degeneration and its further use in staining granular argyrophilic neurons, *Brain Behav. Evol.* 2:213–237.

De Olmos, J.S., and Ingram, W.R., 1972, An improved cupric-silver method for impregnation of axonal and terminal degeneration, *Brain Res.* 33:523–529.

De Olmos, J.S., Ebbesson, S.O.E., and Heimer, L., 1981, Silver methods for impregnation of degenerating axoplasm, in: *Neuroanatomical Tract-Tracing Methods* (L. Heimer and M.J. Robards, eds.), Plenum Press, New York, pp. 117–170.

Desclin, J.C., and Escubi, J., 1974, Effects of 3-acetylpyridine on the central nervous system of the rat, as demonstrated by silver methods, *Brain Res.* 77:349–364.

Deutsch, A., Rosin, D.L., Goldstein, M., and Roth, R.H., 1989, 3-Acetylpyridine-induced degeneration of the nigrostriatal dopamine system: An animal model of olivopontocerebelar atrophy-associated Parkinson's disease, *Exp. Neurol.* 105:1–9.

Deutsch, A., Elsworth, J.D., Roth, R.H., and Goldstein, M., 1990, 3-Acetylpyridine results in degeneration of the extrapyramidal and cerebellar motor systems: Loss of the dorsolateral striatal dopamine innervation, *Brain Res.* 527:96–102.

Fink, R.P., and Heimer, L., 1967, Two methods for selective silver impregnation of degenerating axons and their synaptic endings in the central nervous system, *Brain Res.* 4:369–374.

Forel, A., 1887, Einige hirnanatomische Betruchtungen und Ergebnisse, *Arch. Psychiat. Nervenkr.* 12:162–198.

Fritschy, J.-M., and Grzanna, R., 1989, Immunocytochemical analysis of the neurotoxic effects of DSP-4 identifies two populations of noradrenergic terminals, *Neurosciences* 30:181–197.

Glees, P., 1946, Terminal degeneration within the central nervous system as studied by a new silver method, *J. Neuropath. Exp. Neurol.* 5:54–59.

Glees, P., and Le Gros Clark, W.E., 1941, The termination of optic fibers in the lateral geniculate body of the monkey, *J. Anat. (London)* 75:295–309.

Glees, P., and Nauta, W.J.H., 1955, A critical review of studies on axonal and terminal degeneration, *Monat. Psychiat. Neurol.* 129:73–91.

Grant, G., 1968, Silver impregnation of degenerating dendrites, cells and axons central to axonal transection. II. A Nauta study on spinal motor neurons in kittens, *Exp. Brain Res.* 6:284–293.

Grant, G., 1970, Neuronal changes central to the site of axon transection. A method for the identification of retrograde changes in perikarya, dendrites and axons by silver impregnation, in: *Contemporary Research Methods in Neuroanatomy* (W.J.H. Nauta and S.O.E. Ebbesson, eds.), Springer, Berlin, pp. 173–185.

Grant, G., 1975, Retrograde neuronal degeneration, in: *Golgi Centennial Symposium, Proceedings* (M. Santini, ed.), Raven Press, New York, pp. 195–200.

Grant, G., and Aldskogius, H., 1967, Silver impregnation of degenerating dendrites, cells and axons central to axonal transection. I. A Nauta study on the hypoglossal nerve, *Exp. Brain Res.* 3:150–162.

Grant, G., and Walberg, F., 1979, The light and electron microscopical appearance of anterograde and retrograde neuronal degeneration, in: *Dynamics of Degeneration and Growth in Neurons* (K. Faye, L. Olson, and Y. Zotterman, eds.), Pergamon Press, Oxford, pp. 5–18.

Grant, G., and Westman, J., 1969, The lateral cervical nucleus in the cat. IV. A light and electron microscopical study after midbrain lesions with demonstration of indirect Wallerian degeneration at the ultra-structural level, *Exp. Brain Res.* 7:51–67.

Gudden, B. von, 1870, Experimentaluntersuchungen Über das peripherische und centrale Nervensystem, *Arch. Psychiat. Nervenkr.* 2:693–723.

Guillery, R.W., 1959, Afferent fibers to the dorsomedial thalamic nucleus in the cat, *J. Anat. (London)* 93:403–419.

Hedreen, J.C., and Chalmers, J.P., 1972, Neuronal degeneration in rat brain induced by 6-hydroxydopamine: A histological and biochemical study, *Brain Res.* 47:1–36.

Heimer, L., 1970, Selective silver-impregnation of degenerating axoplasm, in: *Contemporary Research Methods in Neuroanatomy* (W.J.H. Nauta and S.O.E. Ebbesson, eds.), Springer, Berlin, pp. 106–131.

Heimer, L., and Kalil, R., 1978, Rapid transneuronal degeneration and death of cortical neurons following removal of the olfactory bulb in adult rats, *J. Comp. Neurol.* 178:559–609.

Heimer, L., and Peters, A., 1968, An electron microscopic study of a silver stain for degenerating boutons, *Brain Res.* 8:337–346.

Hoff, E.C., 1932, Degeneration of boutons terminaux in the spinal cord, *J. Physiol. (London)* 74:4P–5P.

Holmes, G., and Stewart, T.G., 1908, On the connection of the inferior olives with the cerebellum in man, *Brain* 31:125–137.

Holmes, W., 1943, Silver staining of nerve axons in paraffin sections, *Anat. Rec.* 86:157–187.

Ito, M., Jastreboff, P., and Miyashita, Y., 1980, Retrograde influence of surgical and chemical flocculectomy upon dorsal cap neurons of the inferior olive, *Neurosci. Lett.* 20:45–48.

Jensen, K.F., Miller, D.B., Olin, J.K., and O'Callaghan, J.P., 1990, Evidence for the neurotoxicity of methylenedioxymethamphetamine (MDMA) using a cupric-silver stain for neuronal degeneration, *Neurosci Abst.* 16:256.

Krady, J.K., Oyler, G.A., Balaban, C.D., and Billingsley, M.L., 1990, Use of subtractive hybridization to characterize mRNA common to neurons destroyed by the selective neurotoxicant trimethyltin, *Mol. Brain Res.* 7:287–297.

La Velle, A., and La Velle, F., 1958, Neuronal swelling and chromatolysis as influenced by the state of cell development, *Am. J. Anat.* 102:219–241.

Lieberman, A.R., 1971, The axon reaction: A review of the principal features of perikaryal responses to axon injury, *Int. Rev. Neurobiol.* 14:49–124.

Lieberman, A.R., 1974, Some factors affecting retrograde neuronal responses to axonal loss, in: *Essays on the Nervous System: A Festschrift for Professor J.Z. Young* (R. Bellairs and E.G. Gray, eds.), Clarendon Press, Oxford, pp. 71–105.

Marchi, V., 1891, Sull'origine e decorso dei peduncoli cerebellari, *R. Istituto di Studi Superiori e di Perfezionamento in Firenze*, LeMonnier, Firenze, pp. 1–38.

Miller, D.B., and O'Callaghan, J.P., 1984, Biochemical, functional and morphological indicators of neurotoxicity: Effects of acute administration of trimethyltin to the developing rat, *J. Pharmacol. Exp. Ther.* 231:744–751.

Monakow, C. von, 1882, Weitere Mittheilungen Über durch Exstirpation circumscripter Hirnrindenregionen bedingte Entwickelungschemmungen des Kaninchengehirns, *Arch. Psychiat. Nervenkr.* 12:535–549.

Nauta, W.J.H., 1957, Silver impregnation of degenerating axons, in: *New Research Techniques of Neuroanatomy* (W. Windle, ed.), Charles C. Thomas, Springfield, IL, pp. 17–26.

Nauta, W.J.H., and Gygax, P.A., 1951, Silver impregnation of degenerating axon terminals in the central nervous system. 1. Technique, 2. Chemical notes, *Stain Tech.* 26:5–11.

Nauta, W.J.H., and Gygax, P.A., 1954, Silver impregnation of degenerating axons in the central nervous system: A modified technique, *Stain Tech.* 29:91–93.

Nissl, F., 1892, Ueber die Veränderungen der Ganglionzellen an Facialiskern des Kaninchens nach Ausreissung der Nerven, *Allg. Z. Psychiat. Psych.-gerichtliche Med.* 48:197–198.

Pitres, A., 1884, Recherches anatomo-cliniques sur les scléroses bilatérales del la moelle épinière consécutives a des lésions unilatérales du cerveau, *Arch. Physiol. Norm. Pathol.* 3:142–185.

Potter, H.D., 1975, Distribution and dynamic properties of neurofibrils, in: *Golgi Centennial Symposium, Proceedings* (M. Santini, ed.), Raven Press, New York, pp. 167–175.

Powell, T.P.S., and Cowan, W.M., 1964, A note on retrograde fiber degeneration, *J. Anat. (London)* 98:579–585.

Ricaurte, G.A., Guillery, R.W., Seiden, L.S., Schuster, C.R., and Moore, R.Y., 1982, Dopamine nerve terminal degeneration produced by high doses of methylamphetamine in the rat brain, *Brain Res.* 235:93–103.

Ricaurte, G.A., Seiden, L.S., and Schuster, C.R., 1984, Further evidence that amphetamines produce long-lasting dopamine neurochemical deficits by destroying dopamine nerve fibers, *Brain Res.* 303:359–364.

Ricaurte, G.A., Irwin, I., Forno, L.S., DeLanney, L.E., Langston, E., and Langston, J.W., 1987, Aging and 1-methyl-4-phenyl-1,2,3,6-tetrahydropyridine-induced degeneration of dopaminergic neurons in substantia nigra, *Brain Res.* 403:43–51.

Ricaurte, G.A., DeLanney, L.E., Irwin, I., Witkin, J.M., Katz, J.J., and Langston, J.W., 1989, Evaluation of the neurotoxic potential of N,N-dimethylamphetamine: An illicit analog of methamphetamine, *Brain Res.* 490:301–306.

Sayre, L.M., 1989, Biochemical mechanism of action of the dopaminergic neruotoxin 1-methyl-4-phenyl-1,2,3,6-tetrahydropyridine (MPTP), *Toxicol. Lett.* 48:121–149.

Scallet, A.C., Lipe, G.W., Ali, S.F., Holson, R.R., Frith, C.H., and Slikker, W. Jr., 1988, Neuropathologic evaluation by combined immunohistochemistry and degeneration-specific methods: Application to methylenedioxymethamphetamine, *NeuroToxicology* 9:529–538.

Soury, J., 1899, *Le Système Nerveux Central: Structure et Fonctions, Histoire Critique des Théories et des Doctrines*, Masson, Paris, pp. 1695–1706.

Spencer, P.S., and Schaumberg, H.H., 1984, An expanded classification of neurotoxic responses based on cellular targets of chemical agents, *Acta Neurol. Scand.* 70 (Suppl. 100):9–19.

Swank, R.L., and Davenport, H.A., 1934, Marchi's staining method: II. Fixation. *Stain Technol.* 9:129–135.

Switzer, R., 1991, Strategies for assessing neurotoxicity, *Neurosci. Biobehav. Rev.* 15:21–33.

Tanaka, D., Jr., and Bursian, S.J., 1989, Degeneration patterns in the chicken central nervous system induced by ingestion of the organophosphorus delayed neurotoxin tri-ortho-tolyl phosphate. A silver impregnation study, *Brain Res.* 484(1–2):240–256.

Tanaka, D., Jr., Bursian, S.J., and Lehning, E., 1990, Selective axonal and terminal degeneration in the chicken brainstem and cerebellum following exposure to bis(1-methylethyl)phosphorofluoridate (DFP), *Brain Res.* 519(1–2):200–208.

Tanaka, D., Jr., Bursian, S.J., Lehning, E.J., and Aulerich, R.J., 1990, Exposure to triphenyl phosphite results in widespread degeneration in the mammalian central nervous system, *Brain Res.* 531(1–2):294–298.

van Gehuchten, A., 1903, La dégénérescence dite rétrograde ou dégénérescence Wallérienne indirecte, Nèvraxe 5:1–107.

Vulpian, A., 1866, *Leçons sur la Physiologie Générale et Comparée du Système Nerveux faites au Muséum d'Histoire Naturelle G.*, Ballière, Paris, pp. 237–251.

Walberg, F., 1971, Does silver impregnate normal and degenerating boutons? A study based upon light and electron microscopical observations of the inferior olive, *Brain Res.* 31:47–65.

Walberg, F., 1972, Further studies on silver impregnation of normal and degenerating boutons. A light and electron microscopical investigation of a filamentous degenerating system, *Brain Res.* 36:353–369.

Walker, A.E., 1938, *The Primate Thalamus*, University of Chicago Press, Chicago.

Waller, A., 1850, Experiments on the section of the glossophayngeal and hypoglossal nerves of the frog, and observations of the alterations produced thereby in the structure of their primitive fibers, *Phil. Trans. R. Soc. Lond.* 140:423–409.

Whittington, D.L., Woodruff, M.L., and Baisden, R.H., 1989, The time course of trimethyltin-induced fiber and terminal degeneration in hippocampus, *Neurotoxicol. Teratol.* 11:21–33.

Chapter 11

# Caveats in Hazard Assessment

## Stress and Neurotoxicity

*Diane B. Miller*

## 1. INTRODUCTION AND OVERVIEW

A primary aim of neurotoxicology is to identify agents that impact directly on the nervous system with the ultimate goal of identifying any adverse effects associated with exposure (EPA, 1985; Maurissen and Mattsson, 1989; Reiter, 1978; WHO, 1986). Behavioral, biochemical, electrophysiological, and morphological indicators are all suggested as appropriate means for detecting neurotoxicity (Annau, 1986; DeHaven and Mailman, 1983, 1986; Dyer, 1985; Mattson and Albee, 1988; Miller and Eckerman, 1986; Moser, 1989; O'Callaghan and Miller, 1983; Ross, 1989; Sette, 1989; Spencer and Schaumburg, 1980; Weiss, 1988). Several authors have noted the ways stress can impact on measurements in both pharmacology and toxicology (Pakes, 1990; Rowan, 1990; Vogel, 1987). Interactions between stress and toxicity have been a topic of lively debate in teratology for some time. It has been speculated that certain anomalies produced at a maternally toxic dose of an agent may be due to nonspecific stress (Chernoff *et al.*, 1987, 1989; Khera, 1984).

Although some researchers have expressed concern that systemic toxicity can interfere with neurotoxicity assessment, the interactions between stress and neurotoxicity have not been systematically addressed (Diener, 1987; Gerber and O'Shaughnessy, 1986). Consequently, a general review of the impact of stress or adrenal-axis perturbations on neurotoxicity is not available. This chapter will illustrate how damage to, chemically induced alterations in the secretions of, or activation of the adrenal axis may impact on the endpoints used to assess neurotoxicity. However, it will not exhaustively catalogue all possible interactions between neurotoxicology endpoints and adrenal-axis perturbation.

---

*Diane B. Miller* • Neurotoxicology Division, U.S. Environmental Protection Agency, Research Triangle Park, North Carolina 27711.
*The Vulnerable Brain and Environmental Risks, Volume 1: Malnutrition and Hazard Assessment,* edited by Robert L. Isaacson and Karl F. Jensen. Plenum Press, New York, 1992.

Rather, the intent is to make investigators aware that such interactions occur and may alter their assessment of neurotoxic potential.

In a broad sense *stress* is any change in the organism's environment that disturbs homeostasis. The resulting series of neural and endocrine adaptations are commonly referred to as the *stress response* or *stress cascade*. A *stressor*, broadly defined in an operational sense, is any manipulation capable of disturbing homeostasis. Many of the procedures utilized in the collection of data in toxicology would qualify as stressors using this definition (Table 1). The cascade functions to return the body to homeostasis (Munck et al., 1984; Sapolsky, 1987). One consequence of the release of substances in the stress cascade is an elevation in blood glucose, providing body tissue with the fuel necessary for the increased metabolic demands of an emergency situation. The necessity of the cascade is illustrated by the devastating consequences of stress in individuals suffering from adrenal insufficiency (Addisonian crisis). Symptoms can include confusion, lethargy, and circulatory collapse, followed by death (Forsham, 1968). Prolonged elevations in glucocorticoids also have disturbing consequences and include immunosuppression, osteoporosis, muscle wasting, and steroid diabetes (Forsham, 1968; von Zerssen, 1976).

Most readers will know glucocorticoids are released from the cortex of the adrenal gland as part of the stress cascade (Fig. 1). Corticosterone is the principal glucocorticoid in rodents, while cortisol serves this function in primates, hamsters, and cats. The glucocorticoids have been called carbohydrate-active steroids because of their involvement in carbohydrate metabolism and the mobilization of energy stores. This is in contrast to the role of mineralecorticoids in electrolyte balance. Other components of this negative feedback system are secretions from the adrenal medulla (catecholamines and enkephalins), pituitary [adrenocorticotropin hormone (ACTH) and beta-endorphin], and hypothalamus [corticotropin releasing factor (CRF) and vasopressin], and their actions on the hippocampus (Feldman and Conforti, 1980; Sapolsky et al., 1986). Damage to or interference at any level of the axis will influence the other components because of the reciprocal feedback arrangement. For example, consistent absence of glucocorticoids due to removal or damage of the adrenals or the inhibition of stereoidogenesis results in a

**TABLE 1.** Stress Inducers in Toxicology

Dosing
    Route
        • Inhalation (e.g., nose only)
        • Dermal (e.g., jackets)
        • Gavage (e.g., inexperienced person)
    Maximal tolerated dose (MTD)

Deprivation
    Food or water
    Maternal

Restraint
    For dosing
    For monitoring

Housing conditions
    Group
    Single

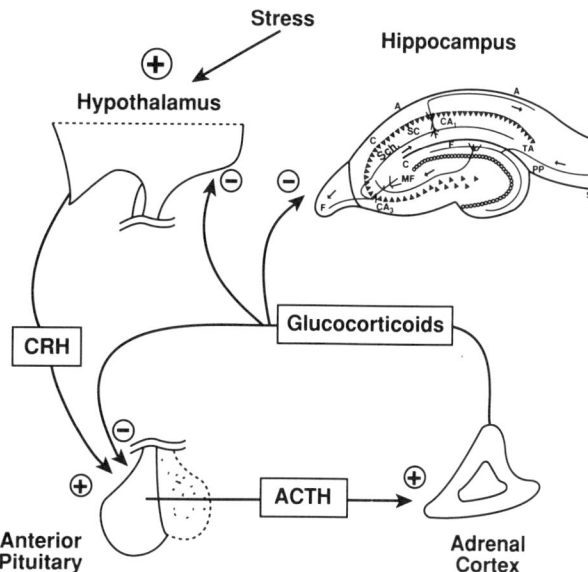

**FIGURE 1.** Schematic of the stress cascade. Adapted from Colby (1988).

compensatory increase in ACTH. The adrenal responds to continued stimulation by ACTH with hyperemia, hypertrophy, and cell proliferation, resulting in a size/weight increase (Pudney *et al.*, 1984). Additionally a number of brain areas, as well as both the adrenal cortex and medulla, are important in coordinating the body's response to the alterations in homeostasis considered under the general heading of stress. Many substances representative of diverse chemical classes (Table 2) can affect the adrenal gland, resulting either in frank damage and a diminution in adrenal hormone secretion or a sustained activation and a resultant increase in the circulating levels of its products (Colby, 1988). The adrenal cortex is well vascularized, providing for easy access of toxicants to

**TABLE 2.** Compounds Producing Lesions in the Adrenal Cortex

| | | |
|---|---|---|
| Acrylonitrile | 7,12-Dimethylbenzanthracene | Polyglutamic acids |
| ACTH | Estrogens | Pyrazole |
| Aflatoxin | Ethanol | Spironolactone |
| Aminoglutethimide | Etomidate | Sulfated mucopolysaccharides |
| Aniline | Fluphenazine | Suramin |
| Carbon tetrachloride | Hexadimetherine bromide | Tamoxifen |
| Chenodeoxycholic acid | Iprindole | Tetrachlorvinphos |
| Chloroform | Ketoconazole | Testosterone |
| Chlorphentermine | Mefloquine | Thioacetamide |
| Clotrimazole | Methanol | Thioguanine |
| Cyproterone | Nitrogen oxides | Toxaphene |
| *op'*-DDD | Parathion | Triparanol |
| Danazol | PBBs, PCBs | Urethane |
| Dilantin | Polyanthosulfonage + aminocaprionic acid | Zimelidine |

From H.D. Colby (1988).

this site (Pudney et al., 1984). One survey (Ribelin, 1984) determined the adrenal to be one of the more vulnerable endocrine glands to toxic insult. Over 90% of the citations concerning toxic damage to endocrine organs consisted of morphological changes or lesions in adrenal gland and testis. The adrenal cortex, responsible for the production of glucocorticoids as well as mineralocorticoids, androgens, and estrogens, was most often affected. Separate zones of the cortex are responsible for these products. This zonation and the complicated negative-feedback control of this endocrine gland may also account for toxic susceptibility. In addition to the central role of the adrenal gland and its secretions during stress, many neuroscientists have come to appreciate the role the adrenal plays in the maintenance of both nervous system function and structure; that is, secretions from the adrenal may serve both a tonic and a regulatory role in the brain, as well as other body systems (Akana et al., 1985; Bohn, 1984; Bohus et al., 1982; Devenport and Devenport, 1983; Henkin, 1970; McEwen et al., 1986; Meyer, 1985; Munck et al., 1984; Sapolsky and Pulsinelli, 1985; Sloviter, 1989). Thus, the regulatory and tonic functions of the adrenal, its vulnerability to toxic insult, and its feedback loops with various brain areas provide for several ways in which the adrenal axis can interact with neurotoxicity. The main focus of this review will be the possible impact of glucocorticoids on endpoints used in neurotoxicology. However, other substances associated with stress and/or the adrenal axis will be discussed when pertinent.

## 2. ADRENAL AXIS INTERACTION WITH BEHAVIORAL MEASURES

The effects of standard laboratory housing, dosing, and handling procedures on endpoints of interest to toxicologists have not been widely studied (Barclay et al., 1988; Brain and Benton, 1979; Gartner et al., 1980; Hirsjarvi and Junnila, 1986; Rowan, 1990). This data gap should be of particular interest to neurotoxicologists because of the demonstrated influence of the adrenal axis on the many behavioral endpoints used for neurotoxicity assessment. For example, the monitoring of motor activity following toxicant exposure has been identified as an method appropriate for the detection of neurotoxicity (EPA, 1985), although the usefulness of this endpoint for this purpose has been questioned (Maurissen and Mattsson, 1989). Placing a rat in a novel environment evokes arousal and activation of the pituitary-adrenal axis (Bohus et al., 1982). The observed increases in locomotor activity may be directly related to release of CRF, the hypothalamic peptide responsible for the release of ACTH from the pituitary (Koob and Bloom, 1985). Adrenalectomy reduces exploratory behavior in the rat, and this reduction appears to be directly related to the loss of corticosterone (Bohus et al., 1982; Veldhuis and De Kloet, 1983; Veldhuis et al., 1982). Extended treatment of adrenalectomized rats with corticosterone will elevate exploratory activity during certain portions of the light cycle (Micco et al., 1980). Various manipulations considered to be stressful (e.g., restraint, shock, type of housing, etc.) will alter exploratory activity in the rat and mouse (Berridge and Dunn, 1989; Katz and Caroll, 1977; Schaefer and Michael, 1991). Housing conditions can alter basal levels of activity and the subsequent acquisition of a learned response (Fig. 2) (Schaefer and Michael, 1991). Further, the behavioral response to such stressors appears to be strain dependent (Badiani and Castellano, 1991; Gentsch et al., 1982). Interestingly, Barclay and colleagues (1988) suggest the use of the "Disturbance Index" (basically movement in an open field) as a way of gauging distress in laboratory animals.

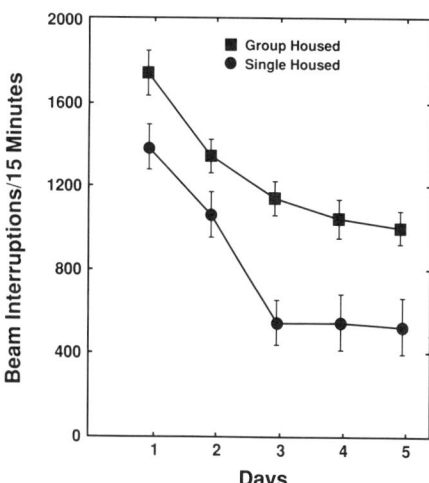

**FIGURE 2.** The role of housing in exploratory motor behavior of rats. Group-housed rats were significantly more active than single-housed rats and also acquired a bar-press response for brain stimulation more readily (not shown). From Schaefer and Michael (1991), with permission.

Such an approach should be viewed with caution because of the complexity of the evaluation of behavior in an open field (Maier et al., 1988).

The demand for increased neurotoxicity testing and attempts to evaluate neurotoxicity utilizing functional and physiological endpoints (EPA, 1985; Lochry, 1987; Moser, 1989) in conjunction with chronic and subchronic toxicity testing provide multiple opportunities for interactions with the adrenal axis. For example, many agents considered to be neurotoxic and/or neuroactive by definition activate the adrenal axis because of the key role of the hippocampus and hypothalamus in pituitary–adrenal function (Ally et al., 1986; Fischer, 1988; Fuller, 1981). In the general toxicology literature, there are many examples of interactions between toxicity and adrenal axis disturbances and a few demonstrations of interactions between neurotoxicants and stress (Lloyd and Franklin, 1991; Uphouse et al., 1982; Vogel, 1987). Brain damage, whether induced physically or by chemicals, is often accompanied by altered function. Thus, neurotoxicity testing strategies incorporating behavioral endpoints would be expected to easily detect such changes. What are considered to be fairly innocuous manipulations, such as daily handling, can alter or prevent the detection of damage when functional endpoints are employed (Fig. 3) (Tilson and Peterson, 1987). Note the daily handling episode altered the motor behavior of only those rats whose hippocampus was damaged with colchicine. Researchers should also not conclude that sham exposure conditions, such as ambient air in inhalation chambers (Cooper et al., 1990) or a series of daily saline injections, are innocuous (Flemmer and Dilsaver, 1989). It is not known if directly adrenotoxic agents or compounds capable of altering adrenal function (e.g., blocking of stereoidogenesis, etc.) (Colby, 1988) will affect the behavioral indices proposed for use in standard neurotoxicity testing. However, a possible role of the adrenal axis should be considered in the interpretation of data. Evidence of chronic adrenal axis activation, such as altered thymus or adrenal weight (Akana et al., 1985), would make such considerations mandatory.

The consequences of manipulations such as handling are also important to consider in developmental neurotoxicity assessment. The exposure of developing rodents to test chemicals often involves daily manipulation of the litter and dam. Some dosing protocols call for removal of the dam from the litter, such as in inhalation exposure procedures,

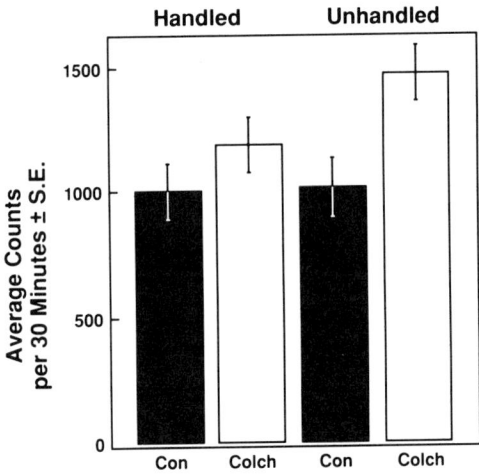

**FIGURE 3.** The effect of handling and a daily injection of saline on the hyperactivity associated with lesioning of the hippocampus with colchicine. From Tilson and Peterson (1987), with permission.

which can call for several hours of separation. The manipulation of litter composition and pup–dam interaction to provide undernourished control litters or to accommodate different dosing protocols (e.g., between- vs. within-litter dose-response assessment) can impact toxicity assessment. Many changes in neural and somatic development, as well as possible changes in the expression of neurotoxicity, can occur as a consequence of such manipulations (Hutchings, 1990; Ruppert et al., 1983; Tonkiss et al., 1988). Tonkiss and colleagues manipulated the litter and dam by several means to effect equivalent reductions in body growth. Despite equivalent body size, brain weights were decreased by differing amounts depending on the undernutrition regimen. Hofer (1978) has suggested the dam serves as a "hidden regulator" of pup physiology. Handling, dosing, and separation from the dam during the developmental period causes the release of glucocorticoids and beta-endorphins (Hennessy and Weinberg, 1990; Iny et al., 1987). It is speculated that many of the growth changes associated with maternal deprivation are not nutritional. Rather, they are mediated through the CNS actions of beta-endorphin; direct injection of this peptide into the CNS will produce the same effects (Greer et al., 1991). Only direct active contact of the dam (licking, etc.) with the rat pup prevents the release of beta-endorphin (Pauk et al., 1986), although corticosterone release can be suppressed by stimuli associated with the dam (e.g., contact with an anesthetized dam) (Stanton and Levine, 1990; Stanton et al., 1987). Simulated maternal contact can normalize early infant development in laboratory animals and humans (Field et al., 1986; Pauk et al., 1986).

Permanent dramatic alterations in the reactivity of the hypothalamic pituitary adrenal (HPA) axis accompany manipulations of the pup–dam relationship (Levine, 1957; Meany et al., 1988a, 1988b, 1989; Wakshlak and Weinstock, 1990). Further, handling in infancy can alter the later response to pharmacological agents throughout the life span (Larson, 1982; Pieretti et al., 1991; Weinberg et al., 1980). This may be important in circumstances where pharmacological challenge is utilized to "uncover" neurotoxic insult (Tilson, 1987; Walsh and Tilson, 1986; Zenick, 1983). Of course, the real concern is that manipulating the pup–dam relationship will alter the neurotoxicity of a suspect compound and cause an over- or underestimation of potency. However, little if any data exist on such interactions. Thus, if prolonged separation of the dam from the litter is necessary during exposure, it may be prudent to incorporate stimuli associated with the dam and home cage into the situation. Such stimuli could include the provision of a surrogate for the mother (e.g., anesthetized lactating rat) (Stanton and Levine, 1990), maintenance of ambient temperature at nest levels (Denenberg et al., 1967; Peters, 1988), and other manipulations designed to diminish the neuroendocrine and/or other responses of the offspring to separation and/or handling.

There are complex interactions between adrenal axis alterations and the scheduling of stressor presentations. A stressor is a stimulus and either habituation or sensitization can occur to it as it does for any other stimuli (Pitman et al., 1990). Thus, repeated exposure to the stressor does not guarantee a reduced secretion (i.e., habituation) of either adrenal gland substances or other substances associated with the stress cascade. The profile of response to repeated presentations of a stimulus (e.g., habituation, no change or sensitization) is related to the intensity of the stimulus (Thompson and Spencer, 1966). For example, frequent exposure to low-intensity stimuli will result in habituation of the glucocorticoid response, but decreasing the frequency of exposure to the same stimulus can result in no adaptation (Pitman et al., 1990). Frequent exposure to a high-intensity stimulus often results in no habituation and in some instances can result in a heightened response or sensitization (Fig. 4) (Konarska et al., 1989; Pitman et al., 1991). Classical conditioning may also play a role in adrenocortical responses exhibited after the repeated presentation of a stressor (Pitman et al., 1986; Stanton and Levine, 1988). It is somewhat problematic to predict the adaptation profiles of possible stressful manipulations employed in toxicology, because the knowledge concerning habituation to a stressor, etc. is based on the ability to alter systematically the stimulus characteristics of that stressor. Much of the data on the relationship between stimulus intensity and adaptation have been obtained with shock, a stimulus more easily quantified than those associated with the handling, housing, dosing, and testing of experimental animals. Few experimenters have attempted to quantify the homeostatic changes associated with the routine manipulations employed in toxicology [but see Rowland et al. (1990), regarding shipping stress and

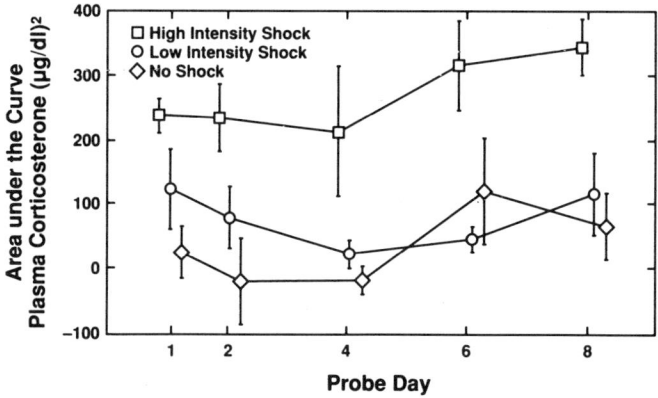

**FIGURE 4.** The profile of adaptation of the glucocorticoid response to a high-intensity and low-intensity stressor—shock. HS, LS, NS stand for high-intensity shock, low-intensity shock, and no shock, respectively. Note the HS group produces more corticosterone in response to shock on day 8 than day 1 (i.e., sensitization). From Pitman et al. (1990), with permission.

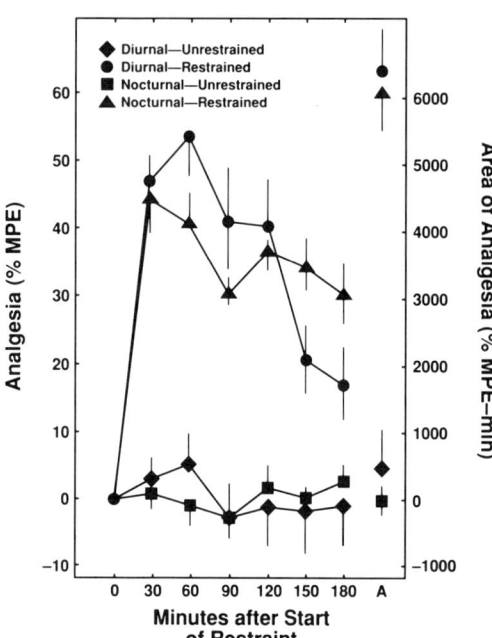

**FIGURE 5.** The effect of restraint on the time to respond to a heat stimulus by a tail-flick response (i.e., analgesia). Note that restraint greatly increases the time to respond to the stimulus; this phenomenon is referred to as stress-induced analgesia. From Miller (1988), with permission.

implantation of osmotic minipumps and Drozdowicz et al. (1990), concerning in-house transport stress]. Because stressors appear to obey the same rules concerning adaptation as other stimuli, it should be possible to gauge the intensity of the stimulation (i.e., stress) associated with many of the procedures used in a toxicological setting. For example, the adaptation profiles for either glucocorticoid or catecholamine secretions could be determined for these types of experimental manipulations as they have been for shock (Natelson et al., 1987). Decisions concerning the intensity of the stimulation associated with a particular manipulation would then be based on the type of adaptation profile obtained.

The restraint of experimental subjects for dosing and the subsequent collection of data and tissue samples is practiced in many areas of toxicology (Pakes, 1990; Wiester et al., 1987), including neurotoxicology (Boyes et al., 1990; Rebert, 1983). Restraint causes a number of physiological and biochemical changes, lasting for many hours (Berridge and Dunn, 1989; Jorgensen et al., 1984; Miller, 1988; Pittman et al., 1988). These can include alterations in body temperature, the levels of physiologically relevant substances, such as glucocorticoids, catecholamines, or endogenous opiates, and pain perception (Fig. 5). Often the degree of physiological alteration (i.e., stress) induced by a particular restraint or confinement procedure and a subsequent habituation to the procedure is inferred by visual inspection of the animal (Weister et al., 1987). Data from Bushnell and colleagues (Bushnell et al., 1979) concerning the pharmacokinetics of lead provide a cautionary note against such an assumption. Primates exposed to lead as infants and placed in unfamiliar test compartments as adults had elevated blood levels of both cortisol and lead. Bone serves as a reservoir for lead in the body, and glucocorticoids at physiological levels can stimulate calcium metabolism (Nishino et al., 1991), with subsequent demineralization

**TABLE 3.** Deprivation

| Treatment | n | Serum corticosterone (means ± SE, nmol/ml) |
|---|---|---|
| Saline (controls) | 19 | 283 ± 26 |
| Starved (24 hrs) | 9 | 746 ± 106[a] |
| Starved (48 hrs) | 11 | 1829 ± 173[a] |

[a]Significant difference ($p < 0.01$) from controls.
From Varma et al. (1988), with permission.

and release of lead. This work also cautions against visual inspection of experimental subjects as a way of determining "stress" levels, as the monkeys displayed normal eating and drinking patterns despite elevated cortisol levels (also see Holden, 1988 for a discussion of this issue in relation to primate research). Obviously, the mobilization of lead from bone stores by substances released during stress can have implications for the screening and evaluation of humans exposed to lead (Pounds et al., 1991).

Procedural manipulations other than handling and restraint may complicate the interpretation of toxicity data. It is a common practice in many areas of toxicology to restrict food availability or to remove food totally for at least 24 hr prior to dosing. An empty gastrointestinal tract facilitates the absorption of orally administered compounds. The circadian patterns of adrenal hormones in blood is partly regulated by food availability. Restricting the food intake of rodents to the morning period will result in high glucocorticoid levels during the morning; the peak elevation normally occurs during the evening (Gray et al., 1978). Food and water intake are closely linked, and the removal of food results in decreased water intake. Incorporation of toxicants into either food or water may also induce decreased intake of both due to taste aversions with a concomitant loss of body weight. Large increases in serum corticosteroid levels (Table 3) (Varma et al., 1988) accompany such manipulations. The role of glucocorticoids in the development of taste aversions is an area of intense research activity (Revusky and Martin, 1988; Revusky and Reilly, 1989; Rondeau et al., 1980). Altered food and water intake, intended or not, can impact on toxicity endpoints (Fig. 6) (Simmons et al., 1990). For a 2-week period rats were offered water containing a mixture of 25 groundwater chemicals at a low concentration. Both food and water intake declined, and a challenge dose of carbon tetrachloride results in significant liver damage. However, data from the group receiving restricted access to water make it apparent that the increased toxicity to carbon tetrachloride is due to the reduced food and/or water intake, rather than the chemical mixture exposure.

In neurotoxicology various schedules of food deprivation are necessary to maintain performance in a variety of learned tasks. Several authors have demonstrated complex interactions between the effects of food deprivation, various schedules of food, or shock motivation used in operant conditioning paradigms and the physiological/neuroendocrine alterations accompanying drug or toxicant exposure (Coveney et al., 1990; Valencia-Flores et al., 1990; Varma, 1988). For example, Valencia-Flores and colleagues showed d-amphetamine would induce drastic body-weight reductions (32.4% of controls) if rats were under chronic water restriction in combination with a schedule of operant water reinforcement involving brief foot shock. The adverse side effects of operant schedules have been noted (Brady and Harris, 1977). The authors theorize this operant schedule is

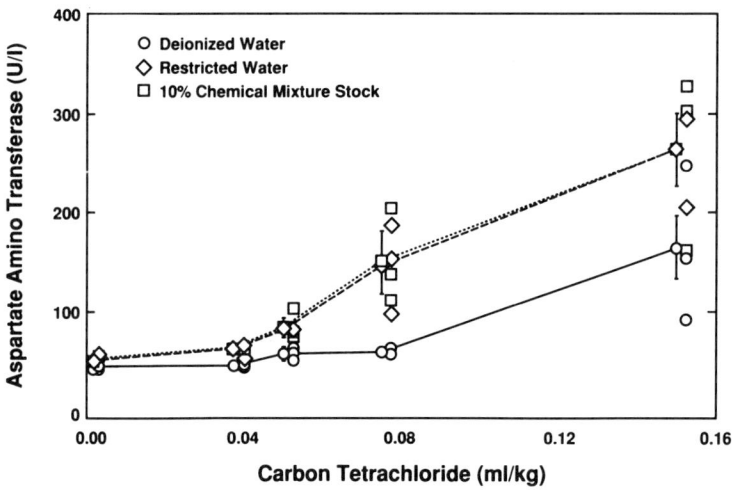

**FIGURE 6.** The effect of reduced food and water intake on the hepatotoxicity of carbon tetrachloride. Note the water-restricted and chemical-mixture group exhibit the same degree of liver toxicity as measured by a dose-related increase in the liver enzyme, aspartate amino transferase. From Simmons *et al.* (1991), with permission.

stressful, and because exposure to it was on an intermittent basis, a sensitization to the somatic effects of d-amphetamine occurred (see preceeding discussion on adaptation to stressors). A sensitization to d-amphetamine has been demonstrated following manipulations generally considered as stressors, including restraint (Antelman and Chiodo, 1983). If extensive information on the toxicity of the amphetamine were not available (as would be the case when evaluating unknown compounds for neurotoxic effects), an ignorance of the possible stressful nature of manipulations involved in the evaluation of its toxicity would lead to an erroneous conclusion regarding the potency of its effects.

Since cognitive dysfunction is often acknowledged as a symptom associated with the exposure of humans to toxic substances, it has been suggested that learning and memory be assessed in the evaluation of compounds for neurotoxicity (Miller and Eckerman, 1986; Peele and Vincent, 1989). It is now acknowledged that hormonal mechanisms, including these of the HPA axis, are an integral component of how the brain codes, stores, and retrieves information (Levine and Levine, 1989; Martinez, 1983; McEwen *et al.*, 1986; Rees and Gray, 1984). Both appetative and aversive conditioning are affected by adrenal steroids. The sympathoadrenal system, in particular, has been implicated generally in the modulation of memory, especially aversively motivated tasks. Support for this role of the adrenal axis comes from work concerning the piracetam-like compounds that are being investigated as possible memory-enhancing agents for use in the treatment of cognitive deficits in Alzehimer's disease, etc. These compounds will improve the retention performance of intact but not adrenalectomized mice (Mondadori and Petschke, 1987). Further, and pertinent to the issue of neurotoxicity assessment, is their finding that retention is also suppressed when adrenal cortex activity is chemically blocked by pretreatment with the steroid synthesis inhibitor, aminoglutethimide (Mondadori *et al.*, 1989). As mentioned previously, adrenal steroids play a prominent role in the development of conditioned taste aversions (Revusky and Martin, 1988). Peripheral catecholamines may also influence learning and memory by modulating central catecholamine systems, particularly norepinephrine (Bellush and Rowland, 1989; Dunn and Kramarcy, 1984; Gold and Stone, 1988). It is certain that exogenous administration of glucocorticoids will affect learning, as does adrenalectomy (McEwen et al., 1986). The extinction of a conditioned avoidance response is hastened by adrenal steroids (Bohus et al., 1982). What is not known is whether changes in the adrenal axis due to toxicant exposure can result in alterations in measures of learning and memory. Certainly manipulations involving the adrenal axis can alter long-term potentiation (see later discussion of this issue), often considered to be a measure of synaptic plasticity and a possible neural substrate for storage of information (Eccles, 1983).

The possible confounds due to stress are not just a problem in laboratory-based evaluations of neurotoxicity. Decreased mental functioning often accompanies brain insult in humans regardless of whether the damage is chemically or nonchemically induced (e.g., stroke, Alzheimer's disease, AIDS). An area of intense study in neurotoxicology is the cognitive abilities of humans following toxicant exposure. Environmental and occupational exposure to toxic substances is often accidental, requiring a rapid response and the development of test strategies. One outcome has been the development of evaluative batteries for field testing of exposed populations. In this way the detection of neurotoxic impairments can be accomplished close to or at the site of exposure (see Gullion and Eckerman, 1986 for a discussion). Often, measures of cognitive function figure prominently in these batteries (Anger, 1989). What should be noted, however, is the problem of stress interactions in the evaluation of neurotoxic impairments after occupational or environmental exposure. In these situations, just the knowledge of exposure can result in crisis-related depression or anxiety reaction (Boxer, 1985; Colligan, 1981; Colligan and Murphy, 1982; Hall and Johnson, 1989). Such reactions are increasingly recognized as a problem in the surrounds of hazardous waste sites (Fiedler, 1990). The constellation of symptoms noted in the vicinity of such sites, and not necessarily directly related to distance from the site, is being referred to as "waste site syndrome" (Neutra et al., 1991). Decrements in test performance may not be related to a direct effect of the compound on the CNS, but caused by the reaction to the suspicion of exposure to a dangerous substance. In such circumstances, cognitive performance can be affected by the "extraneous variables" of mood and motivation, and often there is not a clear relationship between exposure and the change in behavior. Many of the currently available field batteries do not assess affect concurrent with performance (Anger, 1989). Consequently, confounding factors, such as stress may be identified only through the use of appropriate additional validation studies. For example, Brown and Nixon (1979) found a significant deficit in memory performance following exposure to polybrominated biphenyls (PBBs) that was reduced to nonsignificance when the contribution of depression was eliminated. An additional study (Brown et al., 1981) then determined the relation between PBBs, mood alterations, and memory deficits.

## 3. ADRENAL AXIS INTERACTIONS WITH ELECTROPHYSIOLOGICAL MEASURES

Sensory processes concern both the input of sensory information or stimuli, as well as the processing of this information once the stimulus is detected. The adrenal gland interacts with both aspects of sensory processing, and glucocorticoids appear to regulate the detection and recognition of sensory signals (Henkin, 1975; von Zerssen, 1976).

ACTH affects sensory processing by altering attention and mood although the effects appear to be due to the fragment amino acid $ACTH_{4-9}$, and this portion of the whole $ACTH_{1-39}$ does not have adrenal cortical activity (Born et al., 1985, 1987, 1989). An elucidation of the role of glucocorticoids in sensory processing has been accomplished by studying populations in which glucocorticoid levels are altered due to disease (e.g., Addison's or Cushing's patients), by studying normal populations given exogenous glucocorticoids or ACTH, or by studying normal populations at different times during the daily circadian variation in endogenous glucocorticoid level. Much of the early work concerning the role of the adrenal axis and sensory processes was conducted by Henkin (1975) in humans diagnosed as having Addison's disease or Cushing's syndrome. These populations suffer, respectively, from an underproduction or an overabundance of the adrenal secretion, cortisol.

The first step to occur in sensory processing is the detection of the stimulus. Both Addison's disease and Cushing's syndrome cause rather dramatic alterations in taste and smell (Henkin, 1975). Richter (1941) first noted the increased preference of adrenalectomized rats for NaCl and also reported a decrease in threshold for detection of salt as measured behaviorally. Threshold and acuity are reciprocal; when threshold is lowered acuity increases, and alternatively, acuity decreases when threshold is elevated. Humans with adrenal cortical insufficiency have a lower taste detection threshold for NaCl, sucrose, HCl, and urea solutions (representing the four taste classes of salt, sweet, sour, and bitter, respectively) than normal volunteers (Fig. 7) (Henkin et al., 1963). Conversely, an excess of cortisol in Cushing's syndrome results in a higher taste detection threshold (i.e., poorer acuity than normals) (Henkin, 1970). In practical terms this means a person with adrenal insufficiency can tell the difference between water and a 1 mM solution of NaCl, but a normal individual cannot differentiate until the salt solution is at 6 mM. Support for the mediating role of glucocorticoids in taste acuity is the normalization in Addison's patients after treatment with carbohydrate-active steroids (e.g., hydrocortisone, cortisone, or dexamethasone) (Fig. 8). These Na-K active steroids do not normalize

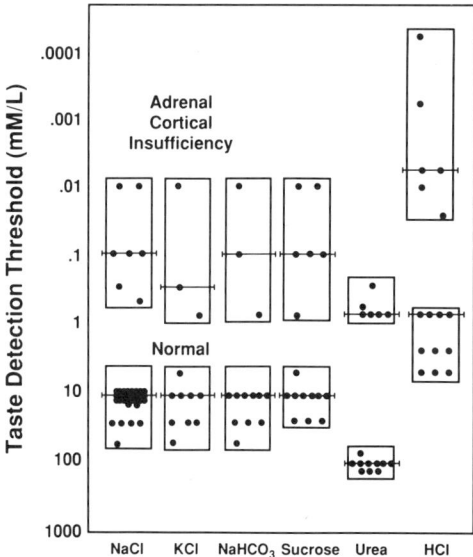

**FIGURE 7.** Adrenal insufficiency alters taste detection thresholds for NaCl, sucrose, HCl, and urea. The lower closed circles, enclosures, and lines represent the individual detection thresholds, range of responses, and median detection thresholds, respectively, in normal volunteers. The upper set represents the same information for patients with untreated adrenal insufficiency. The threshold for persons with insufficient levels of cortisol is lower than that of persons with adequate cortisol. Note the lack of overlap between the two groups. From Henkin et al. (1963), with permission.

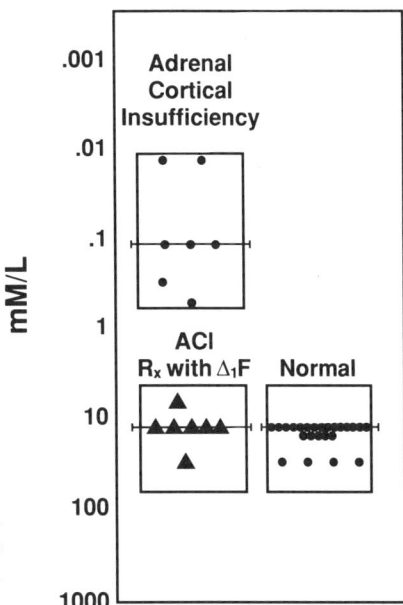

**FIGURE 8.** Normalization of taste acuity following replacement therapy with a carbohydrate-active steroid. Legend the same as Figure 7. $\Delta$, F = prednisolone; ACI = adrenal cortical insufficiency. From Henkin (1970), with permission.

acuity, as might be expected from the observations of increased salt intake in rodents and humans suffering from adrenal insufficiency. Surgical or chemical adrenalectomy lowers cortisol levels and normalizes the response in Cushing's patients (Henkin, 1970). These acuity changes are not limited to taste; increased sensitivity to olfactory, auditory, and nociceptive stimuli also occur in Addison's patients (Kosowicz and Pruszewicz, 1967) and in normals given cortisol (Fehm-Wolfsdorf et al., 1989; Henkin and Daly, 1968; Henkin et al., 1967; Lee and Pfeiffer, 1951). Finally, circadian patterns of taste detection occur in humans and rats (Fujimura et al., 1990; Henkin, 1975). Comparison of detection thresholds at periods when species-specific glucocorticoid levels are at their high or low point show detection thresholds or acuity are the poorest when the glucocorticoid level in blood is high.

The detection threshold (identification of a substance as different from water) can be contrasted to the recognition threshold (identification of the substance as salty, bitter, sweet, or sour). Recognition requires processing after the detection of the stimulus. Adrenal cortical insufficiency results in being able to detect a lower concentration of a substance but poorer processing of information concerning the taste (i.e., decreased recognition acuity). Recognition acuity of Addison's patients is one-fifth to one-tenth that of a normal volunteer but is normalized after treatment with carbohydrate-active steroids. Likewise, Cushing's syndrome results in poorer recognition of the taste. Interestingly, altered taste acuity in adrenal cortical insufficiency is sufficiently robust to serve as a diagnostic criteria for Addison's disease (Kosowicz and Pruszewicz, 1967). The efficacy of a reinforcer, such as food or shock, to a large extent depends on the strength of the reinforcer. Many pharmacological and toxicological agents, as well as various experimental manipulations (e.g., restraint, food deprivation, etc.), elevate corticosterone levels in the rat (Varma et al., 1988; Table 3). It is not known if such an increase or the persistent decrease in corticosterone levels after adrenal damage alter smell and taste acuity in the rodent with concomitant changes in food palatability and reinforcement value.

The preceding discussion concerning the alterations in perception accompanying an increase or decrease in glucocorticoids suggest that any endpoint used to assess sensory function may be impacted by manipulations or treatments resulting in altered hormone levels. Sensory-evoked potentials (SEPs) are electrophysiological measurements considered to be appropriate for determining sensory function in neurotoxicity evaluation (Chapter 9; Dyer, 1985; Rebert, 1983; Ross, 1990). SEPs occur after the presentation of a sensory stimulus and are thought to reflect the activity of neural circuits (i.e., processing of sensory stimulus information in the CNS). It is evident that adrenal insufficiency increases the sensitivity of sensory systems to stimulation and also produces an abnormality in the subsequent processing of the stimuli. Further, an increase in the conduction velocity in peripheral axons accompanies adrenal insufficiency and slows with cortisol treatment (Henkin et al., 1963). Because a threshold is associated with all forms of stimulation, it might be expected that the changes in SEPs associated with Addison's and Cushing's disease, as well as those produced by raising cortisol levels in "normals," should be predictable. However, the limited data available indicate such predictions are not easily made and, considering the degree of processing necessary for perception, this is not surprising. When compared to their control values, the latency of a visual-evoked potential in patients with adrenal insufficiency was decreased when evaluated following cortisol replacement (Ojemann and Henkin, 1967). If just an alteration in threshold occurred with cortisol replacement, an increase in latency might be expected. No consistent changes in latency were observed when Na-K active steroids were given. Directly relevant to the use of sensory evoked potential measures in determining the neurotoxic effects of suspect compounds are reports of altered evoked potentials in humans given cortisol or ACTH. The infusion of cortisol to levels within the physiological range can alter the latency of visual and auditory evoked potentials (Born et al., 1989; Kopell et al., 1970). It has not been determined if other manipulations involved with testing, etc. that induce physiologically relevant elevations in glucocorticoids can affect SEPs in humans. The relationship between SEPs and altered neuroendocrine status does not appear to have been addressed systematically in infrahuman species either. A focused effort to collect such information is quite important, given the emphasis on SEPs in both human and infrahuman neurotoxicity evaluations.

Other electrophysiological processes, such as long-term potentiation (LTP) and kindling, are altered by neuroendocrine status (Cottrell et al., 1984; Foy et al., 1987; McIntyre, 1976; Shors et al., 1990). Such findings suggest that alterations of the adrenal axis, within the physiological range, can have a dramatic impact on electrophysiological measures of brain function. LTP is the increased amplitude of synaptic responses following a train of repetitive stimulation that can persist for weeks. Kindling is a persistent change in the threshold level of electrical stimulation required to induce a seizure following repeated focal stimulation (Goddard, 1983). Kindling is frequently studied in the hippocampus and is considered useful as an experimental model of epilepsy. Stress can totally prevent the induction of LTP in rats (Fig. 9) (Foy et al., 1987). Restraint, or restraint plus tail shock, does not affect general cell excitability, but it does prevent LTP. It might be expected that the ability of stress to block the induction of LTP is due to elevations in glucocorticoid levels, because LTP appears to vary with time of day and the circadian pattern of glucocorticoids (Dana and Martinez, 1984). However, recent work by Shors and colleagues (1990) demonstrates the importance of the adrenal medullary portion of the adrenal axis. Adrenalectomy and adrenal demedullation block the effects of stress on LTP, and this block is not reversed with corticosterone replacement. Adrenalectomy

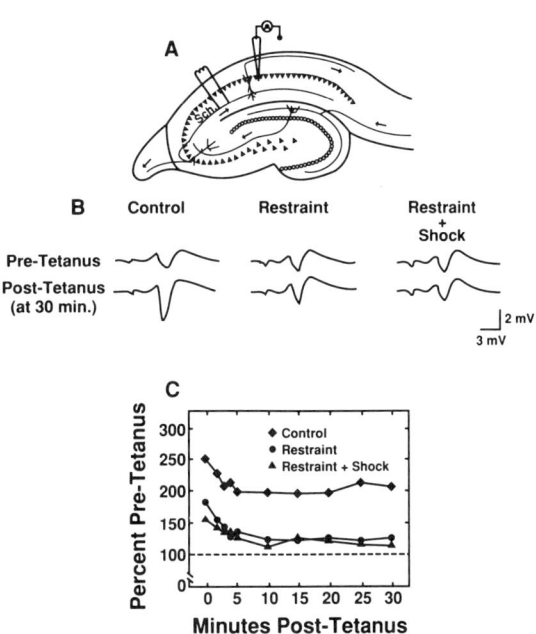

**FIGURE 9.** Exposure to a stressor will prevent long-term potentiation. (A) A transverse section through the hippocampus illustrates the lamellar organization of the slices and placement of the bipolar concentric stimulating electrode in the afferent pathway containing the Schaffer collateral branches (Sch.) of the CA3 pyramidal cell axons. A glass micropipet filled with 2M NaCl was placed in the cell body layer of the CA1 cell field to record field potentials. (B) These representative field potentials from the three treatment groups (control, restraint, restraint and shock) demonstrate that high-frequency stimulation enhanced the population field potential only for the control condition (i.e., an increase of 205% from pre-tetanus to post-tetanus). Field potentials did not change in the other two groups. (C) CA1 hippocampal excitability (expressed as a percentage of pretetanus control). Slices from all groups display a short post-tetanic potentiation but only the slices from the control group display a long-term potentiation (i.e., a significant elevation for the 30 minutes post-tetanus). From Foy et al. (1987).

also reduces the severity of kindled seizures, but these changes can be normalized by corticosterone replacement (Cottrell et al., 1984).

## 4. MORPHOLOGICAL AND BIOCHEMICAL MEASURES USED IN NEUROTOXICITY ASSESSMENT

Intuitively, a perturbation of the adrenal axis would more easily confound the measurement of behavior or a biochemical endpoint such as neurotransmitter levels, as these indices are believed to be more susceptible to alterations in HPA function. Endpoints such as brain morphology measures would be less easily compromised. However, ample data suggest the adrenal axis does play a role in the maintenance of both brain morphology as well as biochemistry and function. Support for this idea includes the following: (1) Morphological changes in brain occur when there are increased circulating levels of glucocorticoids, whether the elevation is due to endogenous or exogenous sources, and (2) morphological changes occur in brain when the adrenal gland is removed. As McEwen (1987) has argued, there is "considerable plasticity in the ability of environmental influences to modify cellular biochemistry and morphology." Thus, any toxicant that alters adrenal steroid levels may impact morphological, functional, or biochemical aspects of the CNS through direct or indirect mechanisms.

Many neurochemical and cellular events are modified by adrenal steroids (McEwen et al., 1986). One of the many prominent actions of glucocorticoids is their impact on growth (Loeb, 1976), and the brain is not exempt from this control. Exposure to excess natural or synthetic glucocorticoids during the developmental period alters brain and body growth (Meyer, 1985). Permanent brain weight reductions result, with the most pronounced deficits occuring in the cerebellum and hippocampus (Cotterrell *et al.*, 1972; Howard, 1968; Howard and Benjamin, 1975; Uno *et al.*, 1990). Glucocorticoids given during brain development cause a suppression of neuronal and/or glial cell proliferation in a number of brain areas, including the cerebrum, cerebellum, hippocampus, and optic nerve. Excessive levels of glucocorticoids also retard myelination, as well as alter dendritic development in cortex (Gumbinas *et al.*, 1973; Oda and Huttenlocher, 1974). ACTH is used to treat infantile spasms and induces a reversible cerebral atrophy, as revealed by computed tomography (Lyen *et al.*, 1979). However, chronic treatment of the developing rat with ACTH has not revealed comparable brain alterations (Ito *et al.*, 1985).

An excess of glucocorticoids can also have catabolic or degenerative consequences throughout the body, including the brain (McEwen *et al.*, 1986). However, all brain areas are not equally susceptible to the degenerative effects of glucocorticoids. Perhaps because of its important regulatory role in the HPA-axis negative-feedback loop, certain areas of the hippocampus appear to be uniquely vulnerable to continuous stress or high circulating levels of glucocorticoids (Sapolsky, 1987; Sapolsky and McEwen, 1986). The hippocampus is a neural target for glucocorticoids and is rich in type 1 and 2 corticosteroid receptors. CA2 and CA3 pyramidal neurons have the highest concentration of glucocorticoid receptors in the brain, and these are the hippocampal pyramidal-cell subfields which are particularily affected by excessive glucocorticoids (McEwen *et al.*, 1975; Sapolsky *et al.*, 1990; Stumpf, 1971). Prolonged exposure to circulating levels of glucocorticoids higher than those required for normal physiological function, whether due to stress or by direct administration, result in hippocampal damage in laboratory rats, guinea pigs, and primates (McEwen *et al.*, 1986; Sapolsky *et al.*, 1984, 1990; Uno *et al.*, 1989). Obviously, the exposure to glucocorticoids is cumulative over the life span, and removal of the adrenals or other means of reducing the total exposure to glucocorticoids can retard the degenerative effects of corticosterone (Landfield *et al.*, 1981; Meaney *et al.*, 1988b). In the aging organism, persistent elevations in glucocorticoids are particularly deleterious to hippocampal pyramidal cells, both in terms of cellular integrity and electroophysiological function (Kerr *et al.*, 1989, 1991; Landfield *et al.*, 1978, 1981; Sapolsky *et al.*, 1986).

An investigator intending to assess the neural damage induced by a known or putative neurotoxicant should be aware that alterations in the adrenal axis can both increase and decrease the degree of neurotoxic insult. The hippocampus has been noted to often be a target of neurotoxicants (Walsh and Emerich, 1991), and interestingly, many of the instances where glucocorticoids enhance neural damage have involved this brain area. Glucocorticoid-enhanced hippocampal damage has been reported after hypoxia–ischemia, excitotoxicity, and metabolic insults. Removal of the adrenals will reduce the degree of induced neural trauma (Morse and Davis, 1990; Sapolsky, 1985, 1986; Sapolsky and Pulsinelli, 1985; Stein and Sapolsky, 1988). Chemical adrenalectomy effected by blocking glucocorticoid synthesis will also protect the hippocampus from ischemic injury (Morse and Davis, 1990). Glucocorticoids also reduce the heterotypic axonal growth (ingrowth of axons utilizing a different neurotransmitter than the one associated with the damaged area) that occurs subsequent to certain types of brain lesions but are necessary for homotypic ingrowth (Scheff and Cotman, 1982; Scheff and DeKosky, 1983; Scheff *et al.*, 1988; Zhou and Azmitia, 1985).

Adrenal secretions also have a protective or maintenance role for one particular area

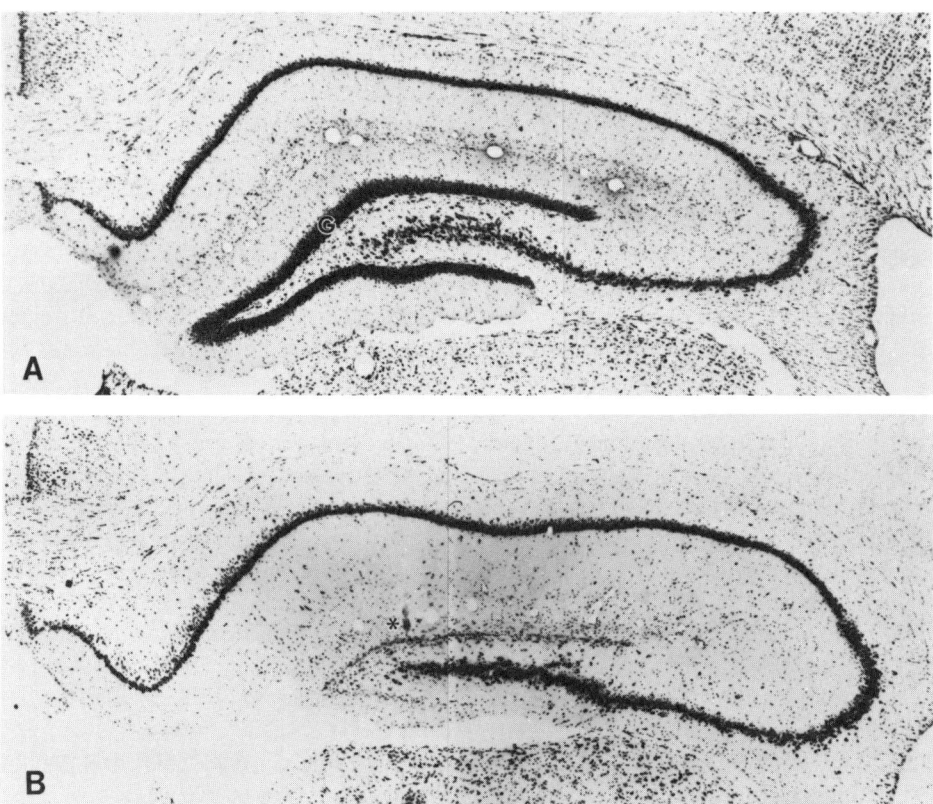

FIGURE 10. Appearance of the hippocampus of the rat (B) following removal of both adrenal glands 3–4 months earlier (A). Note the loss of dentate granule cells. From Sloviter et al. (1989), with permission.

of hippocampus, the dentate gyrus. An almost total degeneration of hippocampal dentate granule cells occurs in rats 3–4 months following adrenalectomy (Fig. 10) (Sloviter et al., 1989). The required substance appears to be corticosterone, as replacement of this hormone will prevent the degeneration. Initially this rather dramatic finding was greeted with skepticism, but severals groups have replicated the effect (McNeill et al., 1991; Roy et al., 1990). Roy and co-workers found a relationship between the completeness of the adrenalectomy and the degree of degeneration. In some instances, enough accessory adrenal tissue, and thus corticosterone, remains following surgery to prevent severe degeneration. The completeness of adrenalectomy can be determined by body weight loss when tap water is substituted for saline. The greater the weight loss, the greater the degree of dentate granule-cell degeneration. As little as 15 ng/ml of serum corticosterone is apparently sufficient to protect dentate granule cells from death (McNeill et al., 1991). Finally, Gould and co-workers (1990) reported the appearance of pyknotic cells within 72 hr after adrenalectomy. Degenerating cells with reduced cellular area and dendritic branch points occurred throughout the dentate gyrus, but not the pyramidal cell layer, and these changes could be ameliorated by corticosterone replacement. A transient "chemical" adrenalectomy can be effected with mitotane (O,P'–DDD) or metyrapone, pharmacological agents that inhibit adrenocortical secretion, and perhaps with other adrenotoxic agents

(Colby, 1988). Whether such a transient decrease in glucocorticoid levels would have a similar impact on the integrity of dentate granule is not known.

Removing the adrenal also impacts on the non-neuronal elements of the brain. An increase in brain size follows adrenalectomy (Devenport, 1979; Devenport and Devenport, 1983; Meyer, 1983). Interestingly, the only other manipulation causing a brain weight increase, other than edema, is environmental enrichment (Bennett et al., 1964; Uphouse and Brown, 1981). Although the adrenal axis is considered to be a possible determinant of the enrichment effects in brain, there is still controversy concerning the mechanism (see Black et al., 1989 for a discussion). Unlike edema, both adrenalectomy and enrichment lead to an increase in tissue mass (Bennett et al., 1964). Further, these brain weight increases occur in the presence of reduced body weight. Total brain weight and the weight of specific brain areas are affected by the removal of adrenal glucocorticoid hormones in developing (Fig. 11) and adult rodents (Devenport, 1979; Devenport and Devenport, 1985; Meyer, 1983, 1987; Meyer and Fairman, 1985; O'Callaghan et al., 1991). Supplementing the adrenalectomized animals with corticosterone, but not mineralocorticoids, will prevent the increase. The increase in brain mass reflects increases in cell division and the production of myelin, at least in animals adrenalectomized before weaning (Meyer, 1983). Neonatal adrenalectomy also alters the dendritic branching of the hippocampal dentate granule cells (Hashimoto et al., 1989). Limited data suggest that the brain-size increase is accompanied by an enhanced learning ability (Yehuda et al., 1988). The brain-weight increase in rats adrenalectomized as adults has not been characterized but may be important in light of the regulatory role of glucocorticoids in the control of brain levels of astrocyte-localized proteins (see O'Callaghan et al., 1991 and the discussion below).

Many studies have been conducted concerning the role glucocorticoids may play in regulating the synthesis of proteins (Nichols et al., 1988; Meyer, 1985). However, the regulation of the astrocyte-associated protein, glial fibrillary acidic protein (GFAP), by the adrenal axis may have important implications in a neurotoxicity context (Nichols et al.,

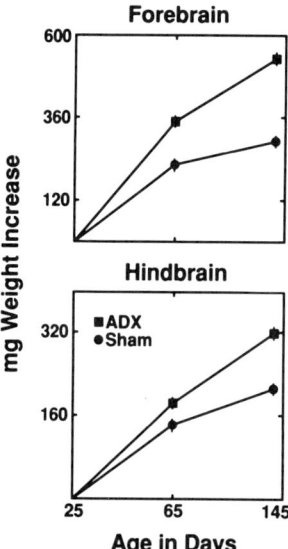

**FIGURE 11.** Increase in wet weight of forebrain and hindbrain of rats following the removal of the adrenals at 25 days of age. From Devenport and Devenport (1983), with permission.

1988, 1990; O'Callaghan et al., 1989, 1991). Removal of the adrenal causes an increased expression of this protein in many brain areas, and supplementation with corticosterone prevents the effect. Further, increased levels of glucocorticoids sufficient to involute the thymus will suppress the synthesis of GFAP. As GFAP synthesis increases in response to injury, the measurement of GFAP has been proposed and utilized as a means for detecting the CNS damage caused by certain neurotoxicants (O'Callaghan, 1988; Reinhard et al., 1988). Because the synthesis of GFAP increases in an adrenalectomized animal, a false positive would occur if an agent causes an increase in GFAP due to a "chemical" adrenalectomy rather than directly damaging the CNS. A brain-wide increase in GFAP synthesis would suggest mediation by an adrenotoxic mechanism. The control of GFAP expression by glucocorticoids does not, however, appear to be a problem in the assessment of compounds that directly damage the CNS. Chronic treatment with corticosterone did not alter the GFAP response elicited by the chemical neurotoxicant, trimethyltin, or the brain injury associated with a stab wound to the cortex (O'Callaghan et al., 1991). Thus, the regulation of the synthesis of GFAP by glucocorticoids and that due to injury are controlled through separate pathways. However, given the usefulness of the GFAP measure in neurotoxicity assessment, further investigations of the interactions between the adrenal axis and the expression of GFAP should be conducted.

Pertinent to the use of interactions between adrenal axis changes and neurotoxicity assessment are examples concerning organophosphate exposure and delayed neuropathy. The chicken is the recommended species for evaluating the delayed neurotoxicity of organophosphates (Bickford, 1982; Gross, 1982; U.S. EPA, 1978). Other species susceptible to this form of delayed neuropathy include humans, nonhuman primates, cats, cows, and water buffaloes, but not rodents or hamsters (Abou-Donia, 1981). Chickens are very

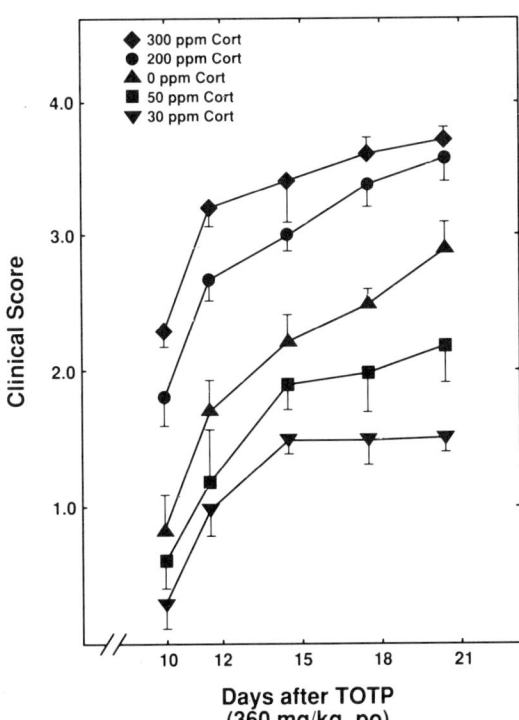

**FIGURE 12.** The effect of high and low doses of corticosterone on the clinical signs of neuropathy induced in the chicken by the organophosphate triorthototyl phosphate. Note that 30 and 50 ppm of corticosterone in food reduce the clinical signs, while they are increased at 200 and 300 ppm. From Ehrich and Gross (1986), with permission.

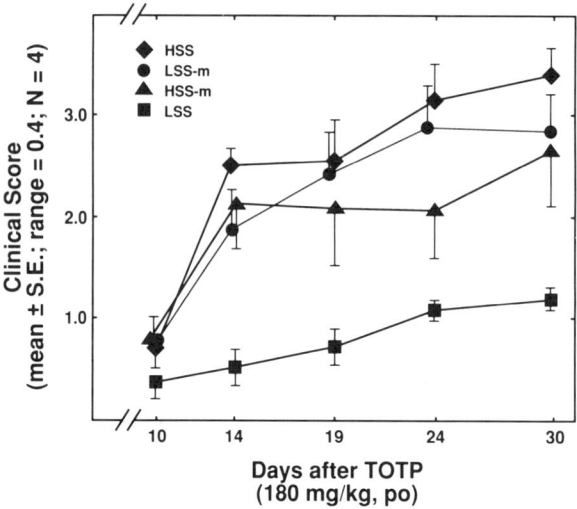

FIGURE 13. Effect of type of housing on the clinical signs of neuropathy induced in the chicken by the organophosphate triorthotolyl phosphate. HSS, LSS, and m stand for high-stress housing, low-stress housing, and moved to the opposite type of housing, respectively. LLS-m and HSS-m chickens were moved immediately prior to dosing, and this is as stressful as maintaining them in HSS housing. From Ehrich and Gross (1983), with permission.

susceptible to stress under certain housing conditions, as indicated by the release of corticosterone and low heterophil/lymphocyte ratios. Alterations in housing can decrease their resistance to various diseases, and this is attributed to the induction of stress by the change in conditions (Gross, 1982; Gross and Colmano, 1969; Hall et al., 1979). Low levels of glucocorticoids given in the food, or by injection, can decrease the severity of the clinical signs associated with the delayed neuropathy (Fig. 12) (Ehrich et al., 1988; Lidsky et al., 1990). However, high doses of corticosterone, whether given exogenously (Fig. 12) or induced by stressful environmental conditions, exacerbated the condition (Fig. 13) and the number of degenerating nerve fibers (Ehrich and Gross, 1983, 1986; Ehrich et al., 1986, 1988). Thus, minor alterations in housing can dramatically alter the amount of compound required to induce neurotoxicity. Also, the exacerbation of delayed neuropathy by glucocorticoids appear to be species specific. High doses of synthetic or natural glucocorticoids will prevent or decrease the behavioral, morphological, and electrophysiological signs of delayed neuropathy in cats exposed to organophosphates (Baker and Stanec, 1985; Baker et al., 1982; Drakontides, 1982). The effects of glucocorticoids and/or stress in other susceptible species and other types of neuropathies is not known. Glucocorticoid therapy is also recommended for certain types of neural trauma, such as spinal cord injury (Hall and Braughler, 1982). However, it has been noted that caution should be exercised in the use of glucocorticoids in all types of neural trauma, given the consequences of excess steroids for the hippocampus (Sapolsky and Pulsinelli, 1985). Interestingly an analogue of $ACTH_{4-9}$, which is without steroidal activity, also has been reported to ameliorate the peripheral neuropathy associated with cisplatin chemotherapy in humans (van der Hoop, 1990).

## 5. SUGGESTIONS

This chapter alerts researchers in neurotoxicology to the interactions between the nervous system and the adrenal axis. A wealth of literature from neuroscience and biology indicate that a variety of neural endpoints are affected by pituitary adrenal hormones. Changes in many of these endpoints regarded as sufficient to demonstrate the presence of neurotoxicity. Thus, the potential effect of a toxicant on the adrenals, or a combined adrenal and direct CNS effect, could influence any of the measures suggested as sufficient to detect neurotoxicity. Importantly, experimental variables such as handling, dosing, and housing procedures may impact neurotoxicity assessment in both adult and developing organisms because of changes induced in HPA function. Laboratory animals are not the "toxicologist's black box" (Calabrese, 1987), and a better understanding of the changes associated with the procedures utilized in toxicity testing will lead to greater confidence in the data provided by such testing. In the meantime, a researcher can take certain steps. If toxicant exposure is accompanied by alterations in food or water intake, the experimenter should be alerted to possible adrenal-axis activation, and a pair-fed group should be included to aid in data interpretation. When possible, adrenal, thymus, and spleen weights should be obtained from experimental subjects utilized for neurotoxicity assessment. In particular, thymus and general body weight are tightly regulated by glucocorticoid levels (Akana *et al.*, 1985). Alteration in their weights may serve to alert investigators to the impact on the adrenal axis of either the chemical treatment itself or of experimental manipulations necessary in the collection of toxicity data. The role of adrenal-axis disturbance in the observed changes should then be considered.

# REFERENCES

Abou-Donia, M.B., 1981, Organophosphorus ester-induced delayed neurotoxicity, *Ann. Rev. Pharmacol.*, 21:511–548.
Akana, S.F., Cascio, C.S., Shinsako, J., and Dallman, M.F., 1985, Corticosterone: Narrow range required for normal body and thymus weight and ACTH, *Am. J. Physiol.* 249:R527–R532.
Ally, A.I., Vieira, L., and Reuhl, K.R., 1986, Trimethyltin as a selective adrenal chemosympatholytic agent in vivo: Effect precedes both clinical and histopathological evidence of toxicity, *Toxicology* 40:215–229.
Anger, K.E., 1989, Human neurobehavioral toxicology testing: Current perspectives, Toxicol. Indust. Health 5:165–180.
Annau, Z., ed., 1986, *Neurobehavioral Toxicology*. The Johns Hopkins University Press, Baltimore.
Antelman, S.M., and Chiodo, L.A., 1983, Amphetamine as a stressor, in: *Stimulants: Neurochemical, Behavioral, and Clinical Perspectives* ( Creese, I., ed.), Raven Press, New York, pp. 269–299.
Antelman, S.M., Eichler, A.J., Black, C.A., and Kocan, D., 1980, Interchangeability of stress and amphetamine in sensitization, *Science* 207:329–331.
Axelrod, J., and Reisine, T.D., 1984, Stress hormones: Their interaction and regulation, *Science* 224:452–459.
Badiani, A., and Castellano, C., 1991, Effects of acute and chronic stress and of genotype on oxotremorine-induced locomotor depression of mice, *Behav. Neural Biol.* 55:123–130.
Baker, T., and Stanec, A., 1985, Methylprednisolone treatment of an organophosphorus induced delayed neuropathy, *Toxicol. Appl. Pharmacol.* 79:397–408.
Baker, T., Drakontides, A.B., and Riker, W.F., Jr., 1982, Prevention of the organophosphorus neuropathy by glucocorticoids, *Exp. Neurol.* 78:397–408.
Barclay, R.J., Herbert, W.J., and Poole, T.B., 1988, *The Disturbance Index: A Behavioural Method of Assessing the Severity of Common Laboratory Procedures on Rodents.* Universities Federation for Animal Welfare, Potters Bar, UK.
Beckwith, B.E., Lerud, K., Antes, J.R., and Reynolds, B.W., 1983, Hydrocortisone reduces auditory sensitivity at high tonal frequencies in adult males, *Pharmacol. Biochem. Behav.* 19:431–433.
Bellush, L.L., and Rowland, N.E., 1989, Stress and behavior in streptozotocin diabetic rats: Biochemical correlates of passive avoidance learning, *Behav. Neurosci.* 103:144–150.
Bennett, E.L., Diamond, M.C., Krech, D., and Rosenzweig, M.R., 1964, Chemical and anatomical plasticity of brain, *Science* 146:610–619.
Berridge, C.W., and Dunn, A.J., 1989, Restraint-stress induced changes in exploratory behavior appear to be mediated by norepinephrine-stimulated release of CRF, *J. Neurosci.*, 9:3513–3521.
Bickford, A.A., 1982, The hen as a test animal for delayed neurotoxicity studies: Introductory comments, *NeuroToxicology* 3:285–286.
Black, J.E., Sirevaag, A.M., Wallace, S.S., Savin, M.H., and Greenough, W.T., 1989, Effects of complex experience on somatic growth and organ development in rats, *Devel. Psychobiol.* 22:727–752.

Bohn, M.C., 1984, Glucocorticoid induced teratologies of the nervous system, in: *Neurobehavioral Teratology* (J. Yanai, ed.), Elsevier Science Publishers, New York, pp. 365–387.

Bohus, B., De Kloet, E.R., and Veldhuis, H.D., 1982, Adrenal steroids and behavioral adaptation: Relationship to brain corticosterone receptors, in: *Current Topics in Neuroendocrinology* (D. Ganten and D. Pfaff, eds.), Springer-Verlag, Berlin, pp. 107–148.

Born, J., Fehm-Wolfsdorf, G., Schiebe, M., Birbaumer, N., Fehm, H.L., and Voigt, H.H., 1985, An ACTH 4-9 analog impairs selective attention in man, *Life Sci.* 36:2117–2125.

Born, J., Fehm, H.L., and Voigt, K.H., 1986, ACTH and attention in humans: A review, Vol. 2, *Neuropsychobiology* 15:165–186.

Born, J., Brauninger, W., Fehm-Wolfsdorf, G., Voiggt, K.H., Pauschinger, P., and Fehm, H.L., 1987, Dose-dependent influences on electrophysiological signs of attention in humans after neuropeptide ACTH 4–10. *Exp. Brain Res.* 67:85–92.

Born, J., Kern, W., Fehm-Wolfssdorf, G., and Fehm, H.L., 1987, Cortisol effects on attentional process in man as indicated by event-related potentials, *Psychophysiology* 24:286–292.

Born, J., Hitzler, V., Pietrowsky, R., Pauschinger, P., and Fehm, H.L., 1989, Influences of cortisol on auditory evoked potentials (AEPs) and mood in humans, *Neuropsychobiology* 20:145–151.

Born, J., Kern, W., Pietrowsky, R., Sittiz, W., and Fehm, H.L., 1989, Fragments of ACTH affect electrophysiological signs of controlled stimulus processing in humans, *Psychopharmacology* 99:439–444.

Born, J., Schwab, R., Pietrowsky, R., Pauschinger, P., and Fehm, H.L., 1989, Glucocorticoid influences on the auditory brain-stem responses in man, *Electroencephalog. Clin. Neurophysiol.* 74:209–16.

Born, J., Unseld, U., Pietrowsky, R., Bickel, U., Voigt, K., and Fehm, H.L., 1990, *Neuroendocrinology* 52:169–174.

Boxer, P., 1985, Occupational mass psychogenic illness: History, prevention and management, *J. Occup. Med.* 27:867–872.

Boyes, W.K., 1990, Proposed Test Guidelines for Using Sensory Evoked Potentials as Measures of Neurotoxicity. U.S. Environmental Protection Agency, Research Triangle Park, NC.

Boyes, W.K., 1992, Testing visual system toxicity using evoked potentials, in: *The Vulnerable Brain and Environmental Risks, Vol. 1: Malnutrition and Hazard Assessment* (R.L. Isaacson and K.F. Jensen, eds.), Plenum Press, New York. pp. 193–222.

Brady, J.V., and Harris, A., 1977, The experimental production of altered physiological states, in: *Handbook of Operant Behavior* (Honig, W.K., Staddon, J.E.R., eds.), Prentice-Hall, Englewood Cliffs, NJ, pp. 595–618.

Brain, P., and Benton, D., 1979, The interpretation of physiological correlates of differential housing in laboratory rats, *Life Sci.* 24:99–116.

Brown, G.G., and Nixon, R.K., 1979, Exposure to polybrominated biphenyls: Some effects on personality and cognitive functioning, *JAMA* 242:523–526.

Brown, G.G., Preisman, R.C., Anderson, M.D., Nixon, R.K., Isbister, J.L., and Price, H.A., 1981, Memory performance of chemical workers exposed to polybrominated biphenyls, *Science* 212:1413–1415.

Buchsbaum, M.S., and Henkin, R.I., 1975, Effects of carbohydrate-active steroids and ACTH on visually-evoked responses in patients with adrenal cortical insufficiency, *Neuroendocrinology* 19:314–322.

Bushnell, P.J., Shelton, S.E., and Bowman, R.E., 1979, Elevation of blood lead concentration by confinement in the rhesus monkey, *Bull. Environm. Contam. Toxicol.* 22:819–826.

Calabrese, E.J., 1987, Animal extrapolation: A look inside the toxicologist's black box, *Environ. Sci. Technol.* 21:618–623.

Chernoff, N., Kavlock, R.J., Beyer, P.E., and Miller, D.B., 1987, The potential relationship of maternal toxicity, general stress, and fetal outcome, *Teratogen. Carcinogen. Mutagen.* 7:241–253.

Chernoff, N., Rogers, J.M., and Kavlock, R.J., 1989, An overview of maternal toxicity and prenatal development: Considerations for developmental toxicity hazard assessments, *Toxicology* 59:111–125.

Colby, H.D., 1988, Adrenal gland toxicity: Chemically induced dysfunction, *J. Am. Coll. Toxicol.* 7:45–69.

Colligan, M., 1981, Mass psychogenic illness: Some clarification and perspectives, *J. Occup. Med.* 23:635–638.

Colligan, M., and Murphy, L., 1982, A review of mass psychogenic illness in work settings, in: *Mass Psychogenic Illness: A Social Psychological Analysis* (M. Colligan, J. Pennebaker, and L. Murphy, eds.), Lawrence Erlbaum Assoc., Hillsdale, NJ.

Cooper, R.L., Mole, M.L., Rehnberg, G.L., Goldman, J.M., McElroy, W.K., Hein, J., and Stoker, T.E., 1992, Effect of inhaled methanol on pituitary and testicular hormones in chamber acclimated and non-acclimated rats, *Toxicology* 71:69–81.

Cotterell, M., Balazs, R., and Johnson, A.L., 1972, Effects of corticosteroids on the biochemical maturation of rat brain: Postnatal cell formation, *J. Neurochem.* 19:2151–2167.

Cottrell, G., Nyakas, C., DeKloet, E.R., and Bohus, B., 1984, Hippocampal kindling: Corticosterone modulation of induced seizures, *Brain Res.* 309:377–381.

Coveney, J.R., Neal, B.S., and Sparber, S.B., 1990, Food deprivation alters behavioral and plasma corticosterone responses to phencyclidine in rats, *Pharmacol. Biochem. Behav.* 36:451–456.

Dana, R., and Martinez, J.L., 1984, Effect of adrenalectomy on the circadian rhythm of LTP, *Brain Res.* 308:392–395.

DeHaven, D.L., and Mailman, R.B., 1983, The uses of radioligand binding techniques in neurotoxicology, *Rev. Biochem. Toxicol.* 5:193–238.

DeHaven, D.L., and Mailman, R.B., 1986, The interactions of behavior and neurochemistry, in: *Neurobehavioral Toxicology* (Z. Annau, ed.), Johns Hopkins University Press, Baltimore, pp. 214–243.

DeKosky, S.T., Scheff, S.W., and Cotman, C.W., 1984, Elevated corticosterone levels: Possible cause of reduced axon sprouting in aged animals, *Neuroendocrinology* 38:33–38.

Denenberg, V.H., Brumaghim, J.T., Haltmeyer, G.C., and Zarrow, M.X., 1967, Increased adrenocortical activity in the neonatal rat following handling, *Endocrinology* 81:1047–1052.
Devenport, L.D., 1979, Adrenal modulation of brain size in adult rats, *Behav. Neural Biol.* 27:218–221.
Devenport, L.D., and Devenport, J.A., 1983, Brain growth: Interactions of maturation with adrenal steroids, *Physiol. Behav.* 30:313–315.
Devenport, L.D., and Devenport, J.A., 1985, Adrenocortical hormones and brain growth: Reversibility and differential sensitivity during development, *Exp. Neurol.* 90:44–52.
Diener, R.M., 1987, Behavioral toxicology: Current industrial viewpoint, *J. Am. Coll. Toxicol.* 6:427–431.
Drakontides, A.B., Baker, T., and Riker, W.F. Jr., 1982, A morphological study of the effect of glucocorticoid treatment on delayed organophosphorus neuropathy, *NeuroToxicology* 3:165–178.
Drozdowicz, C.K., Bowman, T.A., Webb, M.L., and Lang, C.M., 1990, Effect of in-house transport on murine plasma corticosterone concentration and blood lymphocyte populations, *Am. J.Vet. Res.* 5:1841–1846.
Dunn, A.J., and Kramarcy, N.R., 1984, Neurochemical responses in stress: Relationship between the hypothalamic-pituitary-adrenal and catecholamine systems, in: *Handbook of Psychopharmacology*, Vol. 18 (L.L. Iversen, S.D. Iversen, and S.H. Snyder, eds.), Plenum Press, New York, pp. 455–515.
Dunne, M.P., Burnett, P., Lawton, J., and Raphael, B., 1990, The health effects of chemical waste in an urban community, *Med. J. Austral.* 152:592–597.
Dyer, R.S., 1985, The use of sensory-evoked potentials in toxicology, *Fundam. Appl. Toxicol.* 5:24–40.
Dyer, R.S., 1986, The interactions of behavior and neurophysiology, in: *Neurobehavioral Toxicology* (Z. Annau, ed.), Johns Hopkins University Press, Baltimore, pp. 193–213.
Eccles, J., 1983, Calcium in long-term potentiation as a model for memory, *Neuroscience* 10:1071–1081.
Ehlers, C.L., Henriksen, S.J., Wang, M., Rivier, J., Vale, W., and Bloom, F.E., 1983, Corticotropin releasing factor produces increases in brain excitability and convulsive seizures in rats, *Brain Res.* 278:332–336.
Ehrich, M., and Gross, W.B., 1983, Modification of triorthotolyl phosphate toxicity in chickens by stress, *Toxicol. Appl. Pharmacol.* 70:249–254.
Ehrich, M., and Gross, W.B., 1986, Effect of supplemental corticosterone and social stress on orgnophosphorus-induced delayed neuropathy in chickens, *Toxicol. Lett.* 31:9–13.
Ehrich, M., Jortner, B.S., and Gross, W.B., 1986, Dose-related beneficial and adverse effects of dietary corticosterone on organophosphorus-induced delayed neuropathy in chickens, *Toxicol. Appl. Pharmacol.* 83:250–260.
Ehrich, M., Jortner, B.S., and Gross, W.B., 1988, Types of adrenocorticoids and their effect on organophosphorus-induced delayed neuropathy in chickens, *Toxicol. Appl. Pharmacol.* 92:214–223.
Environmental Protection Agency, 1985, Motor activity, *Fed. Reg.* 50(188), 39460, Sect. 798.6200 (b) 1.
Feldman, S., and Conforti, N., 1980, Participation of the dorsal hippocampus in the glucocorticoid feedback effect on adrenocortical activity, *Neuroendocrinology* 30:52–55.
Fehm-Wolfsdorf, G., Scheible, E., Zenz, H., Born, J., and Fehm, H.L., 1989, Taste thresholds in man are differentially influenced by hydrocortisone and dexamethasone, *Psychoneuroendocrinology* 14:433–450.
Fiedler, N., 1990, Understanding stress in hazardous waste workers, *Occup. Med.* 5:101–108.
Field, T.M., Schanberg, S.M., Scafidi, F., Bauer, C.R., Vega-Lahr, N., Garcia, R., Nystrom, J., and Kuhn, C.M., Effects of tactile/kinesthetic stimulation in pre-term neonates, *Pediatrics* 77:654–658.
Fischer, E.G., 1988, Opioid peptides modulate immune functions. A review, *Immunopharmacol. Immunotoxicol.* 10:265–326.
Flemmer, D.D., and Dilsaver, S.C., 1989, Chronic injections of saline produces subsensitivity to nicotine, *Pharmacol. Biochem. Behav.* 34:261–263.
Forsham, P.H., 1968, The adrenals: Part 1, The adrenal cortex, in: *Textbook of Endocrinology* (R.H. Williams, ed.), W.B. Sanders, Philadelphia, pp. 287–379.
Foy, M.R., Stanton, M.E., and Levine, S., 1987, Behavioral stress impairs long-term potentiation in rodent hippocampus, *Behav. Neural Biol.* 48:138–149.
Fujimura, A., Kajiyama, H., Tateishi, T., and Ebihara, A., 1990, Circadian rhythm in recognition threshold of salt taste in healthy subjects, *Am. J. Physiol.* 259 (Regulatory Integrative Comp. Physiol. 28):R931–R935.
Fuller, R.W., 1981, Serotonergic stimulation of pituitary-adrenocortical function in rats, *Neuroendocrinology* 32:118–127.
Gallegos,G., Salazar, L., Ortiz, M., Marquez, W., Davis, A., Sanchez, S., and Conner, D., Simple disturbance of the dam in the neonatal period can alter haloperidol-induced catalepsy in the adult offspring, *Behav. Neural Biol.* 53:172–188.
Gartner, K., Buttner, D., Dohler, K., Friedel, R., Lindena, J., and Trautschold, I., 1980, Stress response of rats to handling and experimental procedures, *Lab. Anim.* 14:267–274.
Gaston, K.E., 1978, Brain mechanisms of conditioned taste aversion learning: A review of the literature, *Physiol. Psychol.* 6:340–353.
Gentsch, C., Lichsteiner, M., Driscoll, P., and Feer, H., 1982, Differential hormonal and physiological responses to stress in Roman high- and low-avoidance rats, *Physiol. Behav.* 28:259–263.
Gerber, G.J., and O'Shaughnessy, D., 1986, Comparison of the behavioral effects of neurotoxic and systemically toxic agents: How discriminatory are behavioral tests of neurotoxicity, *Neurobehav. Toxicol. Teratol.* 8:703–710.
Goddard, G.B., 1983, The kindling model of epilepsy, *TINS* 6:275–279.
Gold, P.E., and Stone, W.S., 1988, Neuroendocrine effects on memory in aged rodents and humans, *Neurobiol. Aging* 9:709–717.
Goldberg, A.L., and Goldspink, D.F., 1975, Influence of food deprivation and adrenal steroids on DNA synthesis in various mammalian tissues, *Am. J. Physiol.* 228:310–317.

Gould, E., Woolley, C.S., and McEwen, B.S., 1990, Short-term glucocorticoid manipulations affect neuronal morphology and survival in the adult dentate gyrus, *Neuroscience* 37:367–375.

Gray, G.D., Bergfors,A.M., Levin, R., and Levine, S., 1978, Comparison of the effects of restricted morning or evening water intake on adrenocortical activity in female rats, *Neuroendocrinology* 25:236–246.

Greer, N.L., Bartolome, J.V., and Schanberg, S.M., 1991, Further evidence for the hypothesis that beta-endorphin mediates maternal deprivation effects, *Life Sci.* 48:643–648.

Gross, W.B., 1982, The transition from hen house to laboratory cage: Problems and pitfalls, *NeuroToxicology* 3:295–298.

Gross, W.B., and Colmano, G., 1969, Effect of social isolation on resistance to some infectious agents, *Poult. Sci.* 48:514–520.

Gullian, C.M., and Eckerman, D.A., 1986, Field testing, in: *Neurobehavioral Toxicology* (Z. Annau, ed.), Johns Hopkins University Press, Baltimore, pp. 288–330.

Gumbinas, M., Oda, M., and Huttenlocher, P., 1973, The effects of corticosteroids on myelination of the developing rat brain, *Biol. Neonate* 22:355–366.

Hall, E.D., and Braughler, J.M., 1982, Glucocorticoid mechanisms in acute spinal cord injury: A review and therapeutic rationale, *Surg. Neurol.* 18:320–327.

Hall, E.M., and Johnson, J.V., 1989, A case study of stress and mass psychogenic illness an industrial workers, *J. Occup. Med.*

Hall, R.D., Gross,W.B., and Turner, E.C., Jr., 1979, Population development of *Ornithonyssus sylviarum* on Leghorn roosters inoculated with steroids and subjected to extremes of social interaction, *Vet. Parasitol.* 5:287–297.

Hashimoto, H., Marystone, J.F., Greenough, W.T., and Bohn, M.C., 1989, Neonatal adrenalectomy alters dendritic branching of hippocampal granule cells, *Exp. Neurol.* 104:62–67.

Henkin, R.I., 1970, The neuroendocrine control of perception, in: *Perception and Its Disorders* (D.A. Hamburg, K.H. Pribram, and A.J. Stunkard, eds.), Williams & Wilkins, Baltimore, 1970; Vol. 48, pp. 270–294.

Henkin, R.I., 1975, The role of adrenal corticosteroids in sensory processes, in: *Handbook of Physiology, Section 7, Endocrinology, Volume VL: Adrenal Gland* (H. Blaschko, G. Sayers, and A.D. Smith, eds.), American Physiological Society, Washington, DC, pp. 209–230.

Henkin, R.I., and Daly, R.L., 1968, Auditory detection and perception in normal man and in patients with adrenal cortical insufficiency, *J. Clin. Invest.* 47:1269–1280.

Henkin, R.I., Gill, J.R. Jr., and Bartter, F.C., 1963, Studies on taste thresholds in normal man and patients with adrenal cortical insufficiency; the effect of adrenocorticosteroids, *J. Clin. Invest.* 42:727–735.

Henkin, R.I., Gill, J.R., Jr., Warmoltz, J.R., Carr, A.A., and Bartter, F.C., 1963, Steroid-dependent increase of neural conduction velocity in adrenal insufficiency, *J. Clin. Invest.* 42:941.

Henkin, R.I., McClone, R.E., Daly, R., and Bartter, F.C., 1967, Studies on auditory thresholds in normal man and in patients with adrenal cortical insufficiency: The role of adrenal cortical steroids, *J. Clin. Invest.* 46:429–435.

Hennessy, M.B., and Weinberg, J., 1990, Adrenocortical activity during conditions of brief social separation in preweaning rats, *Behav. Neural Biol.* 54:42–55.

Hidalgo, J., and Armario, A., 1987, Effect of Cd administration on the pituitary-adrenal axis, *Toxicology* 45:113–116.

Hirsjarvi, P., and Junnila, M., 1986, happy rats—Reliable results, *Acta Physiol. Scand.* 128(Suppl.554): 32.

Hofer, M.A., 1978, Hidden regulatory processes in early social relationships, in: *Perspectives in Ethology: Social Behavior, Vol. 3* (P.P.G. Bateson and P.H. Klopfer, eds.), Plenum Press, New York, pp. 135–166.

Holden, C., 1988, Experts ponder simian well-being, *Science* 241:1753–1755.

Howard, E., 1968, Reduction in size and total DNA of cerebrum and cerebellum in adult mice after corticosterone treatment in infancy, *Exp. Neurol.* 22:191–208.

Howard, E., and Benjamin, J.A., 1975, DNA, ganglioside and sulfatide in brains of rats given corticosterone in infancy with an estimate of cell loss during development, *Brain Res.* 92:73–87.

Hutchings, D.E., 1990, Issues of risk assessment: Lessons from the use and abuse of drugs during pregnancy, *Neurotoxicol. Teratol.* 12:183–189.

Iny, L.J., Gianoulakis, C., Palmour, R.M., and Meaney, M.J., 1987, The beta-endorphin response to stress during postnatal development in the rat, *Dev. Brain Res.* 31:177–181.

Ito, M., Yong, V.W., Perry, T.L., and Singh, V.K., 1985, Chronic treatment with ACTH1-24 does not produce permanent damage to the developing rat brain, *Dev. Brain Res.* 19:315–317.

Jeffreys, D., and Funder, J.W., 1987, Glucocorticoids, adrenal medullary opioids, and the retention of a behavioral response after stress, *Neuroendocrinology* 121:1006–1009.

Jorgensen, H.A., Fasmer, O.B., Gerge, O.G., Tveiten, L., and Hole, K., 1984, Immobilization-induced analgesia: Possible involvement of a non-opioid circulating substance, *Pharmacol. Biochem. Behav.* 20:289–292.

Katz, R.J., and Carroll, B.J., 1977, Endocrine control of psychomotor activity in the rat: Effects of chronic dexamethasone upon general activity, *Physiol. Behav.* 20:25–30.

Kerr, D.S., Campbell, L.W., Hao, S-Y., and Landfield, P.W., 1989, Corticosteroid modulation of hippocampal potentials: Increased effect with aging, *Science* 245:1505–1509.

Kerr, D.S., Campbell, L.W., Applegate, M.D., Brodish, A., and Landfield, P.W., 1991, Chronic stress-induced acceleration of electrophysiologic and morphometric biomarkers of hippocampal aging, *J. Neurosci.* 11:1316–1324.

Khera, K.S., 1984, Maternal toxicity—A possible factor in fetal malformations in mice, *Teratology* 29:411–416.

Konarska, M., Stewart, R.E., and McCarty, R., 1989, Habituation of sympathetic-adrenal medullary responses following exposure to chronic intermittent stress, *Physiol. Behav.* 45:255–261.

Koob, G.F., and Bloom, F.E., 1985, Corticotropin-releasing factor and behavior, *Fed. Proc.* 44:259–263.

Kopell, B.S., Wittner, W.K., Lunde, D., Warrick, G., and Edwards, D., 1970, Cortisol effects on average evoked potential, alpha rhythm, time estimation, and two flash fusion threshold, *Psychosom. Med.* 32:39–49.

Kosowicz, J., and Pruszewicz, A., 1967, The "taste" test in adrenal insufficiency, *J. Clin. Endocrinol. Metab.* 27:214–218.
Krieger, D., 1982, *Cushing's Syndrome*, Springer-Verlag, Berlin.
Landfield, P.W., Lindsey, J.D., and Lynch, G., 1978, Hippocampal aging and adrenocorticoids: Quantitative correlations, *Science* 202:1098–1102.
Landfield, P.W., Baskin, R.K., and Pitler, T.A., 1981, Brain aging correlates: Retardation by hormonal-pharmacological treatments, *Science* 214:581–584.
Larson, A.A., 1982, Nociception in mice after chronic stress and chronic narcotic antagonists during maturation, *Brain Res.* 243:323–328.
Lee, R.E., and Pfeiffer, C.C., 1951, Effects of cortisone and 11-deoxycortisone on pain thresholds in man, *Proc. Soc. Exp. Biol. Med.* 77:752–754.
Levine, R., and Levine, S., 1989, Role of the pituitary-adrenal hormones in the acquisition of schedule-induced polydipsia, *Behav. Neurosci.* 103:621–637.
Levine, S., 1957, Plasma-free corticosteroid response to electric shock in rats stimulated in infancy, *Science* 135:795–796.
Lidsky, T.I., Manetto, C., and Ehrich, M., 1990, Nerve conduction studies in chickens given phenyl saligenin phosphate and corticosterone, *J. Toxicol. Environ. Health* 29:65–75.
Lochry, E.A., 1987, Concurrent use of behavioral/functional testing in existing reproductive and developmental toxicity screens: Practical considerations, *J. Am. Coll. Toxicol.* 6:433–439.
Loeb, J.N., 1976, Corticosteroids and growth, *N. Engl. J. Med.* 295:547–552.
Loyd, S.A., and Franklin, M.R., 1991, Modulation of carbon tetrachloride hepatotoxicity and xenobiotic metabolizing enzymes by corticosterone pretreatment, adrenalectomy and sham surgery, *Toxicol. Lett.* 55:65–75.
Lyen, L.R., Holland, I.M., and Lyen, Y.C., 1979, Reversible cerebral atrophy in infantile spasms caused by corticotropin, *Lancet* 2:37–38.
Maier, S.E., Vandenhoff, P., and Crowne, D.P., 1988, Multivariate analysis of putative measures of activity, exploration, emotionality and spatial behaviour in the hooded rat (*Rattus norvegicus*), *J. Comp. Psychol.* 102:378–387.
Martinez, J.L., Jr., 1983, Endogenous modulators of learning and memory, in: *Theory in Psychopharmacology,* Vol. 2 (S. Cooper, ed.), Academic Press, New York, pp. 47–74.
Masters, J.N., Finch, C.E., and Sapolsky, R.M., 1989, Glucocorticoid endangerment of hippocampal neurons does not involve deoxyribonucleic acid cleavage, *Endocrinology* 124:3083–3088.
Mattsson, J.L., and Albee, R.R., 1988, Sensory evoked potentials in neurotoxicity, *Neurotoxicol. Teratol.* 10:435–443.
Maurissen, J.P.J., and Mattsson, J.L., 1989, Critical assessment of motor activity as a screen for neurotoxicity, *Toxicol. Indust. Health* 5:195–201.
McEwen, B.S., 1987, External factors influencing brain development, in: *The Role of Neuroplasticity in the Response to Drugs* (D.P. Friedman and D.H. Clouet, eds.), NIDA Res. Monogr. 78:1–13.
McEwen, B.S., Gerlach, J.L., and Micco, D.J., 1975, Putative glucocorticoid receptors in hippocampus and other regions of the rat brain, in: *The Hippocampus, Vol. 1* (R.L. Isaacson and K.L. Pribram, eds.), Plenum Press, New York, pp. 375–391.
McEwen, B.S., DeKloet, E.R., and Rostene, W., 1986, Adrenal steroid receptors and actions in the nervous system, *Physiol. Rev.* 66:1121–1188.
McIntyre, D.C., 1976, Adrenalectomy: Protection from kindled emulsion induced amnesia in rats, *Physiol. Behav.* 17:789–795.
McNeill, T.H., Masters, J.N., and Finch, C.E., 1991, Effect of chronic adrenalectomy on neuron loss and distribution of sulfated glycoprotein-2 in the dentate gyrus of prepubertal rats, *Exp. Neurol.* 111:140–144.
Meaney, M.J., Aitken, D.H., Bhatnagar, S., Van Berkel, C., and Sapolsky, R.M., 1988a, Postnatal handling attenuates neuroendocrine, anatomical and cognitive impairments related to the aged hippocampus, *Science* 238:766–768.
Meaney, M.J., Aitken, D.H., van Berkel, C., Bhatnagar, X., and Sapolsky, R.M., 1988b, Effect of neonatal handling on age-related impairments associated with the hippocampus, *Science* 239:766–768.
Meaney, M.J., Aitken, D.H., Viau, V., Sharma, S., and Sarrieau, A., 1989, Neonatal handling alters adrenocortical negative feedback sensitivity and hippocampal type II glucocorticoid receptor binding in the rat, *Neuroendocrinology* 50:597–604.
Meyer, J.S., 1983, Early adrenalectomy stimulates subsequent growth and development of the rat brain, *Exp. Neurol.* 82:432–446.
Meyer, J.S., 1985, Biochemical effects of corticosteroids on neural tissues, *Physiol. Rev.* 65:946–1020.
Meyer, J.S., 1987, Prevention of adrenalectomy-induced brain stimulation by corticosterone, *Physiol. Behav.* 41:391–395.
Meyer, J.S., and Fairman, K.R., 1985, Early adrenalectomy increases myelin content of the rat brain, *Dev. Brain Res.* 17:1–9.
Meyer, J.S., and Fairman, K.R., 1985, Adrenalectomy in the developing rat: Does it cause reduced or increased brain myelination, *Dev. Psychobiol.* 18:349–354.
Micco, D.J., Meyer, J.S., and McEwen, B.S., 1980, Effects of corticosterone replacement on the temporal patterning of activity and sleep in adrenalectomized rats, *Brain Res.* 200:206–212.
Miller, D.B., 1988, Restraint-induced analgesia in the CD-1 mouse: Interactions with morphine and time of day, *Brain Res.* 473:327–335.
Miller, D.B., and Eckerman, D., 1986, Learning and memory measures, in: *Neurobehavioral Toxicology* (Z. Annau, ed.), Johns Hopkins University Press, Baltimore, pp. 94–152.
Morse, J.K., and Davis, J.N., 1990, Regulation of ischemic hippocampal damage in the gerbil: Adrenalectomy alters the rate of CA1 cell disappearance, *Exp. Neurol.* 110:86–92.
Mondadori, C., and Petschke, F., 1987, Do piracetam-like compounds act centrally via peripheral mechanisms? *Brain Res.* 435:310–314.

Mondadori, C., Ducret, T., and Petschke, F., 1989, Block of the nootropic action of piracetam-like nootropics by adrenalectomy: An effect of dosage, *Behav. Brain Res.* 34:155–158.

Moser, V.C., 1989, Screening approaches to neurotoxicity: A functional observation battery, *J. Am. Coll. Toxicol.* 8:85–93.

Munck, A., Guyre, P.M., and Holbrook, N.J., 1984, Physiological functions of glucocorticoids in stress and their relation to pharmacological actions, *Endocrinol. Rev.* 5:25–44.

Natelson, B.H., Creighton, D., McCarty, R., Tapp, W.N., Pitman, D., and Ottenweller, J.E., 1987, Adrenal hormonal indices of stress in laboratory rats, *Physiol. Behav.* 39:117–125.

Neutra, R., Lipscomb, J., Satin, K., and Shusterman, D., 1991, Hypotheses to explain the higher symptom rates observed around hazardous waste sites, *Environ. Hlth. Perspect.* 94:31–38.

Nichols, N.R., Lerner, S.P., Masters, J.N., May, P.C., Millar, S.L., and Finch, C.E., 1988, Rapid corticosterone-induced changes in gene expression in rat hippocampus display type II glucocorticoid receptor specificity, *Mol. Endocrinol.* 2:284–290.

Nichols, N.R., Osterburg, H.H., Masters, J.N., Millar, S.L., and Finch, E.E., 1990, Messenger RNA for glial fibrillary acidic protein is decreased in rat brain following acute and chronic corticosterone treatment, *Mol. Brain Res.* 7:1–7.

Nishino, K., Hirsch, P.F., Mahgoub, A., and Munson, P.L., 1991, Hypocalcemic effect of physiological concentrations of corticosterone in adrenalectomized parathyroidectomized rats, *Endocrinology* 128:2259–2265.

O'Callaghan, J.P., 1988, Neurotypic and gliotypic proteins as biochemical markers of neurotoxicity, *Neurotoxicol. Teratol.* 10:445–452.

O'Callaghan, J.P., and Miller, D.B., 1983, Nervous-system specific proteins as biochemical indicators of neurotoxicity, *TIPS* 4:388–390.

O'Callaghan, J.P., Brinton, R.E., and McEwen, B.S., 1989, Glucocorticoids regulate the concentration of glial fibrillary acidic protein throughout the brain, *Brain Res.* 494:159–161.

O'Callaghan, J.P., Brinton, R.E., and McEwen, B.S., 1991, Glucocorticoids regulate the synthesis of glial fibrillary acidic protein in intact and adrenalectomized rats but do not affect its expression following brain injury, *J. Neurochem.* 57:860–869.

Oda, M.A.S., and Huttenlocher, P.R., 1974, The effect of corticosteroids on dendritic development in the rat brain, *Yale J. Biol. Med.* 3:155–165.

Ojemann, G.A., and Henkin, R.I., 1967, Steroid dependent changes in human visual evoked potentials, *Life Sci., Part 1* 6:327–333.

Pakes, S.P., 1990, Contributions of the laboratory animal veterinarian to refining animal experiments in toxicology, *Fundam. Appl. Toxicol.* 15:17–24.

Pashko, S., and Vogel, W.H., 1980, Factors influencing the plasma levels of amphetamine and its metabolites in catheterized rats, *Biochem. Pharmacol.* 29:221–225.

Pauk, J., Kuhn, C.M., Field, T.M., and Schanberg, S.M., 1986, Positive effects of tactile versus kinesthetic or vestibular stimulation on neuroendocrine and ODC activity in maternally-deprived rat pups, *Life Sci.* 39:2081–2087.

Peele, D.B., and Vincent, A., 1989, Strategies for assessing learning and memory, 1978–1987: A comparison of behavioral toxicology, psychopharmacology, and neurobiology, *Neurosci. Biobehav. Rev.* 13:317–322.

Peters, D.A.V., 1988, Both prenatal and postnatal factors contribute to the effects of maternal stress on offspring behavior and central 5-hydroxytryptamine receptors in the rat, *Pharmacol. Biochem. Behav.* 30:669–673.

Pieretti, S., d'Amore, A., and Loizzo, A., 1991, Long-term changes induced by developmental handling on pain threshold: Effects of morphine and naloxone, *Behav. Neurosci.* 105:215–218.

Pitman, D.L., Ottenweller, J.E., and Natelson, B.H., 1986, Methodological problems in the study of classical aversive conditioning of adrenocortical responses, *Physiol. Behav.* 38:677–685.

Pitman, D.L., Ottenweller, J.E., and Natelson, B.H., 1988, Plasma corticosterone levels during repeated presentation of two intensities of restraint stress: Chronic stress and habituation, *Physiol. Behav.* 43:47–55.

Pitman, D.L., Ottenweller, J.E., and Natelson, B.H., 1990, Effect of stressor intensity on habituation and sensitization of glucocorticoid responses in rats, *Behav. Neurosci.* 104:28–36.

Pounds, J.G., Long, G.J., and Rosen, J.F., 1991, Cellular and molecular toxicity of lead in bone. *Environ. Health Perspect.* 91:17–32.

Preston, S.L., and McMorris, F.A., 1984, Adrenalectomy of rats results in hypomyelination of the central nervous system, *J. Neurochem.* 42:262–267.

Pudney, J., Price, G.M., Whitehouse, B.J., and Vinson, G.P., 1984, Effects of chronic ACTH stimulation on the morphology of the rat adrenal cortex, *Anatom. Rec.* 210:603–615.

Rebert, C.S., 1983, Multisensory evoked potentials in experimental and applied neurotoxicology, *Neurobehav. Toxicol. Teratol.* 5:659–71.

Rees, H.D., and Gray, H.E., 1984, Glucocorticoids and mineralocorticoids: Actions on brain and behavior, in: *Peptides, Hormones, and Behavior* (C.B. Nemeroff and A.J. Dunn, eds.), Spectrum Publications, New York, pp. 579–643.

Reinhard, J.F., Fr., Miller, D.B., and O'Callaghan, J.P., 1988, The neurotoxicant MPTP (1-methyl-4-phenyl-1,2,3,6-tetrahydropyridine) increases glial fibrillary acidic protein and decreases dopamine levels of the mouse striatum: Evidence for glial response to injury, *Neurosci. Lett.* 95:246–251.

Reiter, L.W., 1978, An introduction to neurobehavioral toxicology, *Environ. Health Perspect.* 26:5–7.

Revusky, S., and Martin, G.M., 1988, Glucocorticoids attenuate taste aversions produced by toxins in rats, *Psychopharmacology* 96:400–407.

Revusky, S., and Reilly, S., 1989, Attentuation of conditioned taste aversions by external stressors, *Pharmacol. Biochem. Behav.* 33:219–226.

Ribelin, W.E., 1984, Effects of drugs and chemicals upon the structure of the adrenal gland, *Fundam. Appl. Toxicol.* 4:105–119.

Richter, C.P., 1941, Sodium chloride and dextrose appetite of untreated and treated adrenalectomized rats, *Endocrinology* 29:115–125.

Rondeau, D.B., Jolicoeur, F.G., Merkel, A.D., and Wayner, M.J., 1980, Drugs and taste aversion, *Neurosci. Biobehavioral Rev.* 5:279–294.

Ross, J.F., 1989, Applications of electrophysiology in a neurotoxicity battery, *Toxicol. Indust. Health* 5:221–230.

Rowan, A.N., 1990, Refinement of animal research technique and validity of data, *Fundam. Appl. Toxicol.* 15:25–32.

Rowland, R.R., Reyes, E., Chukwuocha, R., and Tokuda, S., 1990, Corticosteroid and immune response of mice following mini-osmotic pump implantation, *Immunopharmacology* 20:187–190.

Roy, E.J., Lynn, D.M., and Bemm, C.W., 1990, Individual variations in hippocampal dentate degeneration following adrenalectomy, *Behav. Neural Biol.* 54:330–336.

Ruppert, P.H., Dean, K.F., and Reiter, L.W., 1983, Comparative developmental toxicity of triethyltin using split-litter and whole-litter dosing, *J. Toxicol. Environ. Health* 12:73–87.

Sapolsky, R., 1985, A possible mechanism for glucocorticoid toxicity in the hippocampus: Increased vulnerability of neurons to metabolic insults, *J. Neurosci.* 5:1228–1232.

Sapolsky, R., 1986, Glucocorticoid toxicity in the hippocampus: Reversal by supplementation with brain fuels, *J. Neurosci.* 6:2240–2247.

Sapolsky, R.M., 1987, Glucocorticoids and hippocampal damage, *TINS* 10:346–349.

Sapolsky, R.M., and Pulsinelli, W., 1985, Glucocorticoids potentiate ischemic injury to neurons: Therapeutic implications, *Science* 220:1397–1400.

Sapolsky, R.M., Krey, L.C., and McEwen, B.S., 1984, Prolonged glucocorticoid exposure reduced hippocampal neuron number: Implications for aging, *J. Neurosci.* 5:1222–1227.

Sapolsky, RM., Krey, L., and McEwen, B.S., 1986, The neuroendocrinology of stress and aging: The glucocorticoid cascade hypothesis, *Endocrinol. Rev.* 7:284–301.

Sapolsky, R.M., Uno, H., Rebert, C.S., and Finch, C.E., 1990, Hippocampal damage associated with prolonged glucocorticoid exposure in primates, *J. Neurosci.* 10:2897–2902.

Scheff, S.W., and Cotman, C.W., 1982, Chronic glucocorticoid therapy alters axon sprouting in the hippocampal dentate gyrus, *Exp. Neurol.* 76:644–654.

Scheff, S.W., and DeKosky, S.T., 1983, Steroid suppression of axon sprouting in the hippocampal dentate gyrus in the adult rat: Dose-response relationship, *Exp. Neurol.* 82:183–191.

Scheff, S.W., Morse, J.K., and DeKosky, S.T., 1988, Hydrocortisone differentially alters lesion-induced axon sprouting in male and female rats, *Exp. Neurol.* 100:237–241.

Schaefer, G.J., and Michael, R.P., 1991, Housing conditions alter the acquisition of brain self-stimulation and locomotor activity in adult rats, *Physiol. Behav.* 49:635–638.

Sette, W.F., 1989, Adoption of new guidelines and data requirements for more extensive neurotoxicity testing under FIFRA, *Toxicol. Indust. Health* 5:181–194.

Shors, T.J., Levine, S., and Thompson, R.F., 1990, Effect of adrenalectomy and demedullation on the stress-induced impairment of long-term potentiation, *Neuroendocrinology* 51:70–75.

Simmons, J.E., Yang, R.S.H., Svendsgaard, D., Seely, J.C., Thompson, M.B., and McDonald, A., 1990, Effects of a mixture of 25 groundwater contaminants on carbon tetrachloride (CC14) hepatotoxicity. Paper presented at Fourth International Conference on Combined Effects of Environmental Factors, Sept. 30–Oct. 3, Baltimore.

Sloviter, R.S., Valiquette, G., Abrams, G.M., Ronk, E.C., Sollas, A.L., Paul, L.A., and Neubort, A., 1989, Selective loss of hippocampal granule cells in the mature rat brain after adrenalectomy, *Science* 243:535–538.

Spencer, P.S., and Schaumburg, H.H., eds., 1980, *Experimental and Clinical Neurotoxicology*, Williams and Wilkins, Baltimore.

Sprague, G.L., 1987, Be careful what label you use! *Neurotoxicology* 8:637–638.

Stein, B., and Sapolsky, R.M., 1988, Chemical adrenalectomy reduces hippocampal damage induced by kainic acid, *Brain Res.* 473:175–181.

Stanton, M.E., and Levine, S., 1990, Inhibition of infant glucocorticoid stress response: Specific role of maternal cues, *Dev. Psychobiol.* 23:411–426.

Stanton, M.E., and Levine, S., 1988, Pavlovian conditioning of endocrine responses, in: *Experimental Foundations of Behavioral Medicine: Conditioning Approaches* (R. Ader, H. Weiner, and A. Baum, eds.), Lawrence Erlbaum Assoc., Hillsdale, NJ, pp. 25–46.

Stumpf, W.E., 1971, Autoradiographic techniques and the localization of estrogen, androgen and glucocorticoid receptors in the pituitary and brain, *Am. Zool.* 11, 725–739.

Tilson, H.A., 1987, Behavioral indices of neurotoxicity: What can be measured? *Neurotox. Teratol.* 9:427–443.

Tilson, H.A., and Peterson, N.J., 1987, Colchicine as an investigative tool in neurobiology, *Toxicology* 46:159–173.

Thomas, T.L., and Devenport, L.D., 1988, Site specificity of adrenalectomy induced brain growth, *Exp. Neruol.* 102:340–345.

Tonkiss, J., Cohen, C.A., and Sparber, S.B., 1988, Different methods for producing neonatal undernutrition in rats cause different brain changes in the face of equivalent somatic growth parameters, *Dev. Neurosci.* 10:141–151.

Uno, H., Lohmiller, L., Thieme, C., Kemnitz, J.W., Engle, M.J., Roecker, E.B., and Farrell, P.M., 1990, Brain damage induced by prenatal exposure to dexamethasone in fetal rhesus macaques. I. Hippocampus, *Dev. Brain Res.* 53:157–167.
Uno, H., Tarara, R., Else, J., Suleman, M., and Sapolsky, R., 1989, Hippocampal damage associated with prolonged and fatal stress in primates, *J. Neurosci.* 9:1705–1711.
Uphouse, L.L., 1981, Interactions between handling and acrylamide on e striatal dopamine receptor, *Brain Res.* 221:421–424.
Uphouse, L.L., and Brown, H., 1981, Effect of differential rearing on brain, liver and adrenal tissues, *Dev. Psychobiol.* 14:273–278.
U.S. EPA, 1978, Acute delayed neurotoxicity study and subchronic neurotoxicity studies, *Fed. Reg.* 43:37362–37363 and 37374–37375.
Uphouse, L.L., Nemeroff, C.B., Mason, G., Prange, A.J., and Bondy, S.C., 1982, Interactions between "handling" and acrylamide on endocrine responses in rats, *Neurotoxicology* 3:121–125.
Valencia-Flores, M., Velazquez-Martinez, D.N., and Villarreal, J.E., 1990, Super-reactivity to amphetamine toxicity induced by schedule of reinforcement, *Psychopharmacology* 102:136–144.
van der Hoop, R.G., Vecht, C.J., van der Burg, M.E.L., Elderson, A., Boogerd, W., Heimans, J.J., Vries, E.P., van Houwelingen, J.C., Jennekens, F.G.I., Gispen, W.H., and Neijt, J.P., 1990, Prevention of cisplatin neurotoxicity with an ACTH (4–9) analogue in patients with ovarian cancer, *N. Engl. J. Med.* 322:89–94.
Varma, D.R., Ferguson, J.S., and Alarie, Y., 1988, Inhibition of methyl isocyanate toxicity in mice by starvation and dexamethasone but not by sodium thiosulfare, atropine and ethanol, *J. Toxicol. Environ. Health* 24:93–101.
Veldhuis, H.D., and De Kloet, E.R., 1983, Antagonistic effects of aldosterone on corticosterone-mediated changes in exploratory behavior of adrenalectomized rats, *Horm. Behav.* 17:225–232.
Veldhuis, H.D., De Korte, C.C., and De Kloet, E.R., 1982, Adrenalectomy reduces exploratory behavior activity in rat: A specific role of corticosterone, *Horm. Behav.* 16:191–198.
Vogel, W.H., 1987, Stress—the neglected variable in experimental pharmacology and toxicology, *TIPS* 8:35–38.
von Zerssen, D., 1976, Mood and behavioral changes under corticosteroid therapy, in: *Psychotropic Action of Hormones* (T.M. Itil, G. Laudahn, and W.M. Herrmann, eds.), Spectrum, New York, pp. 195–222.
Voronin, L.L., 1983, Long-term potentiation in the hippocampus, *Neuroscience* 10:1051–1069.
Wakshlak, A., and Weinstock, M., 1990, Neonatal handling reverses behavioral abnormalities induced in rats by prenatal stress, *Physiol. Behav.* 48:289–292.
Walsh, T.J., and Emerich, D.F., 1988, The hippocampus as a common target of neurotoxic agents, *Toxicology* 49:137–140.
Walsh, T.J., and Tilson, H.A., 1986, The use of pharmacological challenges, in: *Neurobehavioral Toxicology* (Z. Annau, ed.), Johns Hopkins University Press, Baltimore, pp. 244–267.
Weinberg, J., Smotherman, W.P., and Levine, S., 1980, Early handling effects on the intake of novel substances: Differential behavioral and adrenocortical responses, *Behav. Neur. Biol.* 29:446–452.
Weiss, B., 1988, Neurobehavioral toxicity as a basis for risk assessment, *TIPS* 9:59–62.
Wenk, G.L., 1989, An hypothesis on the role of glucose in the mechanism of action of cognitive enhancers, *Psychopharmacology* 99:431–438.
Wiester, M.J., Tepper, J.S., Weber, M.F., Setzer, C.J., and Schutt, W.A., Jr., 1987, A restraining system for plethysmography in small animals, *Lab. Animal Sci.* 37:235–238.
World Health Organization, 1986, Principles and Methods for the Assessment of Neurotoxicity Associated with Exposure to Chemicals. Environmental Health Criteria 60, WHO, Geneva.
Yehuda, R., and Meyer, J.S., 1991, Regional patterns of brain growth during the first three weeks following early adrenalectomy, *Physiol. Behav.* 49:233–237.
Yehuda, R., McDonald, D., Heller, H., and Meyer, J., 1988, Maze-learning behavior in early adrenalectomized rats, *Physiol. Behav.* 44:373–381.
Yehuda, R., Fairman, K.R., and Meyer, J.S., 1989, Enhanced brain cell proliferation following early adrenalectomy in rats, *J. Neurochem.* 53:241–248.
Zenick, H., 1983, Use of pharmacological challenges to disclose neurobehavioral deficits, *Fed. Proc.* 42:3191–3195.
Zhou, F.C., and Azmitia, E.C., 1985, The effect of adrenalectomy and corticosterone on homotypic collateral sprouting of serotonergic fibers in hippocampus, *Neurosci. Letters* 54:111–116.

# Index

Adrenocorticotropin hormone (ACTH), 240–242, 250, 252
Adrenal axis, 239–259
  adrenocorticotropin hormone (ACTH), 240–242, 250, 252
  behavior and, 242–248
  biochemistry and, 253, 256–258
    glial fibrillary acidic protein (GFAP), 256, 257
  cognitive function and, 248, 249
  electrophysiology and, 252
  glucocorticoids, 240–242, 244–258
  morphological changes and, 253–256
    hippocampus, 254–256
  sensory processing and, 249–252
  stress and, 239–259
Alkaloids, 79–94
Amino acids, 79–82, 95–98
Animal models, 130–146
  common neural substrates, 136–143
  common neurotoxic effects, 140–143, 145
    early detection of, 141, 142, 145
  conceptual/operational approach, 132–135
  developmental profile, 135–137
  neurotoxicant exposure and, 130, 131, 140–144

Benzodiazepines, 71, 72
Brain development, 5–39
  differentiation, 18, 20
  malnutrition effects on, 5–39
  migration, 18, 20
  neurogenesis, 18, 20
  selective vulnerability during, 27–29

Caffeine, 71, 72, 82, 83, 90
Carbon disulfide, 195, 196, 202
Cocaine, 84, 91
Cognitive development, 129–146
  animal models of, 130–146
    neurotoxicant exposure and, 130, 131, 140–145
      triethyltin (TET), 141, 144, 145
      trimethyltin (TMT), 141–143

Dietary nutrients, 67–74
  behavior and, 67, 72, 73
  cholinergic system and, 69, 70, 72, 73
  cognitive function and, 67–73
  types of
    carbohydrates, 70, 71, 73
    fats, 69
    proteins, 68, 73
Dietary (caloric) restriction, 45–62
  aged animals and, 50–60
    behavior, 54–57
    dopaminergic system, 50–56, 60
  feeding regimens and, 48, 49
  neurotoxicity and, 58–61

Fish contamination, 151–169
  animal models of, 152–167
    behavioral effects, 156–167
    developmental effects, 163–167
  consumption of, 152–154, 168
    behavioral effects, 152–154
  Great Lakes, 152–169
Food, 118–122

Glucocorticoids, 240–242, 244–258

Hallucinogens, 85–87
Hippocampal formation, 29–38, 175–188, 254–256
  long-term potentiation, 34
  theta rhythm, 33, 34
Hypothalamic pituitary adrenal (HPA) axis, 244–259

Kindling seizure model, 173–188
  behavioral effects, 174, 181, 183–188
  chemical kindling, 175–188
    endosulfan, 184–187
  clinical relevance of, 187, 188
  electrical kindling, 173–188
  environmental toxins and, 173, 174, 178–188
    convulsions, 174, 178–188

Kindling seizure model (*Cont.*)
  limbic structures and, 175–188
  neuroplasticity and, 178, 181, 182

Lead, 195, 198, 202

Malnutrition, 3–39, 109, 110, 123
  critical period and, 6, 10–15
  developmental effects of
    behavior, 10
    biochemistry, 10
    brain development, 5–29
    mental retardation, 21–27
  developmental types of
    gestational, 5–7, 10, 11, 14–17, 23, 25–27, 34, 37, 38
    postnatal, 5–7, 14–17, 26, 27, 36–38
  factors in
    duration, 4
    environmental stimuli, 3–5, 11
    nutrition, 3–6, 11, 15
    period of development, 4
    severity, 4
  rehabilitation after, 10, 11, 34, 39
Mental retardation, 21–27
  animal models, 25–27
  malnutrition effects on, 21–23
  neuropathology, 21
Methanol, 195, 199, 202
Methylmercury, 195, 199, 202
Molecular configuration, 110–124
  food and, 118–122
    additives, 120, 121
    contaminants, 120, 121
    processing of, 119, 120
  ingestion and, 110–124
  metabolic effects on, 111, 112
  toxicants and, 116–118
Morphine, 83, 92, 94
Monoterpenes, 79, 82, 98–103

Neuronal degeneration, 224–236
  patterns of, 232
  primary, 232, 233
  secondary, 232, 234, 235
  silver stains and, 225–236
  time course of, 232, 233
  types of
    anterograde, 225–227, 232, 233
    retrograde, 225–28, 234
    transneuronal, 225, 226, 229, 234
Nicotine, 82, 83

Plant toxins, 77–105
  alkaloids as, 79–94
    biological action, 80–82, 86, 91, 92
    caffeine, 82, 83, 90
    clinical effects, 85, 91
    cocaine, 84, 91
    convulsants, 85, 88, 89
    hallucinogens, 85–87
    methylxanthines, 82, 83
    morphine, 83, 92, 94
    narcotics, 92
    nicotine, 82, 83
    psychotomimetics, 85–87
    tranquilizers, 92
  amino acids as, 79–82, 95–98
    biological action, 82, 97
    myeloneuropathies related to, 95–97
  monoterpenes as, 79, 82, 98–103
    camphor, 101
    tetrahydrocannabinol, 99
    thujone, 99–101
    turpentine, 100
Psychotomimetics, 85–87

Seizure disorders, 173–188
Silver degeneration stains, 225–236
  selectivity, 230–232
  sensitivity, 230–232
Stress, 239–259

Triethyltin (TET), 141, 144, 145
Trimethyltin (TMT), 141–143

Visual system toxicity, 193–217
  compounds producing, 195–203, 213–216
    carbon disulfide, 195, 196, 202
    lead, 195, 198, 202
    methanol, 195, 199, 202
    methylmercury, 195, 199, 202
  forms of
    direct ocular, 194
    neural, 194
  neurotoxicity testing and, 203, 204
    observation, 203, 204
    motor activity assessment, 203
    neuropathology, 203
  visual evoked potentials (VEPs) and, 204–210, 212–216
    flash evoked, 204–207
    pattern evoked, 206–210

NO LONGER THE PROPERTY
OF THE
UNIVERSITY OF R.I. LIBRARY